THE GUIDE TO

THE HANDLING OF PATIENTS

Introducing A SAFER HANDLING POLICY

4TH EDITION

Illustrations by Kevin Jones

First published 1981
Second edition 1987
Third edition 1992
Reprinted January 1993 with amendments largely in Chapter 2
Fourth edition 1997

Published by National Back Pain Association, 16 Elm Tree Road, Teddington, Middlesex, TW11 8ST.
Telephone: 0181-977 5474 Fax: 0181-943 5318

Design by The HRO'C Group, 53 Church Road, Edgbaston B15 3SJ. Tel: 0121 454 9707.

Printed by Image Publicity, London. Tel: 0181-876 6600.

A catalogue record for this publication is available from the British Library.
ISBN 0 9530582 0 4

Published by NBPA, 16 Elmtree Road, Teddington, Middlesex TW11 8ST.

THE GUIDE TO
THE HANDLING OF PATIENTS
Introducing **A SAFER HANDLING POLICY**

4TH EDITION

CHAIRMAN OF COORDINATING COMMITTEE:
Paul Lloyd, RGN, OHNCert, FRSH, former Adviser in Occupational Health Nursing and Chairman of the Royal College of Nursing Advisory Panel on Back Pain in Nurses.

PRODUCTION TEAM:
Brian Fletcher, Grad Dip Phys, MCSP, Dip I Chor (C), SRP, Member of the Royal College of Nursing Advisory Panel on Back Pain in Nurses; lately District Physiotherapy Adviser, Nottingham Community Health NHS Trust.

Danielle Holmes, RGN, ONC, RNT, Consultant in Patient Handling, DRH Associates.

Christine Tarling, Dip COT, SROT, Care Manager (Occupational Therapist), Social Services Department, Durham County Council.

Moira Tracy, PhD, Dip NEBOSH, MErgS, Member of the RCN Advisory Panel on Back Pain in Nurses, Health and Safety Adviser, Victoria Infirmary NHS Trust, Glasgow.

CONTRIBUTING AUTHORS:
Michael A. Adams, BSc, PhD, Senior Research Fellow, University of Bristol.

Pat Alexander, Grad Dip Phys, MCSP, SRP, Moving and Handling Training Department, West Herts Community NHS Trust

Lesley Crozier, MCSP, Dip TP, and *Sheila Cozens, MCSP, LicAc, MBAcC,* Movement Consultants, Movement Education Services.

Jacqueline Hall, MSc, RNT, SRN, Cert Ed, NNEB, Senior Lecturer, Faculty of Health, Social Work and Education, University of Northumbria at Newcastle.

Philippa Leggett, Dip Biomech, MCSP, SRP, Research Physiotherapist, University of Newcastle-upon-Tyne, and Manual Handling Consultant.

Julie O'Keefe, Dip COT, SROT, Senior Occupational Therapist, Spinal Injuries Unit, Royal National Orthopaedic Hospital, Stanmore.

Stephen Pheasant, PhD, MSc, MA, FEngs, Consultant Ergonomist (Deceased).

Howard Richmond, BA, Solicitor, Deputy Director, Legal Services, The Royal College of Nursing.

Sue Ruszala, BA, MCSP, Dip TP, Manual Handling Adviser, United Bristol Healthcare Trust.

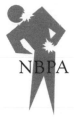

National Back Pain Association
in collaboration with the Royal College of Nursing

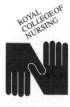

CONTENTS

CONTENTS

Acknowledgements

This fourth edition has built upon the experience and expertise of those who contributed to, and supported, the first three. The indebtedness to them was acknowledged in the third edition, and is due again because, although this edition makes a fresh start, it would not have been possible to do that if the previous work had not been done.

With regard to this edition, it is necessary in particular to mention all those unnamed people, experts in nursing, paramedical, medical, ergonomic and other disciplines, whose guidance has supported the individual authors whose names are given to the chapters for which they are responsible.

Indebtedness continues to past and present members of the RCN Advisory Panel on Back Pain in Nurses, and in particular, in reference to this edition, to Ruth Okumono, RGN, and Rosemary Pearce, RHN; also to Jennifer Klaber Moffett, PhD, MCSP, Senior Lecturer, Rehabilitation, University of Hull; Christine Holmes and Jan Collinge, Members of the Lancashire and Greater Manchester National Back Exchange Group; Angela Carter, Staff Nurse, and Teresa Petherick, Enrolled Nurse, Nottingham; Elaine Fazel, Moving and Handling Coordinator; Marie Hendry, MCSP, SRP, Manager, and Mary Guest, Training and Education Coordinator, and staff of the Disabled Living Centre, Manchester; Professor David Stubbs, PhD, BEd, FEngs, MIOSH, CIBiol, MIBiol, Roben Institute, University of Surrey; Joan Gabbett, Sally Cassar, Noreen Roche.

The National Back Pain Association wishes to acknowledge the help and advice of the Royal College of Nursing, the Back Exchange and the authors, who have helped produce this fourth edition.

We wish to express our sincere appreciation to The Colt Foundation and The Hayward Foundation for their help towards the costs of producing this manual.

Note

The attempt has been made to use the word patient consistently throughout this guide, noting that its title is The Guide to the Handling of Patients, while acknowledging that some workers in health and social services now use the word client instead.

For the same reason – consistency of style and presentation – the male gender form is used as the pronoun for the patient, and the female pronoun for the nurse, or carer.

Disclaimer

In this text it has not been feasible to avoid individual names of products or manufacturers, because of their common usage. In none of these instances should the appearance of such a name be taken to be a recommendation. In most cases, alternative products or manufacturers have or will have to be considered. It is for the reader to seek for guidance: for example from the Disabled Living Foundation's Information Service.

The risks associated with lifting and handling tasks are complex and each situation must be judged on its own merits and it is unreasonable for readers simply to follow instructions in the book without proper assessment of individual circumstances.

Neither the authors nor the publisher can accept responsibility for any consequences which might result from decisions made upon the basis of the advice given therein.

THE GUIDE TO
THE HANDLING OF PATIENTS

Part One:

Introducing a Safer Handling Policy

INTRODUCTION

by Paul Lloyd

This book is for all managers in care services in the public and private sectors whose staff are involved with the moving and handling of people.

This is the fourth edition of the Guide to The Handling of Patients published by the National Back Pain Association in collaboration with The Royal College of Nursing (RCN) Back Pain in Nurses Advisory Panel.

The first edition, published in 1981, set an important landmark in improving standards of training and patient handling methods. It identified the need to reduce the risk of back injury among nurses by increasing awareness, improving training, and emphasising the need to resort to safer methods by making greater use of equipment.

The second and third editions of this guide in 1987 and 1992 set new standards in patient handling activity. Each edition has taken the nursing and other health care professions forward to a situation in which we find ourselves today. We are now ready to commit ourselves to the elimination of manual lifting of patients, except under the direst of emergencies.

Since the third edition was published, several new factors need to be taken into account. The first is the introduction of the Manual Handling Operations Regulations of 1992, introduced on 1st January 1993. This legislation derived from a European Council Directive (90/269/EEC) on minimum health and safety requirements for the manual handling of loads where there is a risk of back injury to workers.

The impact of this legislation on health services has had a mixed response. Generally, managers have not been prepared to implement the necessary changes fully at a time of radical change for care services. The effect of this legislation on health services in both the public and private sectors is dealt with by Howard Richmond in Chapter 1, Legal and Professional Responsibilities.

Pressure of another kind has also emerged. Claims for compensation for nurses' back injuries has been rising steadily following the landmark cases of Williams v Gwent Health Authority, and Moore and Forder v The Norfolk Health Authority in the 1980s.

The RCN has concentrated its resources and efforts in fighting on behalf of its members injured as a result of patient handling accidents where a failure in the duty of care on the part of the employer could be proved in court. Such claims are not hard to win because the principles have now been well established.

Criminal prosecutions also arise for breaches of the Manual Handling Operations Regulations. In one case a health authority was prosecuted by the Health and Safety Executive in a magistrates' court and a fine of £12,000 was imposed because of an unsafe system of work.

In the early 1980s members of the RCN Advisory Panel on Back Pain in Nurses acted as expert witnesses in court. The advisory panel also produced educational material for nurses to try and reduce the risks of injury where such risks were avoidable. Today there is an army of experts on the subject of patient manual handling activity as a result of the many training courses of various kinds which have sprung up in the past two decades. Because there is an urgent need to standardise and harmonise the contents of these training courses, and as a result the joint Inter-professional Curriculum was developed (see Chapter 8).

The level of awareness of the risks of back injury from inappropriate and unsafe patient handling is considerable, as evidenced by the high level of claims still in the legal system. The RCN legal service won more than £8.5 million in compensation for members in 1996, and more than 50 per cent of its personal injury case work load is back pain related.

However, there is little evidence so far that the implementation of the Manual Handling Operations Regulations legislation has had a dramatic impact on the reduction of nurses' back injuries. Nursing is still regarded as a hazardous occupation. A national survey of 4,000 registered nurses in 1992 showed that one in four had time off work due to a work related back injury (Ref 4).

A later survey (Ref 1) in 1996, conducted by the Institute of Employment Studies (IES), which covered nurses working in all areas of practice, revealed that one third of all respondents reported having time off work with back pain or injury, and one in 20 nurses (5 per cent) had time off work with back pain or injury in the previous six months, and the average number of sick days taken was 22. When extrapolated, these figures suggest that no fewer than 14,000 registered nurses in Britain have had time off recently with back pain or injury, and that at least 93,000 registered nurses have had time off due to back pain or injury at some time during their career. The IES survey confirmed that work-related back pain was associated with manual handling at work.

Perhaps one of the reasons for this was the changes occurring in the National Health Service. The problem has moved from the hospital into the community - the Achilles heel of patient handling problems. The challenges in the community are enormous, and the authors contributing to this guide have done their best to try and address these problems.

The NHS is primary care led, with general practitioners taking decisions on how money and other resources will be allocated. Nurses and other professionals working in the community must use their positions to influence spending decisions to ensure that patient handling equipment of the correct type is available when it is needed. This calls for a closer partnership between social service providers, voluntary agencies, and primary care led community health services.

What is new or different about this 4th edition of the guide?

It has been written during a period of enormous change and debate about the best way forward. As a background to these changes, reference is made to the RCN Codes of Practice for the Handling of Patients. In 1993 the RCN code set down as a bench mark that two nurses should not lift a patient who weighed more than 50.8kg (8 stones), and then only under ideal conditions.

This alerted the nursing profession to the conclusion that the manual lifting of patients would eventually have to cease altogether. In the 3rd edition of The Guide to the Handling of Patients, manual lifting techniques, such as the shoulder lift were included, but only as techniques to be used as a last resort measure. Following this, the RCN produced a revised Code of Practice for Patient Handling April 1996 (Ref 3) and at the same time launched a safer patient handling policy with the aim of eliminating hazardous manual handling in all but exceptional life threatening situations. The revised code says: "Manual handling may continue provided that it does not involve lifting most or all of a patient's weight."

Considerable attention has been focused in this edition on the need to employ hoists and sliding aids to move patients. Great efforts have been made by professionals to find ways of moving patients without the need to lift them manually. Manufacturers of lifting and handling equipment have begun to recognise the need to find acceptable and economic solutions to long standing patient handling problems. However, problems still remain, as highlighted in Chapter 21. There are considerable risks of injury to nurses when dealing with patients with learning disabilities, the severely physically disabled, children with behavioural difficulties, and when rehabilitating the patient who is striving to regain independence.

There has been a heated debate about what is acceptable in terms of manual handling when physiotherapists or nurses move patients as part of a rehabilitation programme. Helping an unsteady patient to stand from a seated position or walking a patient as part of a rehabilitative exercise is not free of risk. The authors advocate careful assessment and appropriate methods to keep the risk as low as possible without compromising the patient's rehabilitation.

The intention of this book is to give realistic examples of good practice that works to the benefit of carers and patients in many areas. We also indicate best practice, which is often realistic but may not be applicable at all times due to patients' needs or the time needed to introduce change.

Manufacturers of patient handling equipment will need to address the remaining problems identified in this edition and find acceptable solutions if nurses are not to be obliged to adopt unsafe manual lifting, or act as a crane or prop for a patient unable to take his weight, or who is at risk of falling because he is unsteady and unreliable when on his feet.

Despite all our efforts to harmonise patient handling practice, we are aware that patient handling practice is far behind current teaching and practice in some establishments. The scope of the Manual Handling Regulations applies equally to the best regulated hospital as to the nursing home, the residential home, or the domestic environment, wherever dependent patients or residents need to be moved. Resources must be provided to ensure that whatever equipment is needed it is made available. There can be no excuse on the grounds of lack of resources if this means placing nurses and carers at risk of injury.

The authors hope that this edition will bring about developments that will lead to the elimination of handling practices which are now considered to be unsafe. It must be emphasised that we are not advocating a no handling policy which totally eliminates patient handling, such as supporting or holding a patient or assisting a patient to move himself, or in any other way assisting the patient. We are fully supportive of the nurse's therapeutic touch.

A word of warning. Even when handling equipment is available, users must be aware of the need to use the equipment in accordance with the manufacturer's instructions and agreed local protocols (Ref 2). Even when lifting and sliding equipment has been used, nurses are still being injured. The suitability of the equipment must be assessed and account taken of the individual's capability of using it. Where provided, handles, straps, belts and such like devices, should be used and the patient supervised closely throughout the entire handling procedure.

The manual patient handling techniques which relied on nurses actually lifting patients have been omitted from this edition. Instead, we have concentrated on the alternatives to manual lifting with emphasis on assisted transfers and support procedures to move patients safely and at the same time to minimise the risk of injury to the nurse or carer. We are grateful to the members of the RCN Back Pain Advisory Panel, National Back Exchange, and the many practitioners who have assisted us in compiling this edition. The professions have had five years' experience of working with the Manual Handling Operations Regulations now and much has changed in that time.

Considerable expertise has now been developed by many more practitioners from the nursing, physiotherapy and occupational therapy professions in the safer movement and handling of patients. Using the principles of safer practice as contained in this guide, we hope that these practitioners will continue to develop their expertise of working safely within the regulations and with the new and improved equipment now available.

REFERENCES

1. Hazards of Nursing. RCN. (November 1996). A study commissioned by the RCN conducted by the Institute of Employment Studies using data from a national survey of 6,000 registered nurses in RCN membership.

2. Medical Devices Agency Adverse Incident Centre. Safety Notice MDA.SN 9637.

3. RCN Code of Practice for Patient Handling. (April 1996).

4. Seccombe I., and Ball J., (1992). Back Injured Nurses: A profile. Institute of Manpower Studies.

LEGAL AND PROFESSIONAL RESPONSIBILITIES

by Howard Richmond

INTRODUCTION

The law as it relates to the lifting and handling of patients has two principal objectives, accident prevention and compensation for the injured lifter.

Accident prevention is regulated by statute, principally in the form of the Health and Safety at Work, Etc. Act, 1974 (HSWA 74). (Ref 1).

Compensation for injury to the lifter, at least for accidents taking place on or before 31 December 1992, was provided for by the common law, that is law contained in previous decisions of the courts which assume the force of binding or persuasive precedent. For incidents taking place on or after 1 January 1993 the Manual Handling Operations Regulations 1992 (MHO Regulations) (Ref 2) become relevant to both the regulatory and the compensatory aspects of lifting and handling.

ACCIDENT PREVENTION BY STATUTE

Section 2(1), HSWA 74 imposes a duty on every employer:

> ...to ensure, so far as is reasonably practicable, the health, safety and welfare at work of all his employees.

The scope of the duty is clarified in section 2(2) to include in particular, but only so far as is reasonably practicable:

(a) The provision and maintenance of plant and work systems,that are safe and without health risks

(b) Arrangements for ensuring safety and absence of health risks in the use, handling, storage and transport of articles and substances

(c) Provision of information, instruction, training and supervision necessary to ensure health and safety

(d) Maintenance of any place of work under the employer's control, and all means of access and egress from it in a condition that is safe and without health risks

(e) Provision and maintenance of a working environment that is safe and without risks to health and adequate as regards facilities and arrangements for welfare at work.

Reasonably practicable

With regard to lifting and handling patients, the most relevant requirements are contained in paragraphs

(a) plant and work systems, and

(c) instruction and training

but all of them can apply to some extent.

The duty is not an absolute one. It is qualified by the important words "so far as is reasonably practicable".

An employer needs to comply with this duty only if the cost of providing, say, equipment or training is not grossly disproportionate to the benefit. Were the benefit to be minimal and the cost substantial, an employer might be relieved of complying with the duty (Edwards v. National Coal Board). (Ref 3).

Under Section 7, HSWA 74 the employee is under a corresponding duty to take reasonable care for his or her own health and safety and the health and safety of other people who may be affected by his or her acts or omissions, and to cooperate with the employer in performing the duties under the Act.

Where it is reasonably practicable to comply with one of these duties and the employer fails to do so, enforcement action can be taken by the Health and Safety Executive (HSE). HSE inspectors have a right of entry to conduct inspections and a power to serve Improvement Notices specifying particulars of the breach of health and safety law which has been contravened and specifying a time within which the breach should be remedied.

An example might be to require provision of suitable lifting equipment in an orthopaedic ward with heavy, highly dependent patients, where there is no hoist available.

An inspector has the additional power to serve a prohibition notice preventing activities being carried out if there is a risk of serious personal injury.

Failure to comply with improvement or prohibition notices, or commission of a breach of the general duties in Section 2(2)(a)-(e) in, or any regulations made under HSWA 74, can give rise to a criminal prosecution.

On conviction:

in the Crown Court the maximum penalties in the most serious cases are two years' imprisonment and an unlimited fine

in the Magistrates' Court, where most cases are heard, the maximum fine is £20,000, and where the conviction relates to failure to comply with prohibition or improvement notices, up to six months' imprisonment

Where an offence is committed by a corporate body, senior managers or directors can also be made individually liable where the offence was committed with the consent or connivance of that manager or is attributable to that manager's neglect.

ACCIDENT PREVENTION BY REGULATION AND GUIDANCE

The HSWA 74 is a general enabling Act which allows the Secretary of State to make regulations and allows the Health and Safety Commission (HSC) to issue codes of practice and guidance notes.

The Manual Handling Operations Regulations 1992 (MHO Regulations) (Ref 2) govern the lifting and handling of patients in the workplace.

The Management of Health and Safety at Work Regulations 1992 (M of HSW Regulations 92) (Ref 4), the Provision and Use of Work Equipment Regulations 1992 (Ref 5), and the Workplace (Health, Safety and Welfare) Regulations 1992 (Ref 6) also apply, but to a lesser extent.

These regulations aim to translate into domestic law the UK's obligations under various European Community directives relevant to health and safety law. These directives are discussed more fully later in this chapter under the heading The 1992 European Directives.

As with accident prevention by statute, a breach of

any provision in these regulations can ultimately lead to a prosecution being brought by the HSE.

Regulation 3(1) of the M of HSW Regulations 92 requires employers to make a suitable and sufficient assessment of all the risks to the health and safety of their employees while at work. When this general assessment indicates the possibility of risks to employees from the manual handling of loads, the provisions of regulation 4 of the MHO Regulations come into play.

The employer is required to follow a three stage procedure:

first, to avoid manual handling operations involving a risk of injury, so far as is reasonably practicable

second, where hazardous manual handling operations cannot with reasonable practicability be avoided, to assess them, taking into account the task, the load, the working environment, and the individual capabilities of the lifters as set out in Appendix 1 to the MHO Regulations which are almost identical to the reference factors set out in an Annex of the Official Journal of the European Communities (see page 21)

third, on the basis of the information supplied by the assessment, the employer must reduce the risk of injury to the lowest level that is reasonably practicable.

The assessment must be kept up to date, and the employee must be given a general indication of and, where reasonably practicable, precise information on, the weight of the load.

The assessment should be recorded and readily available.

The Manual Handling Operations Regulations 1992: HSE Guidance

The MHO Regulations 1992 are accompanied by HSE guidance which does not have the force of law. Nevertheless, HSE inspectors can take it into account when considering whether there is compliance with the regulations.

For instance Appendix 1, paragraph 10 of the guidance note contains a diagram of guideline weight figures. Although it is stressed that these are not weight or force limits, these figures indicate the threshold beyond which there is a risk of the employee being injured.

A failure on the part of an employer to carry out an assessment of manual handling operations before the guideline figures were exceeded might be evidence of a breach of the MHO Regulations 1992 but it would be for a court to decide.

Paragraph 42 of the guidance note indicates that an assessment made at the last minute is unlikely to be suitable and sufficient as required by the regulations; employers must look in a considered way at the whole range of manual handling operations required of employees.

Generic assessments drawing together common threads from a range of broadly similar operations are considered acceptable.

The Management of Health and Safety at Work Regulations 1992: Code of Practice

The M of HSW Regulations 1992 are accompanied by an Approved Code of Practice (ACoP). In any prosecution where it is proved that there has been a failure to observe a relevant provision in an ACoP, the defendant must show that the regulations are satisfied in some way other than by observing the ACoP.

Guidance on manual handling

The Health Services Advisory Committee to the Health and Safety Commission originally published guidance, The Lifting of Patients in the Health Services, in 1984 (Ref 7) and this was updated in its Guidance on manual handling of loads in the Health Services 1992 (Ref 8).

This guidance can be taken into account by a court but only as assistance in considering whether there is evidence of a breach.

A suitable analogy might be with the Highway Code (Ref 9). A breach of the Highway Code might be evidence of an offence under the Road Traffic Acts or of negligence in civil law, but not conclusively.

There is also guidance of an unofficial nature; this volume itself, for instance; or the Code of Practice for the Handling of Patients, first issued by the Royal College of Nursing in 1982 (Ref 10), updated in March 1993 (Ref 12) and then in April 1996 (Ref 12).

The status of these documents is that of expert opinion. Such opinion may be persuasive in that it represents the consensus of foremost experts in the field and, in the case of the Code of Practice, endorsed by the leading professional nursing organisation in the UK. However, such opinion is no more than potentially persuasive on any aspect until accepted by a court, and it would be open to any defendant in court proceedings to bring expert evidence to the contrary.

These documents are not admissible in court proceedings on their own; they have to be drawn on and supported by an expert witness in each case, a point discussed in more detail in the following section on compensation.

COMPENSATION FOR THE INJURED LIFTER

The employer's responsibility

Section 47 HSWA 74 states that breach of the general duties in Section 2(2)(a)-(e) HSWA 74 does not give rise to civil liability, that is, that breach of these general duties does not entitle an employee to compensation for an injury from a lifting and handling accident. However, this is a distinction without a difference in practice, since the common law places equivalent duties on the employer to take reasonable care for the safety of the employees and to carry out operations so as not to subject employees to unnecessary risk. This is a personal responsibility which cannot be delegated.

The modern authority for the employer's duty is set out in a House of Lords case (Wilsons and Clyde Coal Limited v. English) (Ref 14) which requires that all employers provide and maintain, so far as is reasonable:

(a) a safe place of work with safe means of access and egress

(b) safe appliances, equipment, and plant for doing work

(c) a safe system for doing work

(d) competent and safety conscious personnel.

In addition, the employer is responsible for the negligence of employees even if the employer is not at fault. This is known as vicarious liability, a legal principle which often causes confusion to lay people. It is discussed further, under Problem Areas, later in this chapter.

Claims for compensation for injury, usually injury arising from the lifting and handling of patients, are most often pursued on the basis of the employer's failure to provide a safe system of work, although a failure to provide equipment, a safe place of work, or competent fellow personnel can also be factors. The plaintiff has to prove that the employer has breached the duty in one of the above respects, and that this breach of duty caused the injury.

Each case is argued on its particular merits and expert evidence is required to prove what reasonably safe system of work, whether in design or implementation, and having regard to what the employer knew or ought to have known at that time, could have avoided the accident

in what respects the employer fell short of that duty in the particular case before the court.

Previous editions of The Handling of Patients assisted courts to decide on the standard to be attained. For instance, in the case of Edwards v. Waltham Forest Health Authority (1989) (Ref 15) Mr. Justice Potts stated:

"I have reached the conclusion that the standards set out in page 5 of The Handling of Patients, A Guide for Nurse Managers, and the measures to be adopted on bath transfers as described at page 35 (which provides that lifting a patient manually out of a bath should only be necessary in an emergency if a patient is taken ill or helpless and under no other circumstances) were well known in the nursing profession in April 1982. I am also satisfied upon the evidence that I have heard that those standards and measures were entirely proper and were the standards and measures that could and should have been adopted by all competent employers for their employees. I have to say that I am surprised that in this case, on the evidence, no responsible person at (the) hospital seems to have applied his or her mind to what is set out in this volume, and in particular to those parts mentioned".

It should not be assumed that The Handling of Patients sets the standard to be achieved in all circumstances. Although it embodies the opinion of several foremost experts in the field, its application to the facts of any particular case must be proved by an expert witness; a defendant could bring other experts to argue that in any particular set of circumstances the advice given was not appropriate or reasonable.

The landmark case is that of Williams v. Gwent Health Authority (1982) (Ref 16) where the defendant was held to be liable for having an unsafe system of work in allowing the drag lift to be used.

Since that time plaintiffs have recovered compensation where unsafe systems have been found in the use of the orthodox lift (Moore v. Norfolk Health Authority (1982) (Ref 17) in respect of falling patients (Bayley v. Bloomsbury Health Authority (1987) (Ref 18) in respect of a district nurse lifting a patient on her own (Hammond v. Cornwall and Isles of Scilly Health Authority (1986) (Ref 19), and in respect of the use of the Australian lift on a heavy patient where a hoist should have been used (Munro v. Plymouth Health Authority (1991)) (Ref 20).

In addition, a health authority has been found vicariously liable where a co-lifter failed to lift on the count of three, injuring the lifter taking the lead (Page v. Enfield and Haringey Health Authority (1985)) (Ref 21).

Courts are reluctant to find breach of duty on the ground of staff shortages alone (Stewart v. Highland Health Board (1987)) (Ref 22).

Civil liability

As said at the start of this section on compensation, breach of the general duties in Section 2(2)(a)-(e) HSWA 74 does not give rise to civil liability. However, breaches of provisions in regulations made under HSWA 74 can give rise to civil liability for what is called breach of statutory duty, unless the regulations provide otherwise.

Regulation 15 of the M of HSW Regulations 92 states that a breach of the duty imposed by those regulations does not confer a right of any action in any civil proceedings (although this may not prevent the duties set out in the parent Framework Directive 891391/EEC being directly effective, for which see the section headed The 1992 European Directives, below).

There is no such exclusion in the MHO Regulations. This means that a breach of any duty in regulation 4 setting out the assessment procedure can be invoked in a civil claim. In this context it should be noted that the duty to carry out an assessment where there is a risk of injury is almost absolute, that is to say, there will be no defence to a failure to carry out an assessment except perhaps to plead that there was no risk of injury at all.

The application of the findings of the assessment is subject to the test of reasonable practicability. The employing organisation will only be relieved of liability if it can show that the cost of putting into effect the findings of the assessment would have been grossly disproportionate to the benefits.

Further, such cost benefit calculations must have been made before the incident giving rise to the claim. In principle, therefore, the MHO Regulations should make it easier for a plaintiff to prove breach of duty.

Proving the injury

As well as proving the breach of duty itself, the plaintiff has to prove, with the assistance of expert medical evidence, that the breach of duty caused the injury sustained. This is by no means straight forward, since lifters can often be shown to have vulnerable backs, either resulting from naturally occurring degenerative changes, or from previous back injuries, or from the effects of cumulative strain from regular heavy lifting.

It is difficult to obtain the evidence necessary to pursue a claim based on cumulative strain alone. In most cases one is considering the injury caused by a particular lifting incident and the effect that incident may have in aggravating and/or accelerating existing injury, albeit symptom free, until that incident occurred.

Most people show signs of degenerative change in the spine, especially towards their middle years. There is no proven connection between the appearance of signs of this, and symptoms of pain. Consultants tend to rely upon their clinical experience and can come to greatly differing opinions as to the extent to which an accident has accelerated symptoms, say by two years as against 20 years in any one case. At the end of the period of acceleration the effects of the accident cease, so compensation for loss of past and future earnings, indeed all the considerations that influence the amount of compensation, crucially depend on the length of the period of acceleration.

There is no easy answer to these conflicts of evidence, although the fact that statistically the incidence of back pain peaks between the ages of 45 and 50 can provide good arguments against short acceleration periods in the case of younger plaintiffs. For example, there would have to be fairly convincing evidence in support of a two year as against a 20 year acceleration period for a 25 year old plaintiff. These conflicts cause difficulties for all concerned, including the courts. The problem is caused by a lack of scientific knowledge.

A concept which can cause confusion in back injury claims is that of "functional overlay", that is, exaggerated or inappropriate responses to injury. Functional overlay can be diagnosed by specific tests which can be made while the person is being examined and which are mainly intended to avoid unnecessary surgery. However, as long as the pain is shown to be genuine, even if overlaid by the plaintiff's over-sensitive personality or response to pain, compensation should not be affected.

The legal principle is that a defendant must take a victim as it finds him or her, even if the plaintiff has an unduly vulnerable personality which the defendant did not know about or foresee. The House of Lords, in the case of Page v. Smith (1995) (Ref 23) held that a defendant is legally responsible as long as it could be reasonably foreseen that the conduct would expose the plaintiff to the risk of personal injury of some kind, whether physical or psychological.

In many cases of soft tissue injury, no organic cause for pain can be discovered, even using up to date scanning techniques. There may be possible physical causes from scar tissue or changes in the nervous system causing chronic pain syndrome, which cannot be physically verified. However, as long as the plaintiff's pain is considered to be genuine and caused by the accident in question, on the balance of probabilities the fact that it may be psychological in nature will not help the defendant. The defendant will be relieved of legal responsibility only if it can be proved that the plaintiff is malingering, that is consciously inventing or exaggerating pain symptoms with a view to obtaining compensation. Such conduct is rare and is usually identified by covert video surveillance.

Much interest has been generated by the case of Walker v. Northumberland County Council (1995) (Ref 24) where a social worker recovered compensation for stress related illness caused by overwork. The heavy physical work involved in manual lifting can be stressful, particularly when staffing levels are inadequate. Chronic stress puts a person at risk of back pain. Stress can also contribute to many work related accidents since the person under stress can be distracted, and be more prone to error and consequently vulnerable to injury. Even in the absence of specific injury the strong possibility of sustaining injury can itself be stressful.

A management response

Safer lifting policies are suitable management responses to tackle the stress and ill-health caused by heavy manual lifting, as well as reducing the incidence of musculo-skeletal injury. Employers must identify any sources of occupational stress when making the risk assessment required by regulation 3 (1) of the M of HSW Regulations 92, taking into account the HSE booklet Stress at Work, a Guide for Employers (1995) (Ref 25).

Assessing damages and cash awards

Although the plaintiff in a civil claim has to prove negligence, namely that the breach of duty caused the injury, this is not an end in itself, it is only a means to an end - compensation. The aim of financial compensation is to put the plaintiff back into the position he or she would have been in if the accident had not happened. Where loss of earnings and extra expense are incurred, the arithmetic at least can be fairly straightforward. Lawyers call these special damages.

Financial compensation for pain and suffering, restricted life style, or a destroyed career whose path can only be guessed at, are more difficult and controversial. The trial judge has some discretion in assessing these so-called general damages within a framework of principles set down in previously decided cases.

Awards for pain and suffering and loss of amenity made by English courts are considered by many to be too low. Back injuries attract awards in the range of £1,000 to £20,000 depending on the degree of severity.

However, where a lifter's career is destroyed by the accident, awards can be greatly boosted by compensation for past and future loss of earnings, and recent awards have been in the range of £150,000 to £345,000. Although such sums can seem large it must be remembered that the capital sum plus income generated (for which the courts assume a rate of return of 4.5 per cent a year) are intended to replace many years' earnings and are often not as generous as the headline figures might suggest.

Thus, although compensation claims are not intended to be punitive, the amounts which can be ordered to be paid are many times higher than any fines which might be levied under the HSWA 74, and in this regard compensation claims could be considered to have an indirect deterrent effect. In 1995, 33 trades unions recovered £304 million for members suffering from workplace injury and ill health, whereas fines for prosecutions for breaches of health and safety law did not exceed £4 million. In addition, the unsuccessful party, usually the employer, will have to pay the successful party's legal costs as well as its own. In smaller cases, costs can amount to as much as the compensation, and where a claim proceeds as far as trial, costs can be in the tens of thousands of pounds.

The value of potential claims should form part of the risk benefit calculation which might lead employers to decide to allocate more resources to carry out their duties.

Contributory negligence

Defendants routinely allege that plaintiffs are partly to blame for the accident; this is called contributory negligence. A finding of contributory negligence does not defeat the claim, but reduces the compensation. For example, a plaintiff found to be 25 per cent to blame would have the compensation reduced by 25 per cent. Experience shows that courts have been reluctant to make such findings in nurse lifting cases.

Procedural delays

Over the years there has been continuing concern about delays in civil procedures, particularly personal injury claims. Changes to the court rules made in 1991 which were designed to speed things up have had mixed success. They have created a lot more work for the courts and the parties, particularly the requirement to exchange all evidence before trial in the form of detailed witness statements.

Lord Woolf's reports to the Lord Chancellor on the civil justice system in England and Wales, in June 1995 (Ref 26) and July 1996 (Ref 27), will change all civil procedures. Of particular relevance to personal injury claims will be the emphasis on court management of the proceedings, with the amount of legal work being restricted so as to be proportional to the value or importance of the claim. There will also be restrictions on the use of expert witnesses. Where there is a substantially established area of knowledge, for instance occupational therapist's assessments on a plaintiff, the court may appoint a single expert. By contrast, where there are several tenable schools of thought, or where the boundaries of knowledge are being extended, a single expert may not be appropriate. Therefore where experts in the handling of patients, or medical experts, disagree, this second provision is likely to apply. Implementation of the Woolf recommendations in full is planned by October 1998.

For claims worth under £10,000 there will be a fast track procedure with a fixed date for trial being fixed at the outset, expert evidence being given on paper only, and fixed legal costs. The more adversarial aspects of civil litigation should be tamed and more and earlier settlements reached.

Sick pay and other benefits

Although emphasis has been placed on compensation which can be recovered through bringing a civil action, it must be mentioned that compensation is available from other sources where an employee is incapable of working through sickness or accident.

There may be an entitlement to sick pay from the employer, but only if provided for in the contract of employment. Employers also administer the Statutory Sick Pay Scheme which provides benefits for the first 28 weeks of sickness.

Beyond that, Sickness/Incapacity Benefit may be available from the Department of Social Security. Of particular relevance is the Industrial Injuries scheme which provides Disablement Benefit to compensate those who have suffered disablement from a loss of physical or mental faculty caused by an industrial accident. However, benefit is only payable where the loss of faculty amounts to 14 per cent or more.

Of particular interest to National Health Service employees is the NHS Injury Benefits Scheme, which should be better known than it is. Benefit is payable to all NHS employees, regardless of length of employment, who suffer an injury because of NHS employment. There are separate schemes for those absent temporarily through injury and those whose employment is terminated. The aim is to compensate for reduction of earning ability caused by the injury and, depending on length of service and degree of reduction in earning ability, benefits can be awarded up to a maximum of 85 per cent of pre-injury pay, together with entitlement to a lump sum on termination of employment. Where compensation is recovered in a civil action, NHS Injury Benefit payments have to be repaid or adjusted. In this respect they can be considered to be payments on account of compensation although no fault need be proved.

With regard to Social Security benefits, all payments made to injured employees for accidents after 1 January 1989 must be repaid by the employer to the Department of Social Security where compensation is agreed or ordered to be paid in excess of £2,500. This provision, subject to much criticism, has had adverse effects on plaintiffs. The Social Security (Recovery of Benefits) Act 1997, due to come into effect on 1 October 1997, is intended to mitigate some of the harsher effects of the recoupment of benefits upon plaintiffs. Its principal effect is to ring fence general damages for the injury and for future financial loss while abolishing the £2,500 exemption threshold. The indirect deterrent effects on employers, who bear some of the costs of supporting injured employees previously borne by the tax payer, will remain.

DISABILITY DISCRIMINATION ACT 1995

It is often remarked upon how seemingly reluctant the health services are to redeploy injured staff. Insurance companies, mindful that claims for future loss of earnings form the largest element in compensation awards, are now more interested in schemes designed to get injured employees back to work. The Disability Discrimination Act 1995 (Ref 28) transforms what was previously good practice into a legal duty.

To qualify as disabled under the Act, a person must have a physical or mental impairment which adversely affects their ability to carry out normal day to day activities, and the adverse effect must be both substantial and long term. Many employees suffering from chronic lower back pain caused by lifting and handling accidents should qualify.

It will be unlawful for an employer to discriminate against a disabled person in recruitment. More importantly, there is a duty on an employer to make reasonable adjustment to working arrangements which have an impact on disabled employees. Examples of steps which an employer may have to take include transferring a person to fill an existing vacancy, altering working hours, allowing an employee to be absent during working hours for rehabilitation assessment or treatment, and acquiring or modifying equipment.

It will be interesting to see how the courts interpret what adjustments might be reasonable in the light of the duties in the MHO Regulations. The question is, if a safer handling policy is reasonably practicable under health and safety legislation, cannot it also be argued that such a policy can lead to a reasonable adjustment to allow more injured employees to continue working? Many medical reports on injured nurses advise that they should avoid work which involves lifting or bending. Reasonable adjustments which enable such nurses to continue working are, it will be submitted, reasonably practicable. Provided suitable and sufficient risk assessments are made, safe systems of work implemented, and suitable equipment provided as recommended throughout this guide, many work injured nurses should be able to continue working.

EMPLOYMENT

An employee owes a duty to the employer to obey reasonable and lawful instructions and to act with reasonable care and skill. Thus a failure to perform as trained or instructed could render the employee liable to disciplinary proceedings and ultimately to dismissal. However, it is only a refusal to obey an employer's lawful instructions that can amount to misconduct leading to dismissal, for either refusal by an employee to do something which would be a breach of health and safety regulations, or a refusal to cooperate in the employer's breach, cannot amount to conduct that would justify dismissal.

Where the employer has complied fully with the health and safety obligations there are now specific duties amplifying the general duty under Section 7 HSWA 74 under which the employee is under a duty to take reasonable care for his or her own health and safety, and for the health and safety of those who may be affected by his or her act or omission, when handling and lifting - principally the patient, but also fellow members of staff.

Regulation 12 of the M of HSW Regulations 92 requires an employee to use all work equipment and safety devices provided by the employer in accordance with the training and instruction which the employer is obliged to provide.

In relation to handling and lifting, Regulation 5 of MHO Regulations obliges each employee, while at work, to make full and proper use of any system of work provided for the employee's use by the employer in complying with the duty to reduce the risk of injury to employees to the lowest level reasonably practicable, where it is not reasonably practicable to avoid manual handling operations altogether.

This duty is absolute and an employee's breach of the employer's instructions and procedures for safer lifting would bring the prospect of disciplinary proceedings. If injured, the employee would face a reduction in the compensation as a consequence of his or her contributory negligence to the extent that a court would consider just and equitable having regard to the employer's share in the responsibility for the damage.

Where the employer has complied with the obligations under the MHO Regulations by, in effect, providing a work place, work equipment, and systems of work to avoid lifting in all but exceptional or life threatening situations, there should be no problem for the employee.

The problem arises when the employer has not complied with these obligations and the employee has to cope. Is the employee entitled to refuse to lift in such circumstances? One can argue that an instruction to lift in circumstances likely to cause injury where it is reasonably practicable to avoid that risk altogether, is an unlawful instruction entitling the employee to refuse. It is a brave employee who courts disciplinary proceedings, and proceedings in the industrial tribunal following dismissal, even if he or she is ultimately successful. Compensation is no substitute for a job. In any case, where patient well being is at stake, the transition to a safer handling policy has to be planned using the framework of law which now puts obligations on employees and also provides them with some degree of protection. However, where the employee is required to continue to work where an employer has not complied with its obligations, albeit during a phased period of implementation by the employer, the employer cannot plead the employee's acquiescence as a defence to a personal injury claim.

Since paragraph 42 of the guidance note to the MHO Regulations indicates that an assessment made at the last minute is unlikely to be suitable and sufficient as required by the regulations, and that employers should look in a considered way at the whole range of manual handling operations required of employees, employees should approach the problem in an equally considered and systematic way, preferably through their safety representatives.

There is a duty on all employees under Regulation 12 (2) M of HSW Regulations 92 to inform the employer of any work situation the employee reasonably considers to represent either a serious and immediate danger to health and safety, or a shortcoming in the employer's health and safety arrangements, as long as that situation arises out of that employee's own activity, and has not been previously reported to the employer. This is an absolute duty. Every employee should therefore be advised to remind their line manager if there is no safer handling policy in operation.

While not suggesting that the implementation of this absolute duty by the employee would bring sanctions from the employer, the employee has protection under sections 22A and 57A of the Employment Rights Act 1996 (Ref 29) which was amended to implement rights granted in the EU Framework Directive (89/391/EEC) (Ref 32). These provisions give employees the right not to suffer any detriment, which could be a failure to investigate safety concerns reported by that employee if a failure to do so impinged upon that employee, or be dismissed.

The protection is in the first instance granted to health and safety representatives, safety committee members, or other employees carrying out statutory or agreed health and safety functions. The protection is granted to employees where either there is no safety representative or safety committee, or it was not reasonably practicable to raise the concerns through such channels, and the employee used reasonable means to draw attention to work circumstances which the employee reasonably believed were harmful or potentially harmful to health and safety.

There are further rights granted to employees where they reasonably believe themselves to be in serious and imminent danger. In such circumstances the employee has a right to leave the work place or to take appropriate steps to protect him or herself. Such circumstances are rare in the context of handling.

The so-called Working Time Directive 93/014/EC (Ref 30) survived a challenge by the UK government in the European Court on 12 November 1996, and became binding on all European member states from 23 November 1996. From that date onwards the UK was in breach of its obligations to introduce domestic legislation to implement the directive although consultations over proposed regulations started soon thereafter. The main provisions of the directive are: a minimum daily rest period of 11 hours; entitlement to a rest period where the working day exceeds six hours; a weekly continuous rest period of 35 hours; and a maximum weekly working time of 48 hours.

The directive is complex. It gives flexibility both to the member state in legislation and to employers and employees who can agree jointly to contract out of certain provisions. If fully implemented it would substantially effect the working patterns of nurses and carers. To the extent that long working hours of handling patients without breaks increases the risk of injury, this directive has the potential to give further protection to the employee. Perhaps negotiators could use it as a factor in negotiating for a safer lifting policy?

PROFESSIONAL CONDUCT

Some professional people involved in lifting and handling are subject to codes of conduct. For instance, a nurse who refused to carry out what she considered was an unsafe lift was referred to the United Kingdom Central Council Professional Conduct Committee, but was found not guilty of conduct unbefitting a nurse (UKCC v. Lalis Lillian Grant (Nursing Standard 18/2/89).

The UKCC has indicated that it will always look at any cases of refusal to lift on an individual basis, and has stressed the importance of recording the reasons for making that decision. Although the most important consideration must be the patient's safety and well being, this must not be at the expense of the nurse's health and safety. In most circumstances of this kind, it would be unlikely for the Professional Conduct Committee to find against a nurse (Nursing Times 10 April 1996, page 29).

Clause 13 of the 3rd edition (June 1992) (Ref 31) of the Code of Professional Conduct for the Nurse, Midwife and Health Visitor states:

> "Report to an appropriate person or authority where it appears that the health or safety of colleagues is at risk, as such circumstances may compromise standards of care and practice".

It is therefore conceivable that a senior nurse with responsibility for standards of safety regarding lifting and handling could be accountable to the nursing professional body as well as to the court. Also, all nurses have a professional duty to report their concerns.

THE 1992 EUROPEAN DIRECTIVES

Important changes in health and safety were brought about as a result of the completion of the single market in the European Community (EC) on 31 December 1992.

The aim of the legislation was to harmonise health and safety standards throughout the EC so that undertakings operating in a country which might otherwise have lower health and safety standards, and consequently lower costs, do not have an unfair competitive advantage. This process is described in the jargon of bureaucracy as the creation of a level playing field.

Authority for the legislation arises principally from Article 118a of the Treaty of Rome 1957 (amended by the Single European Act, 1987) which has the objective of harmonising health and safety standards in the EC and encouraging and maintaining improvements in those standards. Article 100a which aims to remove technical barriers to trade is also relevant.

The main instrument by which these aims are translated into domestic law is through the directive. A directive places obligations on a member state as to the result to be achieved by domestic legislation, but leaves open to each state the form and method of implementation as long as this is done within a stated time limit. Problems have arisen where directives have not been complied with either at all, or insufficiently.

Recent decisions of the European Court, and of the UK House of Lords, have had the effect of upgrading the status and force of EC directives. The arguments are complex and will continue to be litigated over the next few years. However, there is a significant force of legal opinion behind the following propositions in respect of the force and effect of directives:

1. that where directives are sufficiently clear and precise, unconditional, and leave no room for discretion in implementation, that they are binding on EC members' national courts in relation to civil claims at least, whether or not the plaintiff relies on them

2. that they must be enforced by national courts against all classes of defendant whether in the public or private sector

3. that breach of provisions in directives relating to health and safety can constitute breaches of duty in English common law negligence or breach of statutory duty regardless of implementation in domestic law, because national courts are now compelled to interpret existing domestic law in the light of directives

4. that in interpreting EC law national courts must adopt the purposive approach of the continental civil law tradition, to be contrasted with the much narrower textual approach of the English common law, stressing as it does the meaning of words

5. that if the domestic law falls short of the requirements of any directive the national court must interpret the domestic law in the light of the wording of the directive and if necessary re-write it to rectify the omission, and

6. that an individual who has been harmed as a result of the failure of a member state to take all necessary steps to achieve the result required by a directive can, subject to certain conditions, sue the member state for compensation.

In the light of these principles it is best to concentrate on the provisions of the relevant directives, rather than the regulations made under the HSWA 74, as the text of the directive is likely to prevail where there is any inconsistency with the wording in the regulation.

Regarding lifting and handling, these are principally:

the Council Directive of 12 June 1989 (89/391/EEC) (Ref 32) on the introduction of measures to encourage improvements in the safety and health of workers at work, the so-called Framework Directive, intended to be implemented by the M of HSW Regulations 92

the Council Directive of 29 May 1990 (90/269/EEC) (Ref 33) on the minimum health and safety requirements for the manual handling of loads where there is a risk particularly of back injury to workers, the Manual Handling of Loads Directive intended to be implemented by the MHO Regulations 1992.

The Manual Handling of Loads Directive is subsidiary to the Framework Directive and should be interpreted in the light of it.

Article 5.1 of the Framework Directive provides that:

the employer shall have a duty to ensure the safety and health of workers in every aspect related to the work.

Articles 6.1 and 6.2 provide:

1. Within the context of his responsibilities the employer shall take measures necessary for the safety and health protection of workers, including prevention of occupational risks and provision of information and training, as well as provision of the necessary organisation and means. The employer shall be alert to the need to adjust these measures to take account of changing circumstances and aim to improve existing situations.

2. The employer shall implement the measures referred to ... (above) ... on the basis of the following general principles on prevention:

(a) avoiding risks

(b) evaluating the risks which cannot be avoided

(c) combating the risks at source

(d) adapting the work to the individual, especially as regards the design of work places, the choice of work equipment and the choice of working and production methods, with a view, in particular, to alleviating monotonous work and work at a predetermined work rate and to reducing their effect on health

(e) adapting to technical progress

(f) replacing the dangerous by the non-dangerous or the less dangerous

(g) developing a coherent overall prevention policy which covers technology, organisation of work, working conditions, social relationships and the influence of factors related to the working environment

(h) giving collective protective measures priority over individual protective measures

(i) giving appropriate instructions to the workers

These general obligations do not contain the limitation, familiar from the HSWA, to exercise duties "so far as is reasonably practicable" or to take only "reasonable" care as required by common law. The only limitation permitted under the Framework Directive is in Article 5.4 which provides:

This directive shall not restrict the option of member states to provide for the exclusion or the limitation of the employer's responsibility where occurrences are due to unusual and unforeseeable circumstances, beyond the employer's control, or to exceptional events, the consequences of which could not have been avoided despite the exercise of all due care.

It will be argued that the effect of the Framework Directive is to impose a higher duty on employers closer to that of "Practicability" rather than "Reasonable practicability." This means that a duty must be performed if it is capable of being performed in the technical sense, economic considerations not being relevant.

As indicated above, the M of HSW Regulations 92 (Ref 4) cannot be invoked in support of a civil compensation claim. Further, they relegate the obligations in article 6.2(a)-(i) to paragraph 27 of the accompanying Approved Code of Practice. Both devices arguably amount to an insufficient implementation of the Framework Directive.

The Manual Handling of Loads Directive, which must be read in the light of the Framework Directive, provides in Articles 3 and 4:

3.1. The employer shall take appropriate organisational measures, or shall use the appropriate means, in particular mechanical equipment, in order to avoid the need for the manual handling of loads by workers.

3.2 Where the need for the manual handling of loads by workers cannot be avoided the employer shall take the appropriate organisational measures, use the appropriate means, or provide workers with such means in order to reduce the risk involved in the manual handling of such loads, having regard to ... (various reference factors set out in an annex relating to the characteristics of the load, the physical effort required, the characteristics of the working environment, and the requirements of the activity – see table 1).

4. Wherever the need for manual handling of loads by workers cannot be avoided, the employer shall organise work stations in such a way as to make such handling as safe and healthy as possible, and:

(a) assess in advance if possible the health and safety conditions of the type of work involved, and in particular examine the characteristics of loads taking account of ... (the reference factors in the annex referred to above).

(b) take care to avoid or reduce the risk particularly of back injury to workers, by taking appropriate measures, considering in particular the characteristics of the working environment and the requirements of the activity, taking account of ... (the reference factors in the annex referred to above).

Again, the extent of the duty which article 3.1 imposes on employers is arguably higher than the standard of reasonable practicability required by the MHO Regulations (Ref 2).

However, paragraph 108 of the guidance note to the MHO Regulations itself emphasises the ergonomic approach advocated by previous editions of The Handling of Patients. Further, the HSE emphasises that the costs of mechanising lifting procedures, although expensive, will lead to productivity gains and to cost savings from reducing injury.

It is therefore likely that regardless of whether the Framework and Manual Handling of Loads directives conflict with the M of HSW Regulations 92 and/or the MHO Regulations, employers will be required to provide hoists and/or other appropriate equipment for lifting patients heavier than the guideline figures, and that a failure to do so may lead to legal consequences as regards regulation and as regards compensation.

The main change brought fully into effect in the MHO Regulations is the requirement to make an assessment before lifting or handling any patients where the lifting or handling manoeuvre carries a risk of injury which cannot otherwise be avoided. Of particular relevance to a hospital ward situation is Article 6.1.2(d) of the Framework Directive quoted above relating to the rate of work which might have significant implications for ward routines.

SAFER HANDLING POLICIES

Regulation 4 of the MHO Regulations (Ref 2) applies only to handling operations involving a risk of injury. When that risk has been established, and only then, does the duty either to avoid or reduce the risk come into play. The question, is when does the lifting and handling of patients involve a risk of injury under the regulations?

In its March 1993 Code of Practice (Ref 12), the Royal College of Nursing, through its Advisory Panel for Back Pain in Nurses, provided an answer. It advised that no two nurses should, even under ideal conditions, take the full weight of a patient weighting more than 50kg (8 stones). This figure was arrived at by applying the guideline figures for lifting and lowering set out in paragraphs 9 – 11 and figure 1 of appendix 1 to the MHO Regulations. Whilst emphasising, as the appendix does, that no threshold is safe, the code of practice arrived at this figure by reducing the guideline figures by one third as is recommended for women – for 90 per cent of nurses are women. Thus, the guideline figure for one nurse lifting close to the body is 17kg (38lbs).

Paragraph 8 of the appendix recommends that once these guideline figures are exceeded, the requirement for an assessment under regulation 4 (1)(b)(i), and the duty to reduce the risk of injury applying the test of reasonable practicability under regulation 4 (i)(b)(ii), are triggered, and, that once the guideline figures are exceeded by more than a factor of two, that any operations should come under very close scrutiny. The guideline figure for one female nurse lifting close to the stomach in ideal conditions is 17kg, or 22kg for two female nurses. This implies that lifting should be avoided with almost all patients. But is that reasonably practicable? A safer handling policy would cost money, time and trouble, to quote Lord Justice Asquith in Edwards v. National Coal Board (Ref 3) when defining the meaning of reasonable practicability.

The evidence now accumulating and set out in the Royal College of Nursing publication, introducing a

Safer Patient Handling Policy (April 1996) (Ref 34), suggests that it is. It appears that the largest item of expenditure, the cost of lifting equipment, amounts to a once only cost of about 0.3 per cent of the employer's budget, with a recurring cost for maintenance and replacement of about 0.3 per cent a year afterwards.

To justify not spending such sums the employer would have to be able to show that such cost was grossly disproportionate – several times greater than – the size of the risk, and the indirect and direct costs of sickness and injury attributable to the manual handling of patients. The items of expenditure which can be attributable to a handling accident in the NHS can include:

contractual and statutory sick pay of injured staff

social security benefits repayable to the Compensation Recovery Unit of the Department of Social Security

the cost to the NHS of treating injured staff

the additional care costs of any injured patients

cost of arranging for and paying temporary staff

recruitment costs of replacement staff

training and induction of replacement staff

the wasted cost of training the nurse who has to retire early because of injury

the cost of NHS Permanent Injury Benefit and/or increased cost to pension fund caused by early retirement

the costs of defending legal actions from injured patients and staff and the damages awarded to them

the effect of negative publicity on morale, productivity and corporate image

the cost of management time in dealing with this substantial list.

For a rough estimate of the likely cost one can look to a study by the HSE in 1991 of a National Health Service trust hospital. The figure which emerged for the direct and indirect costs of all accidents and ill health among staff was 5 per cent of annual running costs. Whatever proportion of this figure can be attributable to handling injuries (and the HSE has estimated nearly 50 per cent – see paragraph 6 of HSAC Guidance on Manual Handling of Loads in the Health Services 1992), it is likely to exceed 0.3 percent.

If anything, it may be that the cost of taking no action is disproportionate to the cost of establishing a safer handling policy. Wigan and Leigh Health Services NHS Trust calculated the financial loss caused by lifting related injuries, 42 per cent of all lost hours due to work related injury, at £0.5m. After having a safer handling policy in operation for one year the number of lost hours due to manual handling injuries fell by more than 80 per cent, a saving of £400,000 a year (Nursing Times 10 April 1996 page 28).

From figures like these it seems likely that an employer would be hard pressed to mount a defence to criminal or civil proceedings brought under regulation 4 of the MHO Regulations, for the burden of proof is on the employer to show that the cost is several times the risk.

It is important to note that the employer's calculations must have been made at a point in time before the accident to which the proceedings relate. (Edwards v. National Coal Board) (Ref 3). Further, in a civil claim, the Manual Handling of Loads Directive can be invoked as an aid to the interpretation of the MHO Regulations especially in so far as they fail adequately to implement the wording and purpose of the directive.

The provisions of Article 3.1, the text of which is set out above, arguably sets out a stricter standard than that of what is reasonably practicable. It is likely the directive, which makes specific reference to the use of mechanical equipment, imposes a duty to avoid manual handling if it is technically possible and suggests that cost, time and trouble would not be taken into account.

It is now fairly clear that it is reasonably practicable for employers to have safer handling policies in compliance with regulation 4(1)(a) MHO Regulations in all but exceptional or life threatening situations (see Chapter 7). Because nurses and carers are dealing with human beings, not loads, the need to assess and reduce risk under regulation 4(1)(b) will not disappear even though the need to lift and take the full weight of the patient will. Handling will remain, and will still have its attendant risks for the patient and the handler. The requirement for instruction, training, and the provision of safe systems of work will also continue.

EQUIPMENT

Since legal developments are likely to lead to increased use of equipment and other aids, it is appropriate to mention the employer's duties as regards work equipment. The common law duty and the general duty under the Health and Safety at

Work Act are similar, namely, to provide and maintain work equipment in so far as is reasonably practicable. The employer can seek to ensure proper maintenance of and training for the use of equipment, but may not be able to avoid a hidden defect in its manufacture. However, where an employee sustains personal injury because of a defect in equipment provided by the employer, and the defect is the fault of another party, for example, the manufacturer or maintenance contractor, the injury is still deemed to be attributable to the fault of the employer (Employers Liability (Defective Equipment) Act, 1969) (Ref 35). This means that the employer cannot defend a claim of negligence even though entirely blameless. The employer may have a claim against the third party, be it manufacturer or contractor, but is still primarily responsible for compensating the injured employee if the third party is proved or admitted to be negligent.

Alternatively, the injured employee may be able to claim compensation under Part I of the Consumer Protection Act, 1987 (Ref 36). A product is defective if the safety of the product is "not such as persons generally are entitled to expect." There is an advantage here in that fault need not be shown. However, the employee can only claim against the employer if the manufacturer cannot be identified.

Work equipment is now regulated under the Provision and Use of Work Equipment Regulations 1992 (Ref 37) (PUWE Regulations 92) which implement a EC directive of 30 November 1989 concerning the minimal health and safety requirements for the use of work equipment by workers (89/655/EEC) (Ref 38).

The regulations came into force on 1 January 1993 for all work equipment first provided after 1 January 1993, and came fully into force for all work equipment whenever provided on 1 January 1997. The duty falling on the employer, which is an absolute duty, is to ensure that work equipment is so constructed or adapted as to be suitable for the purpose for which it is used. A hoist would not be suitable for lifting a patient who was heavier than the maximum weight specified by the manufacturers.

An employee bringing a claim for injury caused by using unsuitable work equipment will be able to rely on this strict duty. Work equipment must not only be suitable when first introduced, but must be maintained in an efficient state, in efficient working order, and in good repair. Paragraph 70 of the guidance note to this regulation emphasises that "efficient" relates to how the condition of the equipment might affect health and safety and is not concerned with productivity. The absolute duty to maintain is linked to a duty to keep any maintenance log up to date.

There are also absolute duties to provide employees with adequate health and safety information, and where appropriate, written instructions. Those instructions should include any foreseeable abnormal situation and any conclusions to be drawn from experience in using the equipment. For example, any problems in using a hoist should be noted in writing by some means attached to the hoist.

Every employer is under an absolute duty to ensure that all persons who use work equipment have received adequate training for the purposes of health and safety, including any risks which may be entailed in using it, and the precautions to be taken. Breach of any or all of these duties can be invoked where injury is the consequence.

The employer is also under a duty to consult with safety representatives in good time concerning the introduction of new technologies into the work place. This would apply to much of the equipment involved in safer patient handling.

THE WORK PLACE

Emphasis on the suitable equipment required to introduce a safer patient handling policy should not detract from the importance of a safer work place. Schedule 1, paragraph 3 to the MHO Regulations concerning the factors to which the employer must have regard, and the questions which must be considered in carrying out manual handling assessments, emphasises the importance of the working environment.

The Workplace (Health, Safety and Welfare) Regulations 1992 (Ref 6) came into full effect on 1 January 1996 after three years during which they applied only to new, extended or modified work places. There are provisions requiring:

adequate ventilation (Regulation 6)

a reasonable temperature (at least 16 degrees Centigrade) with sufficient thermometers to monitor it (Regulation 7)

suitable and sufficient lighting (Regulation 8)

every room to have sufficient floor area, height and space for the purposes of health and safety (Regulation 10)

work stations (which arguably can include beds) to be arranged so that they are at a suitable height and can be reached without undue bending or stretching (Regulation 11).

Slipping and tripping accidents are a significant risk in the health services, second only to lifting accidents. In some lifting accidents there is an element of slipping. Under Regulation 12 W(HS & W) Regulations 92 relating to the condition of floors and traffic routes, there is an absolute duty from 1 January 1996 to ensure that every floor in a work place is suitable for its purpose, and in particular should have no hole, slope, or be uneven or slippery, so as to expose any person to a risk to their health and safety. Further, every floor shall be kept free from obstructions or any article or substance which may cause a person to slip, trip or fall.

This duty is subject to the qualification "so far as is reasonably practicable," so an employer can seek to defend a claim by arguing that the cost of complying with this duty was grossly disproportionate to the risk.

The EC directive giving rise to these regulations imposes a stricter duty. It remains to be seen whether the English courts will find that the stricter duty in the directive should be preferred to the qualified duty in the regulations. Precedent suggests that they will.

PROBLEM AREAS

The legal responsibilities of the lifting trainer

The lifting trainer owes a duty to provide proper instruction and supervision to trainees, so far as is reasonable, and the more inexperienced the trainees, the greater is that duty. In the case of Beattie v. West Dorset Health Authority (1990) (Ref 40) the plaintiff was injured during a training session. She and a co-trainee, who was seven and a half inches taller than her, were practising the use of the Cradle or Orthodox lift. Another trainee weighing ten and a half stones acted as the patient. The court held that the trainer was negligent in pairing the plaintiff with a totally inexperienced and significantly taller partner without instructing that partner in how to compensate for the height difference, and in failing to intervene to prevent them from practising a hazardous lift.

Where the trainer is acting in the course of employment, the employer must meet any claim by providing legal representation, satisfying any court judgment, or paying any compensation which may be agreed between the parties. The employer's obligation stems from the doctrine of vicarious liability mentioned above. It applies regardless of whether the employer is negligent by, for instance, failing to train the trainer fully. The employee trainer is always wise to ensure that the precise scope of training duties is set out in writing in the contract of employment or job description.

The doctrine of vicarious liability applies only to events taking place in the course of employment and not to acts committed by employees who are, in the delightful phraseology used by the courts "off on a frolic of their own."

Where the lifting trainer is not an employee but an independent contractor, the employer's duty to provide a safe system for training in the lifting and handling of patients, so far as is reasonable, remains. The employer can delegate the performance of the duties to provide a safe system, but never the responsibility. The employer can discharge responsibility by taking reasonable care in the selection of independent contractors. In future, the scope of this duty may be significantly tightened by the impact of Article 5.2 of the Framework Directive which provides that where the employer enlists competent external services or persons to comply with the employer's obligations under the directive, this shall not "discharge him from his responsibilities in this area."

Agency workers

This leads to the situation of the agency worker contracted to form part of a lifting and handling team. It is arguable that the employer must take reasonable steps to ensure that any outside contractor has been trained and assessed as competent in lifting and handling patients, and that failure to do so is in breach of duty to the employees who may be injured as a result of that contractor's lifting error. However, the combined effects of Articles 5.2 and 5.4 of the Framework Directive would suggest that employers may be legally responsible for the failures of outside contractors, regardless of fault, in most circumstances.

If the agency worker is injured, her position is at first sight less favourable than that of the employee. This is because the duties under Regulation 4 of the MHO Regulations are expressed as those of the employer towards the employee. Non-employees who are injured can invoke the general law of negligence which in theory imposes duties less onerous than those imposed by the MHO Regulations.

The courts have appreciated the trend towards self employment but will not allow that trend to assist employers in avoiding their health and safety obligations. In the case of a skilled person, the question is: whose business is it to be responsible for that person's health and safety – is the agency nurse carrying out her own business or that of the contractor? Agency nurses are indistinguishable from their full time employed colleagues, apart from being self employed for income tax purposes, being required, for instance, to observe ward routines and procedures. They are almost certain to be treated as employees and to be owed the duties under the MHO Regulations (Lane v. Shire Roofing (Oxford) Ltd [1995]) (Ref 41).

Disclaimers

Occasionally health care providers attempt to limit their legal responsibilities for injury to their employees by the use of exclusion clauses or disclaimers. An example would be an attempt to relieve the employer or lifting trainer from any responsibility for injury caused to the employee or another party by asking the employee to sign a disclaimer along the following lines:

> *At the conclusion of this training I was competent to handle manually as taught. Accordingly, I disclaim any responsibility on my place of work or trainer for any subsequent injury after training.*

Where an employee might make a claim for personal injury despite having signed a disclaimer of this kind, the disclaimer would be rendered ineffective by Section 2 (1) of the Unfair Contract Terms Act 1977 which provides that a contract term or notice cannot restrict any person's legal responsibility for death or personal injury resulting from his or her negligence.

Where third parties may make a claim for personal injury against an employee who had signed a disclaimer, the employer is not relieved from the legal responsibility for the negligence of the employee, under the doctrine of vicarious liability. This means that the employer must meet any claim against an employee where that employee is acting in the course of employment, and this rule operates regardless of any fault on the part of the employer. An employer may also be legally responsible for the negligence of self employed persons acting under the employer's control. The Employer's Liability (Compulsory Insurance) Act 1969 requires employers, with some exceptions, to take out insurance to cover claims by their own employees, and it is a criminal offence to fail to do so. The exceptions include public bodies such as NHS trusts and local authorities who will have sufficient resources to meet claims from their own funds.

More generally, English courts have always been reluctant to attach legal responsibility to authors whose negligent misstatements have allegedly caused loss to readers who have relied on them. To be able to sue for wrong advice, a person has to show the adviser knew that the advice would be relied upon and that it was reasonable in the circumstances for such reliance to be placed in the adviser. Where there is a close relationship between the parties, and the recipient of the advice is an individual or a small identifiable group, for instance between an occupational health nurse as consultant and the nurses employed by a NHS trust, it is more likely that legal responsibility will arise. Any disclaimer of legal responsibility in a contract would not be effective unless it passed the "reasonableness" test in the Unfair Contract Terms Act 1977. In an ordinary contract for the supply of professional services it would be difficult to justify an exclusion of liability for negligence.

The professional and the carer in the community

The problems arising from the lifting and handling of patients in the community are far greater, because the health care provider has only limited control over conditions in the patient's home, while still under an obligation to provide a reasonably safe system of work for employees who lift and handle patients in their own home.

One problem that can arise is when patients or relatives refuse a hoist where risk assessment indicates this is necessary to minimise risk of injury to the community nurse. Where all reasonable efforts have been made to achieve acceptance of such recommendations, it would be reasonable of management to inform the patient that services might have to be withdrawn. (see Chapter 2).

Lifting and handling often involves securing the assistance of carers who are family members and who may often, themselves, be elderly or disabled. It can be said that the community or district nurse has a duty to teach such carers to handle safely, by assessing their ability to handle, and by teaching them the principles of safe handling and assessing their level of competence. This would apply both to manual techniques and to the use of any appropriate lifting aids which may be provided.

A carer who is injured may have a claim against the provider of community care services if such training can be proved to have fallen below the standard of training which expert opinion considers a carer should receive. However, since there is no employer/employee relationship between the carer and the health care provider the claim would be made under the general law of professional negligence; as such it would face problems of foreseeability, standard of care to be expected, causation and the reluctance of the courts to "open the floodgates" to new categories of claims.

It should be remembered that in assessing the need for handling equipment in the patient's home, the MHO Regulations must be complied with. Self employed people must take the same steps to protect themselves as an employer should for employees. The patient's needs will be assessed under the provisions of Section 47 (1)(a) of the NHS and Community Care Act 1990 (Ref 44).

The carer's role has also been formalised under the Carers (Recognition and Services) Act 1995 (Ref 45). The local authority, if asked by the carer, is required to assess the carer's ability to provide care, and to take account of that assessment in making any decision. The ability of the carer to cope with the handling needs of the patient will be relevant. The assessment must balance the interests of the patient and the lay and professional carers, but standards and quality of care and health and safety concerns need not normally come into conflict.

Regulation 9 of the Management of Health and Safety at Work Regulations 92 (Ref 4) requires cooperation and coordination where two or more employers share a workplace. This would include a patient's home where the local authority social services department and an NHS trust were both involved in providing services.

OFFICIAL JOURNAL OF THE EUROPEAN COMMUNITIES

No.1. 156/12   21.6.90

Annex 1

Reference Factors

(Article 3 (2), Article 4 (a) and (b) and Article 6 (2))

1. Characteristics of the load
The manual handling of a load may present a risk particularly of back injury if it is:

- too heavy or too large

- unwieldy or difficult to grasp

- unstable or has contents likely to shift

- positioned in a manner requiring it to be held or manipulated at a distance from the trunk, or with a bending of twisting of the trunk

- likely, because of its contours and/or consistency, to result in injury to workers, particularly in the

- event of a collision.

2. Physical effort required
A physical effort may present a risk particularly of back injury if it is:

- too strenuous

- only achieved by a twisting movement of the trunk

- likely to result in a sudden movement of the load

- made with the body in an unstable posture.

3. Characteristics of the working environment
The characteristics of the work environment may increase a risk particularly of back injury if:

- there is not enough room, in particular vertically, to carry out the activity

- the floor is uneven, thus presenting tripping hazards, or is slippery in relation to the worker's footwear

- the place of work or the working environment prevents the handling of loads at a safe height or with good posture by the worker

- there are variations in the level of the floor or the working surface, requiring the load to be manipulated on different levels

- the floor or foot rest is unstable

- the temperature, humidity or ventilation is unsuitable.

4. Requirements of the activity
The activity may present a risk particularly of back injury if it entails one or more of the following requirements:

- over frequent or over prolonged physical effort involving in particular the spine

- an insufficient bodily rest or recovery period

- excessive lifting, lowering or carrying distances

- a rate of work imposed by a process which cannot be altered by the worker.

From EC Directive 90/269/EEC. Reproduced with the permission of the Commission of the European Communities.

REFERENCES

1. Health and Safety at Work etc. Act 1974, HMSO

2 Manual Handling Operations Regulations 1992, and Guidance on Regulations L23, HMSO 1992

3. Edwards -v- National Coal Board [1949] 1 All ER 743

4. The Management of Health and Safety at Work Regulations 1992 and Approved Code of Practice L21, HMSO 1992

5. Provision and Use of Work Equipment Regulations 1992 and Guidance on Regulations L22, HMSO 1992

6. Workplace (Health, Safety and Welfare) Regulations 1992 and Approved Code of Practice L24, HMSO 1992.

7. The Lifting of Patients in the Health Services, Health Services Advisory Committee to the Health and Safety Commission 1984

8. Guidance on manual handling of loads in the Health Services, Health Services Advisory Committee to the Health and Safety Commission 1992

9. The Highway Code . HMSO

10. Code of Practice for the Handling of Patients , Royal College of Nursing, 1982

11. Code of Practice for the Handling of Patients Royal College of Nursing, 1992

12. Code of Practice for the Handling of Patients Royal College of Nursing March, 1993

13. Code of Practice for the Handling of Patients Royal College of Nursing April, 1996

14. Wilsons & Clyde Coal Limited -v- English [1938] AC 57

15. Edwards v. Waltham Forest Health Authority (1989) Unreported

16. Williams v. Gwent Health Authority [1983] C.L.Y. 2551

17. Moore -v- Norfolk Health Authority (1982) Unreported

18. Bayley v. Bloomsbury Health Authority (1987) Unreported

19. Hammond v. Cornwall and Isles of Scilly Health Authority (1986). Unreported

20. Munro v. Plymouth Health Authority (1991) Unreported

21. Page v. Enfield and Haringey Health Authority (1985) Unreported

22. Stewart v. Highland Health Board (1987) Unreported

23. Page v. Smith [1995] 2 All ER 736

24. Walker v. Northumberland County Council [1995] 1 All ER 737

25. Stress at Work, a Guide for Employers (1995). HSE

26. Access to Justice - Interim Report to the Lord Chancellor on the civil justice system in England and Wales by the Right Honourable Lord Woolf. HMSO June 1995

27. Access to Justice - Final Report by the Right Honourable Lord Woolf 1996. HMSO July 1996

28. Disability Discrimination Act 1995. HMSO

29. Employment Rights Act 1996. HMSO

30. Council Directive (93/014/EC)of 23 November 1993 concerning certain aspects of the organisation of working time.

31. Code of Professional Conduct for the Nurse, Midwife and Health Visitor 3rd edition (June 1992). United Kingdom Central Council for Nursing Midwifery and Health Visiting.

32. Council Directive of 12 June 1989 (89/391/EEC) on the introduction of measures to encourage improvements in the safety and health of workers at work.

33. Council Directive of 29 May 1990 (90/269/EEC) on the minimum health and safety requirements for the manual handling of loads where there is a risk particularly of back injury to workers (fourth individual Directive within the meaning of Article 16 (1) of Directive 89/391/EEC)

34. Introducing a Safer Patient Handling Policy Royal College of Nursing(April 1996)

35. Employers Liability (Defective Equipment) Act, 1969. HMSO

36. Consumer Protection Act, 1987.HMSO

37. Provision and Use of Work Equipment Regulations 1992

38. Council Directive of 30 November 1989 concerning the minimal health and safety requirements for the use of work equipment by workers (second individual Directive within the meaning of Article 16(1) of Directive 89/391/EEC) (89/655/EEC).

39. The Costs of Accidents at Work. HSE 1993

40. Beattie v. West Dorset Health Authority (1990) Unreported

41. Lane v. Shire Roofing (Oxford) Ltd [1995] IRLR.

42. Unfair Contract Terms Act 1977. HMSO

43. The Employer's Liability (Compulsory Insurance) Act 1969. HMSO

44. NHS and Community Care Act 1990.HMSO

45. Carers (Recognition and Services) Act 1995. HMSO

INTRODUCING A SAFER HANDLING POLICY

by Moira Tracy and Sue Ruszala

SUMMARY

No-one working in a hospital, nursing home or a patient's own home, should need to lift patients any more. Yet manual lifting still continues to be done and because of it, carers have back pain and other musculo-skeletal disorders. Hoists, sliding aids, and other specialised equipment should now be used routinely to move patients without manual lifting.

This chapter is for all managers and care staff, and shows how practices are to be changed. It draws on the experience of people in wards or NHS trusts which have introduced a safer handling policy.

INTRODUCTION

A safer handling policy

The greatest risk of back pain at work comes from heavy lifting. Other tasks or postures also put stress on the back, shoulders, and so on, and these are very important, but in nursing, the first priority to reduce back pain is to eliminate heavy lifting. Organisations increasingly try to reduce the risks with a safer handling policy, sometimes called no-lifting or minimal lifting policies. This benefits patients as well as staff.

A safer handling policy requires a risk assessment to be made for handling tasks, and the risk to be reduced to the lowest level that is reasonably practicable, as stated in the Manual Handling Operations Regulations (Ref 3). According to a safer handling policy:

> patients are never lifted manually

> patients are encouraged to assist in their own transfers

> appropriate equipment and furniture is used to reduce the risk of musculo-skeletal disorders.

In stating that patients are never lifted manually, the policy refers to lifting the whole, or a large part of, the weight of a patient. The policy does not prevent a nurse from giving a patient some assistance, or using pushing, pulling, upward or downward forces. But this is only acceptable if forces are as low as is reasonably practicable

(Manual Handling Operations Regulations (1992) and Chapter 1), taking into account alternative methods and equipment. For instance, if a patient needs the help of a nurse to stand (see Chapter 15), the nurse may exert considerable force. A proper risk assessment should identify the need for a safer handling method. All tasks, whether lifting, sliding or just assistant, must be done with the equipment, and in an environment and system of work, that reduce the risk to the lowest level that is reasonably practicable.

There are situations in which an exception can be made to a safer handling policy, in which a patient may be lifted manually:

Emergencies

Chapter 21 explains that there are few emergencies which cannot be foreseen. A safe system of work must be planned for foreseeable emergency situations: the risk must be reduced to the lowest level that is reasonably practicable.

There are few situations in which a victim must be moved to safety immediately and there is not enough time to obtain equipment or plan the move. Staff may find themselves taking rapid decisions in which they compromise their own safety. This is unavoidable and no blame should be implied. However, staff should apply principles of safer handling where ever possible, bearing in mind that if they are injured while moving a patient during an emergency, they may not be able to carry out further life saving activities such as resuscitation.

Conflicts with a patient's needs

There is rarely conflict between the needs of the patient and the safety of the nurse, where it becomes acceptable not to use handling equipment and to resort to manual lifting.

For example, when helping a patient to stand, nurses and physiotherapists may run a high risk of injury if the patient falls unexpectedly. But if a good assessment has been made and the carers position themselves properly or use suitable equipment (see Chapter 15), the risk to the carers is low.

If the patient's needs are genuinely so complicated that there is a true conflict of interest, a formal risk assessment must be done with great care. When deciding what is reasonably practicable, the risk to the patient from how elements of care are given or withheld, and his needs, must be taken into account as well as the risks to the nurse. A balance must be found where one party's benefit does not significantly increase the other party's risk.

Babies

Units which deal with babies and children should not concern themselves with rules not to lift, and should avoid the complications of trying to set weight limits for lifting. They should concentrate on avoiding or reducing the risk of injury, based on risk assessments and on the numerical guidelines in the Appendix to the Manual Handling Operations Regulations. For instance, the design of a cot can be more significant than the weight of the baby inside it. (see Chapter 19).

The Manual Handling Operations Regulations 1992 describe the responsibilities of the employer and the employee and define the phrase 'reasonably practicable.' The regulations are dealt with fully in Chapter 1.

THE SAFER HANDLING POLICY IN PRACTICE

Many patients can contribute to a move. Where it is assessed as safe to do so, patients should be encouraged and shown how to move themselves, and it is to their benefit.

Hoists can move non-weight-bearing patients on and off a chair, bed, bath, toilet, and floor.

Rigid or fabric sliding devices assist with transfers on to bed or trolley, and with moves up, down and around the bed.

Profiling beds, which are powered by an electric motor and can be controlled by the patient, can reduce much of the need for patient handling.

There is a great deal of handling equipment which can be purchased, leased, or hired at short notice. A comprehensive guide is published by the Disabled Living Foundation (Ref 2).

Handling techniques have improved. For example, patients can often be rolled instead of lifted.

When the patient refuses

Rarely, a patient may refuse to be moved with equipment, or a patient at home may refuse to have a hoist brought in and furniture moved. When this happens, seek help from someone such as a handling trainer, as the explanation may be:

> that a carer has allowed the patient to detect a sense of insecurity over the use of equipment,

> or

> the patient has been hurt in the past by the clumsy application of slings.

The benefits to the patient and relatives should be pointed out.

A solution can be to use another method or piece of equipment.

If the patient still refuses, a manager must consider:

> the risk of injury to staff from manual handling

> balanced against

> the risk to the patient if a procedure is not carried out.

The result of this assessment is usually to change an element of care, for example, to nurse a patient in bed.

The cost

Manual lifting can cost more – time lost through back pain, claims for negligence, and so on – than time and money spent on training and equipment for safer handling.

The cost of equipment to make a safer handling policy possible need not be great, and modifications of facilities, such as the widening of a toilet area, are often affordable.

Costs need to be estimated and budgets allocated, possibly over several years, to put a safer handling policy into effect.

The total equipment value of hoists, sliding aids, special baths, and so on, may be expected to be about 0.3 per cent of the annual budget.

In these examples, the figures have been rounded.

A HOSPITAL GROUP

This describes a 1991 estimate for a group of hospitals which employed 30,000 people, had 10,000 beds, and an annual budget of £600 million.

The typical needs for each medical ward were considered to be on average:

2 hoists

1 height adjustable bath

1 lateral transfer sliding aid

handling equipment, such as sliding sheets and rope ladders

Similar estimates were made for each type of patient care area.

The hospitals already had some hoists, special baths, transfer aids and small handling equipment, about one-third of what was needed to put the policy into effect. The cost of the extra equipment was 0.3 per cent of the annual budget.

This equipment usually lasts for up to 15 years so the average yearly cost was between 0.03 per cent and 0.04 per cent, including the cost of maintenance. The passage of time showed that these estimates were probably too high by 10 per cent.

THE VICTORIA INFIRMARY NHS TRUST, GLASGOW

This describes the trust's situation in 1995. More equipment is regularly bought.

The trust's annual budget is £60 million. It employs 2,400 people and has 450 beds in its general hospital, 260 beds in its geriatric hospital, and 100 beds in its maternity hospital. Its hoists and slings, sliding aids, and small handling equipment, cost about £120,000, or 0.2 per cent of its annual budget. Its height adjustable and tiltable baths cost £35,000.

Most of this is usable for at least 10 to 15 years, and the cost of maintaining it is £14,000 to £19,000 a year, or 0.02 per cent to 0.03 per cent of the annual budget; this cost includes a maintenance contract of about £90 a year for each hoist. This quantity of equipment was acquired gradually.

Between 1991 and 1994, the trust allocated about £20,000 each year, and in addition the wards bought extra slings and small handling equipment, and a few were donated.

In 1994, £37,000 was spent to launch a minimal lifting policy.

Some toilets and associated bathrooms were upgraded to improve patient care and handling at a cost of £3,000 each, which includes knocking down walls, replacing a shower cubicle with a sink unit, removing steps to the shower and to the toilet, re-flooring with a less slippery surface, and re-decorating.

Hoists and other aids are deployed as follows:

Most wards in the trust have a full-length sliding aid for bed-to-trolley transfers and several fabric sliding aids for bed moves.

The 260-bed geriatric hospital has 23 hoists, of which five are standing/sitting hoists. Long-term wards with 32 patients use three hoists each, whereas rehabilitation wards generally have two hoists.

The 450-bed general hospital averages one hoist in each ward, and has 23 hoists, of which three are standing/sitting. This includes x-ray and outpatients, which need one hoist each. Wards which only occasionally have dependent patients share with other wards on the same floor.

The maternity hospital has some small handling equipment but does not use a hoist.

THE POLICY THAT MAKES THINGS HAPPEN

Lifting patients is a major cause of carers' back pain and other musculo-skeletal disorders.

Managers often despair at the sight of hoists collecting dust in cupboards, and nurses may become frustrated at a failure to get a partition wall knocked down in a small bathroom.

Planning for a safer handling policy is a catalyst for change. It forces carers to change their habits, and they usually say they would never go back to former practices. It also commits an organisation to provide whatever is needed – such as handling equipment and training – to reduce risk.

Anything less breaks the law

An organisation that is not working to a safer handling policy is not complying with the EEC Directive (Ref 1) or the Manual Handling Operations Regulations 1992 (Ref 3) (see Chapter 1). Health care organisations may become liable to fines and costs for failing to make risk assessments and reduce risks, and may have to meet civil claims for negligence.

A safer handling policy enables managers to demand good handling practices and is an important means of protection from liability. Employer's liability insurance premiums should reduce accordingly.

However, the policy must be credible: a trust cannot maintain that an injured nurse should have used a hoist, according to policy, if there was not reasonable access to a hoist.

Anything less is more expensive

In addition to insurance premiums, anything less brings the unnecessary costs of sickness, treatment, lost time, replacement, induction and training, redeployment, premature retirement, reduced efficiency, low morale, and so on.

> The Wigan and Leigh Health Services NHS Trust introduced a safer patient handling policy in 1994. The reduction in sickness absence which had been due to unsafe handling saved the trust £400,000 in one year (see Chapter 10).

Good for patients

Safer handling often adds to the quality of care a patient receives. Encouraging self-help stimulates patients physically and mentally, it reduces side effects associated with immobility, and contributes towards their physical rehabilitation.

Most dependent patients accept the use of a hoist as routine safe practice, appreciating increased comfort it gives or recognising the advantages to themselves and the carer. Obese patients may feel less reticent about asking carers to move them.

Good for carers

A safer handling policy should lead to a reduction in accidents as well as in sick leave. It should convert nurses' heavy jobs into jobs that are merely physically active. Injury rates should, in theory, go down to one-tenth of their former levels, to become similar to the rate among other workers whose jobs require only a moderate amount of physical activity.

The Victoria Infirmary NHS Trust of Glasgow has reduced its manual handling injuries by half since 1992 when the use of equipment was gradually increased. One immediately recognised effect is that nurses are less tired by the end of their shift. The Wigan and Leigh Trust reduced sickness absence due to handling by 84 per cent.

This seems to confirm that a safer handling policy can reduce the prevalence of back pain by as much as nine-tenths: Chapter 3 describes a study that showed that people in heavy occupations are 10 times more likely to have back pain than people in jobs involving medium workloads.

PLANNING THE POLICY

A safer handling policy requires the following to be in place:

sufficient and suitable handling equipment and furniture is provided

there is room and space for the equipment and furniture to be used properly and safely

the environment is appropriate - good floors, space in toilets, hand rails, for example

carers have been trained how to handle patients, how to assess patients, and how to use the equipment.

The first steps:

- make the risk assessments required by the Manual Handling Operations Regulations 1992

- work out the costs of supplying what is needed

- work out acceptable solutions to problems (reducing risk to the lowest level that is reasonably practicable), as, for example, when a bathroom cannot be made more spacious

- make the money available, possibly over several years.

When solutions cannot be introduced immediately, short term measures must be put in place to reduce risk to the lowest level that is reasonably practicable during the interim period.

Alternative methods

Carers should continually assess the needs and capabilities of their patients, and devise the best handling methods accordingly.

A safer handling policy restricts their choice of methods to those which the organisation considers acceptable.

Although a carer may feel competent to select another method, the policy should not allow her to do so: employees have to comply with established safe systems of work. Exceptions should be made for rare, genuine emergencies (see Chapter 21). If for any reason a ward or a group of carers feel the need to deviate from the organisation's methods, this should be agreed with the manager and handling co-ordinator: the risk assessment and alternative safe system of work must be documented.

Monitoring

The policy is worthless unless carers are required to comply with it and it is strictly enforced so as to bring benefits to patients, carers, and the organisation. Experience has shown that rules are no defence against a claim for negligence unless they are enforced.

The success of a safer handling policy will be measured through incident or accident reports, the number of absences through sickness, reports to the occupational health department, and the number of civil claims against the organisation. A review of risk assessments should be made following incidents, accidents, near misses, or when conditions change.

Before taking disciplinary action against someone who has not complied with the policy, the reasons for non-compliance should be examined: for example, there may not be enough readily available handling equipment.

One way to monitor compliance is to check the patient care plans. These should indicate

>   the capabilities of the patient

>   the equipment and handling methods used

The usual patient care plans do not make it easy for carers to write enough detail, so they may need to be changed - not just for monitoring, but to make sure that the results of a patient's assessment are there to be seen by all the professionals caring for the patient.

CASE STUDIES

ONE OF THE FIRST SAFER HANDLING POLICIES: BROOMHILL HOSPITAL, GLASGOW.

>   About 10 years ago, a ward sister at Broomhill hospital started a no-lifting policy in her ward, after getting an abandoned hoist repaired. The policy worked well, and when she became the hospital's nursing officer, she extended the policy to all wards and departments. Broomhill catered for severely disabled people, nearly all of whom required lifting.

>   Most nurses worked in accord with the policy, but some did not and were threatened with disciplinary action. Before the policy was fully introduced, staff at the hospital had about 30 back injuries a year. These went down to 10, three, then no injuries at all in subsequent years.

>   After some years, injuries began to occur again. Staff believed this was due to the policy not being enforced following a change in management. They also blamed staff cuts. However one sister continued to apply the policy in her ward, which had no more back injuries:

>   this ward had two ambulifts, one bathing stretcher and one height adjustable bath. The bathroom was difficult to get into with a hoist, but even so staff did not lift manually.

UNITED BRISTOL HEALTHCARE NHS TRUST

>   The United Bristol Healthcare NHS trust employs 6,500 staff in 50 wards and in the community. It set up a minimal lifting policy in January 1994. The policy requires:

>>   improving poor working postures

>>   minimising all potentially hazardous manual lifting

>>   no patient lifting in all but exceptional or life threatening circumstances.

>   A commitment to risk management has supported the adequate provision of handling equipment, environmental improvements, and suitable training for staff. An improved uniform design allows greater freedom of movement. In total, the trust spent less than £250,000 on additional equipment and ergonomic improvements to put the policy into effect. Further improvements and provision or replacement of equipment is continuing and is met out of directorate funds.

>   Each department is responsible for reviewing work practices, identifying improvements and introducing control measures. Training and specialist advice supports the departmental team. The trust's Link Trainer programme has helped to change staff attitudes, question traditional handling methods, and empower staff to put into effect safer handling practices in their departments. Reporting of back pain incidents is encouraged, and this highlights the need to review risk assessments in a work area or activity. A small initial rise in the reporting of back pain incidents, due to increased awareness, was anticipated, and occurred.

>   The emphasis has been on increasing the use of handling equipment and self help methods for patients. Pre-admission information to patients has facilitated this approach. For example, patients have been told:

>>   Wherever possible you will be asked to move yourself. If this is not possible nurses need to use a variety of aids and equipment to minimise injury;

>   and this is reinforced on admission. Managers support the use of handling equipment to lift patients where indicated, in both the hospital and the community.

THE VICTORIA INFIRMARY NHS TRUST, GLASGOW

At the end of 1992, ward sisters were told about the Manual Handling Operations Regulations, and were told to use handling equipment whenever possible. Around the same time, more staff were becoming aware of the benefits, with a large proportion of nurses completing training in patient handling.

Writing manual handling risk assessments also made sisters aware of their responsibilities. There was not enough handling equipment at the time to stop manual lifting occurring in all wards, but several ward sisters declared their own wards had a no-lifting policy. Benefits were quickly found, with staff saying they were less tired. Other wards increased their use of equipment. During 1993, most wards claimed to have stopped manually lifting non-weight-bearing patients.

However, contradictions were found in places: for example, they still lifted up the bed manually, using the shoulder lift, which caused several injuries. Also, only when some injuries had occurred while staff were straight-lifting hip-replacement patients was the practice questioned. Physiotherapists knew of a ward or two where patients were still draglifted.

In 1994, the hospital managers accepted and supported the idea of a policy when they realised that only a little more equipment was needed.

When the required hoists were in place, and every ward had been given sliding aids to avoid manual lifting up and down the bed, the policy was launched.

Nurses were given a new section of the care plan to cover handling in more detail. Also provided were pictures of moves they had learned on handling courses, partly in order to give names to moves which could be written in the care plan.

The announcement of the policy did not cause any controversy: when questioned, nurses said they were doing it anyway.

Nurses' back injuries diminished by half over the following four years.

SAFER HANDLING IN A GYNAECOLOGY UNIT

The Link Trainer programme in United Bristol Healthcare NHS trust stimulated one staff nurse to review the handling practices in her gynaecology unit. She realised that staff lifted patients everywhere, and even able-bodied pre-operative patients were lifted from bed to trolley, despite the fact that they had walked to the toilet five minutes earlier. Various reasons were given:

established practice

patient dignity

risk prevention following pre-medication

easier and more convenient for staff.

The unit raised awareness about legislation and the sharing of ideas on reducing lifting. A number of practices changed:

handling issues are recorded in the care plans

patients are allowed to move themselves on to trolleys or a sliding device is used

patients for minor surgery walk to the theatre accompanied by a nurse

a hoist is available where needed

more effective pain control increases the patients' independent movement

pre-admission evenings include a practical session on how patients can move themselves post-operatively – this is reinforced pre-operatively on the ward.

Patients responded well. They reported feeling a sense of achievement at being able to move themselves, and relieved at not feeling so dependent. It takes more time to allow patients to move at their own pace, but they should not feel so disempowered as to have to wait for a nurse to move them.

SAFER HANDLING IN DAY SURGERY AND OUTPATIENT DEPARTMENTS

United Bristol Healthcare NHS Trust's day surgery and outpatient departments improved their handling practices and reduced the amount of manual handling that was done. The improvements include:

providing height adjustable trolleys, tables and treatment couches to allow staff to have better working postures, to promote the use of handling equipment, and to allow patients to transfer themselves where they are able

replacement of operating tables with special height adjustable operating trolleys making hoists available where needed

examining or treating patients in wheelchairs or transport chairs where appropriate

encouraging the taking of blood samples or other specimens in a lying position (this has significantly reduced the incidence of fainting in one clinic)

providing a special frame to hold patients' limbs in different positions for plastering

providing a variety of chair heights and styles – an appropriate chair makes it easier for people to move independently

identifying handling needs at the time of booking.

ACKNOWLEDGEMENTS

This chapter expands and updates the Royal College of Nursing's booklet (April 1996): 'Introducing a Safer Patient Handling Policy.'

The authors are grateful for the contributions from staff at the Victoria Infirmary NHS Trust (Glasgow) and at United Bristol Healthcare NHS Trust, and for long conversations with Mrs. Margaret Milne and Sister Ann Cartlin regarding the no lifting policy in Broomhill Hospital, Glasgow.

REFERENCES

1. EEC Council Directive: Article 16(1) of Directive 89/391EEC (90/269/EEC) 29 May 1990

2. Handling people: equipment, advice and information, The Disabled Living Foundation, 380-384 Harrow Road, London W9 2HU

3. Health and Safety Executive, 'Manual Handling Operations Regulations 1992: Guidance on Regulations', HMSO, 1992

BACK INJURY IN NURSES- ERGONOMICS AND EPIDEMIOLOGY

by Stephen Pheasant

SUMMARY

Ergonomics is the science of work:

> of the people who do it and the ways in which it is done

> the tools and equipment that they use

> the places they work in

> the way they feel about their working lives.

Ergonomics is more concerned with fitting the job to the person than fitting the person to the job. It is concerned with the design of safe systems of work.

INTRODUCTION

This chapter looks at the problem of back injury in nurses from a standpoint of what might be called common-sense ergonomics. Ergonomics is not an arcane and mysterious science. There are those who say it is mainly common sense - and there is truth in this. This chapter adds some exact science to what ought to be apparent from common sense.

THE RISKS OF LIFTING

Lifting and handling tasks entail three sorts of risks:

> risks of accidental injury

> risks of over exertion

> risks of cumulative over use.

Examples:

Accidental injury

Two nurses are lifting, or moving, a patient. One slips on a wet patch on the floor, falls awkwardly and injures her back.

This is an accidental injury – an accident being an unplanned, unanticipated, or uncontrolled event. This is not to say that nobody is to blame. It was presumably someone's responsibility to ensure that spillages on floors are cleaned up – and indeed the nurse might have done well to check this before moving the patient.

An overexertion injury

Two nurses are lifting a heavy and dependent patient up the bed, using the so-called orthodox or cradle-lift, which violates the elementary principles of safer lifting and has been condemned for many years. As they take the weight of the patient, one nurse feels a sudden sharp pain in her back.

This is not an accident – here is no unexpected event which interrupts the planned action other than the pain itself. This is an over exertion injury.

What happened? Some anatomical structure in the nurse's back failed under load – because the force applied to that structure exceeded its mechanical strength.

It may be that this nurse had lifted this patient in this way many times before. Why should she injure herself on this particular occasion? Perhaps the two nurses did not get their timing quite right, or perhaps the injured nurse was in some way more vulnerable on this occasion.

It is becoming increasingly clear that the process of back injury very often has a cumulative component.

An over use injury

Over use injuries occur when the rate of cumulative damage to some bodily structure exceeds that structure's natural capacity for healing and repair. Sports injuries are often like this – tendinitis in runners is an example – and it would be surprising if the same did not apply to the nurse's back.

A second week student nurse is a week or so into her placement for care of the elderly. She has to lift and handle heavy and highly dependent patients. Toward the end of an arduous shift she feels a dull ache in her back. That evening, while she is resting and doing nothing in particular her back becomes intensely painful, or she feels a sudden sharp pain in her back when she sneezes. Investigations reveal a prolapsed disc. Was this disc lesion caused by her work? Or the sneeze? Or did it happen spontaneously?

Common sense points to the work. So does the science of biomechanics (see Chapter 4). Laboratory experiments on segments of vertebral column taken from people who do not need them any more have reproduced the phenomenon of fatigue failure of the intervertebral disc or gradual disc prolapse (Ref 1).

There are good physiological reasons for thinking that this kind of injury is most likely to occur in young people – the disc dries out with age and fails in a different way. This injury was caused by cumulative trauma.

There are other ways in which the back may be damaged by cumulative trauma. The example given is of an injury occurring as a result of the cumulative effect of the stresses to which the nurse's back was exposed for a short period. The cumulative wear and tear on the spine which result from heavy lifting, or from working in bent or twisted postures, may have an effect over a longer time scale.

People in heavy manual jobs are about twice as likely to show signs of advanced disc degeneration, by the time they are in their 50s, as people in lighter work (Ref 12). Long term injury processes of this kind probably account for many of the cases of disabling back trouble which come on progressively in the later years of working life.

The long term effects of heavy lifting

A 45 year old nurse has spent her nursing career working with highly dependent patients on poorly staffed and equipped wards. She has suffered several over exertion injuries to her back, and an accidental injury. Additionally to these acute incidents, she undertook significant and regular heavy patient handling – cumulative load. At the age of 45 years another incident ends her career in nursing and she is medically retired.

The concept of cumulative damage is not new and layman's language has been used to describe the notion of wear and tear as being a particular problem in dock workers (Ref 13). Typically, in older dockers an acute insult is superimposed upon a long term effect of load handling. The analogy with nursing of the notion of wear and tear is appropriate, and the above example illustrates how the concept can be applied to nursing.

Nurses may spend, on average, some 22 per cent of their working day in a stooped position, and stooping for this length of time has been found to be associated with an increased risk of back pain (Ref 4).

Further, it is argued that an interaction occurs between the static loading on the spine when stooping and the dynamic loading on the spine when lifting, this contributing to the cumulative risk to the nurse's back.

EPIDEMIOLOGY OF BACK TROUBLE

Epidemiology is the branch of medical science which deals with the statistics of disease. It seeks to identify the risk factors which are statistically associated with the onset and development of diseases, to find out who is at risk and for what reasons.

Back trouble is difficult to study epidemiologically, for a number of reasons.

Back trouble has a diverse pathophysiology; the back can go wrong in a number of different ways

Back trouble has a multifactorial aetiology: a person may be at risk for a number of different reasons. Some of these risk factors are external to the individual concerned – most importantly, the nature of his or her work. Others are idiosyncratic to that individual – for example, risks stemming from that person's lifestyle, physical makeup and genetic endowment. These are called exogenous and endogenous risk factors respectively. These may interact in various complex ways, and may contribute to the different pathologies which may affect the back.

Back trouble has a diverse natural history. Many episodes of back trouble are short lived. They may be precursors of something worse to come. Some are little worse than the aches and pains of every day life. There is a danger that the results of surveys based on the self reporting of symptoms may be swamped by these relatively trivial episodes - and the risk factors which are associated with more serious back trouble may be hidden.

The results of the most extensive epidemiology investigation of back trouble in nurses reported to date (Ref 25) are summarised in table 1. They are compared with the results of a more recent but more limited study of nurses (Ref 19) and some equivalent figures for the general population of this country (Ref 11). The three surveys were conducted in 1979, 1992 and 1993 respectively.

One should always be cautious about conclusions drawn from comparisons between different surveys.

Taken at face value however, these three sets of figures point to two important conclusions:

that the incidence and prevalence of back pain in nurses is significantly higher than that of the general population

that the incidence and prevalence of back pain in nurses has climbed dramatically during the last decade or so.

Nurses reading this will have their own views as to why the latter should be the case.

Table 1

Incidence and prevalence of back pain in the general population

	POINT PREVALENCE (1)	ANNUAL PREVALENCE (2)	ANNUAL INCIDENCE (3)
NURSES (Ref 27)	17%	43%	8%
NURSES (Ref 19)	24%	59%	15%
GENERAL POPULATION (Ref 11) Men	12%	36%	7%
Women	15%	38%	8%

Notes:

(1) The point prevalence of a condition is the percentage of people in a sample who are suffering from that condition at the time of the survey.

(2) The annual prevalence is the percentage suffering the condition some time during the previous year.

(3) The annual incidence is the percentage suffering it for the first time during the previous year.

The data from surveys (refs 25 and 27) shows the percentage of nurses who attribute the back pain they have suffered during the previous year to various causes. Thus 37 per cent of all episodes of back trouble are episodes of acute onset associated with patient handling procedures.

Given a total annual prevalence of 43 per cent, this leads to a figure of 16 per cent for the proportion of nurses suffering acute back trouble as a result of patient handling each year - or more than one nurse in six. If the data (Ref 19) are correct, the figure today would be around 22 per cent, or more than one nurse in five. These figures almost certainly underestimate the true magnitude of the problem, however, in that they include accidental injuries and injuries due to acute over exertion, but not injuries occurring as a result of cumulative over use as might lead to back trouble of insidious onset.

One of the most interesting and extensive epidemiological studies of low back trouble

reported (Ref 21) was based on a survey of men and women drawn from many different walks of life, including nurses, who were asked many questions about their work. In essence the results of this study show that two distinct groups of people are likely to suffer from low back trouble: those whose work is physically very heavy and those whose work is totally sedentary.

But those whose work is moderately physically demanding but not excessively so, and who spend some time sitting and some time standing - have a strikingly low prevalence of back trouble. The difference in prevalence level, between those in this middle category and those at either extreme, was about ten to one.

Magora's findings seem to indicate that the curve which relates the physical demands of work to the risk of suffering back trouble is U-shaped or, J-shaped (Figure A page 47). This has been confirmed in an elegant study of the signs of physical injury in a sample of cadaveric spines of people for whom both occupational and medical histories were available (Ref 32).

It is not suggested that nurses suffer with their backs because they spend too long sitting down at work. It follows therefore that the task to be done is to move the work of the nurse from the far right of the J-shaped curve back into the middle low risk zone. This, in principle, ought to be achievable by eliminating the excessive degree of heavy lifting which nursing work entails.

The most detailed study reported to date, of the risk of cumulative injury to the spine by frequent and repeated heavy lifting, (Ref 18) was a study of Canadian institutional aids (nursing auxiliaries) who were mostly women and had an average age of 38, plus or minus five years. The investigators took a detailed lifetime occupational history of them and analysed the physical demands of the various jobs which they had held, using biomechanical techniques of considerable sophistication. This enabled them to calculate an index of the loading on the spine which these jobs had entailed. This figure was then summated across the jobs to yield a cumulative lifetime exposure measure.

This cumulative measure was significantly higher in those institutional aids who suffered with back trouble: the more heavy lifting performed throughout the years, the more likely a person is to have trouble with the back at the age of 40, or thereabouts.

The role of lifting and carrying at work was investigated as part of an extensive investigation of the epidemiology of acute prolapsed lumbar intervertebral disc, which took into account a host of occupational and other risk factors (Ref 16). The risk of suffering a disc prolapse increased with the amount of lifting and carrying which the person did; reaching a relative risk of 3.5 in subjects who lifted more than 11kgs (25lbs) more than 25 times per day. This means that people who do this amount of lifting are 3.5 times more likely to have a disc prolapse than people in occupations that involve only moderate handling.

Finally, higher levels of risk were associated with lifting while twisting; either with the knees bent (relative risk of 2.7) or with the knees straight (relative risk of 6.1).

An interesting and unusual study was made of Swedish nursing aids who worked on two geriatric wards (Ref 20). The care needs of the patients on these wards were the same. One of them they described as a traditional ward. It had three mobile hoists for 59 patients and working conditions were cramped, particularly as regards lavatory arrangements.

The other, which they called the modern ward, was spacious, and half the beds had ceiling mounted electric hoists. The researchers used wooden boots which had devices mounted in them to measure the vertical lifting forces which the nursing aids had to exert.

The aids on the traditional ward did about twice as much lifting per shift and their annual incidence of back injuries was exactly twice as high. This was despite the fact that the number of staff for each patient on the traditional ward was also twice as high.

A study of Australian nurses (Ref 2) found that the one-month prevalence of back trouble, the percentage of people in the sample reporting symptoms during the previous month, increased with the frequency of lifting patients; from 29 per cent for no lifts per shift to 55 per cent for more than 11 lifts for each shift.

An interesting feature of this study was that the amount of lifting undertaken by these nurses decreased with age, as did the prevalence of back trouble. For the population as a whole the prevalence of back trouble tends to increase with age at least until the middle years of life.

The high level of risk in young student nurses has recently been confirmed in this country (Ref 17). But an earlier study (Ref 8) showed a double peak in the annual incidence of back trouble in nurses, with those starting out in the profession being in a high risk category, as were those who had been nursing for around 20 years.

A 1984 study (Ref 31) reported a higher one-month prevalence of back trouble in nursing aids than in qualified nurses, and the aids had heavier jobs, as measured by the amount of lifting they said they did and the time spent in bent or twisted positions. This was confirmed by a study in 1987 (Ref 10) which found that the incidence of acute back injury was highest in aids, followed closely by student nurses and then by staff nurses. The injury rate was negligible in ward sisters.

The annual incidence of acute back injury occurring while lifting patients was analysed by the ward or department on which the nurse was working at the time (Ref 23). The results are shown in table 2. The highest injury rates were found where the patient dependency was greatest, such as in geriatric wards and in the community.

Table 2

Annual prevalence of back pain of acute onset associated with patient handling as a function of ward of specialty

	PREVELANCE %
Significantly higher than average (p≤0.01) General medicine	37
Geriatrics	34
Orthopaedics	34
District nursing	27
Overall rate for all nurses	19
Significantly lower than average (p≤0.10) Obstetrics	6
Outpatients	4
Accident and emergency	2
Administration	1

Note:
Prevalence figures are for whole time equivalents (Ref 23)

To summarise: the more lifting that a nurse - or anyone else - does, the more likely she is to injure her back, either as a result of accidental injury or acute over exertion, or as a result of cumulative over use, or by some combination of these.

PERSONAL RISK FACTORS

Some nurses will be more at risk than others. Back trouble tends to be recurrent. So the single most important personal risk factor, predicting whether a person is likely to suffer from back trouble in the future, is whether that person suffered from it in the past. Physical fitness is also important. This was shown in a study of Los Angeles fire fighters (Ref 7) and there is no reason to think that it would not hold for nurses (see also Chapter 4).

Smokers are more likely to suffer a prolapsed disc than non-smokers. The level of risk rises with how much a person smokes (Ref 15). This is thought to be due to the effects of nicotine on the blood supply to the spine. There is also evidence that disc lesions run in families (Ref 3) – from which it may be supposed that some people's discs are genetically predisposed to fail more easily under loading than others – although the reason is not known.

Pregnancy and motherhood carry a constellation of risk factors. Women who have more children have more prolapsed discs (Ref 14).

It is important to stress, however, that these endogenous or personal risk factors which place an individual at risk of developing back trouble, interact with those exogenous or occupational risk factors to which the person is exposed in the course of his or her work.

This is expressed in the equation:

$$\text{total risk} = \frac{\text{exogenous}}{\text{risk exposure}} \times \frac{\text{endogenous}}{\text{"at riskness"}}$$

The nurse who is at risk because of her genetic make up or life style will not necessarily develop back trouble unless she is placed in a high risk work situation, or may not suffer with her back early in life.

Psychosocial factors

Some features of back trouble have a psychological or psychosocial component. This touches upon very difficult territory. Whether or not a person reports having suffered from a back injury will depend to some extent on how she feels about her work, how she feels about herself and so on - at least if the injury is not a very serious one. This has been confirmed in a much quoted epidemiological study (Ref 14).

But this is not interesting or important when trying to find out how back injuries occur. What has been shown, more importantly, is that psychological factors are probably just as significant as physical ones in determining whether an acute episode of back trouble progresses into something involving long term chronic pain and disability (Ref 6).

This is not the same as saying that the injury itself has a psychological component. Too much is often made of the so-called psychosocial aspects of musculoskeletal injury at work. Psychosocial factors are important in the reporting of injury and in determining whether the resulting condition progresses to chronicity. But the injury itself is a physical event. A person is not injured (in this sense) merely because she says she is or believes herself to be.

It may be however that a person is more likely to injure herself if she is stressed because of fatigue, moves differently, takes short cuts, and so on. This does not mean that the psychological experience of being stressed has caused the injury, only that excessive workload can lead to both psychological stress and physical injury.

SAFE SYSTEMS OF WORK - THE ERGONOMIC APPROACH

The law requires employers to avoid hazardous lifting and handling procedures so far as is reasonably practicable, and to reduce the level of risk of those which cannot be avoided, so far as is reasonably practicable. A reasonably practicable measure is one which does not entail a cost (wether in money time or trouble) which is in gross disproportion to the degree of risk (see Chapter 1). There is no burden on the employer to devise systems of work which are free of risk.

This would be impossible as people cannot go about the ordinary activities of everyday life without exposing themselves to some measure of risk.

But the employer must take steps to ensure that the collective risks of accidental injury, over exertion and injury resulting from cumulative over use, are as low as is reasonably practicable. This is sometimes called the ALARP principle.

The ALARP principle points clearly and unequivocally to the need for such bodies corporate as employ nurses – trusts, nursing homes and so on – to take steps towards implementing a Safer Handling Policy as a matter of priority.

For simplicity it is convenient to deal with the risks of handling the patient load under five headings:

    the patient

    the procedure

    the working area and the equipment used

    the nurse or nurses

    the system as a whole.

The Patient

Common sense tells us that it is more hazardous to handle heavy patients than light patients.

What is heavy? Figure B, page 47, shows what a statistician call a cumulative distribution of body weight in the adult population of men and women this country. Half the population weigh more than 66kg (10stone 5lbs) and about 90 per cent weigh something between 49kg (7stone 10lbs) and 90kg, (14stone 2lbs) although 5 per cent weigh more or less than these figures.

A careful study of the graph shows that it is not symmetrical about its mid-point. This is because there are more abnormally heavy people in the population than abnormally light ones, obesity being more survivable in the short term than emaciation, which is often a sign of impending death. This being so, it is sometimes necessary to devise an acceptably safe system of work for caring for a 222kg (35stone) patient who is developing bed sores (see Chapter 14).

The Procedure

There has been a major revolution in the way risks associated with handling the human load are perceived. This is illustrated by the positions taken on this issue in the earlier editions of this book. The first (Ref 29) edition condemned the drag lift but considered the orthodox or cradle lift to be acceptable under certain circumstances.

The second (Ref 28) edition explicitly condemned both, but considered the three person lift for transferring an unconscious patient from bed to trolley to be acceptable under certain circumstances.

The third (Ref 30) edition regarded all of these as unacceptable, regarded the poles and canvas transfer as acceptable but undesirable, and regarded the hammock lift for transferring a patient from bed to chair as acceptable. Nowadays these are all regarded as unsafe.

It is easier to be specific about the relative level of risk which a procedure entails when compared with other procedures, than it is to be specific about how risky a particular procedure is in any absolute sense.

Table 3 summarises the results of a series of experiments in which the intra abdominal pressure (IAP) resulting from various lifts was measured. These are presented in the form of a league table of risk.

In addition, they allow an estimate to be made that the orthodox or cradle lift is almost 40 times more likely to cause injury than the Australian or shoulder lift (Ref 23). But the level of scientific understanding is not sufficient to enable an estimate to be made of how likely it is that a nurse will injure herself lifting a patient of a particular weight by a particular method.

A relatively safer procedure like the shoulder lift up the bed is not altogether risk free. The calculations tell, for example, that for the heaviest people – 1 to 2 per cent of patients – there is a better than even chance that the shoulder lift will entail levels of truncal stress of a potentially injurious magnitude, although it may not cause injury on a particular occasion.

Table 3	WL50 (kg)	% exc
PROCEDURE		
Cradle (orthodox) lift	58	75
Hammock lift	62	62
Three person lift	66	51
MODERATE		
Hammock lift	69	42
Under arm drag	71	37
LOWER RISK		
Pivot turn 180°	97	2
Shoulder (Australian) lift	96	2
(both feet on the floor)		
Pivot turn 90°	108	<1
Shoulder lift (knee on bed)	110	<1

Note: WL50 is the weight of patient beyond which there is a better than even chance of the procedure resulting in a truncal stress (as indicated by intra abdominal pressure) of potentially injurious magnitude.

% exc is the percentage of adult patients who are heavier than this weight.

Note that these figures are for comparative purposes only and should not be used as weight limits. They do not take into account stresses on other joints or the effect on the spine of twisting or sideways bending.

Even if this lift is performed only on light weight or average weight patients, it could lead to cumulative strain. Different people performing this lift get themselves into all sorts of different positions. It is not an easy procedure to learn and bad habits creep in easily. Experience tells us that, when performing this lift, some people will be more at risk than others.

Applying the ALARP principle, the bodily lifting of the whole of the human load is usually avoidable. Most of the transfer procedures achieved by manual lifting can be performed with less physical effort by the use of a sliding aid (see Chapter 13). It will generally be safer to slide than to lift.

This reduces the level of risk, particularly the risk of injury by cumulative over use. Such aids are inexpensive. It is thus reasonably practicable to eliminate even one of the lower risk lifts, such as the shoulder lift up the bed, by sliding the patient instead.

However, things can go wrong with sliding procedures. So there will be occasions when it is safer to hoist the patient than slide him. And there is, for example, no acceptably safe way of getting a fallen patient up off the floor without using a hoist unless the patient can offer a high degree of assistance, (see Chapter 20).

Hoists are more expensive than sliding aids, perhaps a couple of thousand pounds as against a couple of hundred. The design of hoists is improving all the time – so the cost of using a hoist in terms of time and trouble is going down. An example is the two Swedish geriatric wards mentioned earlier (Ref 13).

Where potentially hazardous transfers are performed frequently and repeatedly in the same place, the ALARP principle points to the ceiling mounted hoist as the handling method of choice.

The Working Area

"The nurse must be able to get easily to both sides of the bed, and reach easily any part of the patient without stretching... a thing impossible if the bed be too wide or too high." *Florence Nightingale 1859.*

It is not possible to handle patients safely in working areas which do not permit the nurse full and unhampered freedom of movement, or where the furniture and equipment in use present unnecessary obstacles to be overcome or force the nurse to adopt an unsatisfactory working position.

Consider the working area around the bed by way of example. Current norms recommend a minimum bed spacing of 2.5 metres, as measured between bed centres (Ref 22). Converting this to Imperial units this works out (in round numbers) as eight feet. This is what Florence Nightingale recommended. Ergonomics being largely a matter of common sense, and Florence Nightingale being a woman of great common sense, the figure is probably just about right in ergonomic terms. It will allow adequate space for a hospital bed of standard width, a chair and a locker, and should allow enough room in which to manoeuvre a mobile hoist.

Problems may arise in two ways. The norm is sometimes violated in the interests of cramming as many beds as possible into the available space. If this is done in the interests of economic expediency then it is reprehensible – in that it compromises both the well being of the patient and the safety of the nurse. Alternatively the available space may be taken up with another piece of furniture or equipment. This is largely a matter for good housekeeping.

The importance of having a clear working area before starting any patient handling procedure cannot be overstated. This includes things like clearing up spillages and other slipping or tripping hazards. A piece of paper or plastic bag can be a slipping hazard.

In ergonomic terms the hospital bed is a working surface. It is the nurses' work bench. The correct height of a working surface will depend in part on the task for which it is used and in part upon the height and bodily proportions of the user. Since the

tasks which the nurse must perform at the patient's bedside are diverse, it necessarily follows that the work of the nurse cannot be performed safely at a bed of fixed height. Even the task of making a bed can be performed with a good deal less strain on the back if the bed is first raised up to the correct level. The continued use of non-adjustable beds for patients requiring more than an absolutely minimal degree of nursing care cannot be condoned.

Experience shows that the easier it is to adjust the height of a bed – or any other piece of furniture - the more likely it is to be adjusted. Pedal operated adjustment mechanisms are preferred over hand cranks, motorised adjustment mechanisms are the design of choice, particularly in high risk areas for back injury such as care of the elderly wards. For more about beds, see Chapter 14.

The problems of handling patients in the bathroom or lavatory are dealt with in Chapters 16 and 17.

The Nurse or Nurses

Nurses come in all shapes and sizes. About 90 per cent are women. Evidence seems to indicate that the 10 per cent or so who are men are just as likely to suffer from back injuries as the women, and possibly even more so (Ref 24). This is puzzling since common sense and physiology indicate that when other factors are equal, size and strength are an advantage when lifting and handling loads. It may be that male nurses tend to be given the heavier jobs to do, or possibly that male nurses tend to move towards high risk situations.

Where two or more nurses together are to handle patients it is important that they should be well matched in height. If they are not, the chance of some accidental mishap occurring during the course of the procedure, or of one nurse taking an undue portion of the strain, will increase.

Nurses with back trouble, or a recent history of serious back problems, should not be placed in situations of risk. Given the high prevalence of back trouble in nurses this may not be an altogether simple matter. But it is a problem which needs to be positively addressed in the interests of all concerned.

The safety of a nurse who is pregnant also needs to be considered. There is evidence that heavy lifting during the first trimester of pregnancy carries an increased risk of spontaneous abortion (Ref 9). In the stages of pregnancy from around six months onwards or thereabouts, the prospective mother's exercise tolerance will tend to diminish and hormonal changes leading to the slackening of her ligaments and other connective tissues, particularly the sacroiliac ligament, will tend to render her vulnerable to back injury. Assuming female nurses to be a random sample of women then one may estimate that some 2 per cent of all nurses of child bearing age will be pregnant at any time.

If ten women nurses of child bearing age are on a ward, the chance of one being pregnant is one in five, the chance of two being pregnant is one in 25, and of three, it is one in 125. By the laws of chance alone there will sometimes be a cluster of pregnant nurses working in the same area. This again is a possibility which needs to be taken into account.

Nurses wear uniforms. The national uniform, introduced in the early 1970s, was not satisfactory in ergonomic terms. A study of the limitations on movement that this uniform caused (Ref 26) found that there were situations in which it would preclude safer methods from being adopted. Fortunately it is now disappearing from hospitals and being replaced with more functional alternatives – but where it is still in use it should be phased out.

The working system as a whole

The ergonomic approach to the design of work is sometimes characterised as being systems oriented. To optimise the match between the job and the worker the system needs to be looked at as a whole, not just the individual parts. This means asking questions like:

> are the various items of equipment in the ward compatible with each other?

> does the mobile hoist fit in the bathroom?

> has it got the right slings?

> what facilities are available for storage?

> are sensible quantities of supplies being stored?

> are deliveries from central stores made in a satisfactory way?

> how is the heavy work of the ward distributed among the staff?

> are there periods of peak workload during the day which could be avoided by adopting different ways of working?

REFERENCES

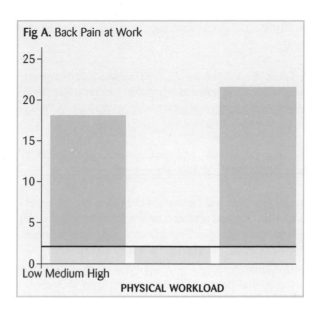

Fig A. Back Pain at Work

PHYSICAL WORKLOAD

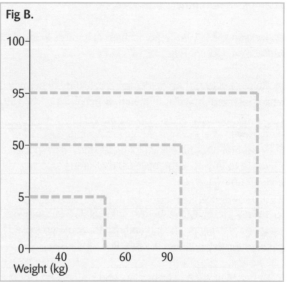

Fig B.

Weight (kg)

1. Adams M.A., and Hutton W.C.,(1985). Gradual disc prolapse. Spine, 10,524-531

2. Arad D., and Ryan M.D.,(1986). The incidence and prevalence in nurses of low back pain. Aust. Nurs. J., 16. 1,44-48

3. Battie M.C., Videman T., Gibbons L.E., Fisher L.D., Manninen H., and Gill K.,(1995). Determinants of lumbar disc degeneration. A study relating lifetime exposures and MRI findings in identical twins. Spine, 20,24,2601-2612

4. Baty D., and Stubbs D.A.,(1987). Postural stress in geriatric nursing. Int. J. Nurs. Studies, 24,339-344

5. Bigos S.J., et al,(1991). A prospective study of work perceptions and psychosocial factors affecting the report of back injury. Spine, 16,1,1-6

6. Burton A.K., Tillotson K.M., Main C.J., and Hollis S.,(1995). Psychosocial predictors of outcome in acute and sub-chronic low back trouble. Spine, 20, 722-728

7. Cady L.D., Bischoff D.P., O'Connell E.R., Thomas P., and Allan J.H.,(1979). Strength and fitness and subsequent back injuries of firefighters. J. Occup. Med., 21,269-272

8. Cust G.,(1976). Low back pain in nurses. Queens Nurs. J., 19,6-8

9. Goulet L., and Theriault G.,(1987). Association between spontaneous abortion and ergonomic factors. A literature review of the epidemiological evidence. Scand. J. of Work Env. and Health 13,399-403.

10. Heap D.C.,(1987). Low back injuries in nursing staff. J. Soc. Occup. Med., 37,66-70

11. Hickman M., and Mason V., (1994) The Prevalence of Back Pain: a report prepared for the Department of Health by the Office of Population Censuses and Surveys, Social Survey Division, based on the omnibus survey March, April, June, 1993.

12. Hunt L., (1954). Cervical, dorsal and lumbar spinal syndrome. Acto. Orthop. Scand. Suppl., 17

13. Jackson J.M., (1968). Biomechanical hazards in the dock worker. Am. Occup. Hyg., 11,147-157

14. Kelsey J., (1975). An epidemiological study of hermated lumbar intervertebral discs. Rheum. & Rehab., 14,144-159

15. Kelsey J., et al,(1984b). Acute prolapse lumbar intervertebral disc. An epidemiological study with special reference to driving automobiles and cigarette smoking. Spine, 9,608-613

16. Kelsey J.L., et al,(1984a). An epidemiological study of lifting and twisting on the job and risk for acute prolapsed lumbar intervertebral disc. J. Orth. Res., 2 61-66

17. Klaber Moffatt J.A., Hughes T.I., and Griffiths P.,(1993). A longitudinal study of low back pain in student nurses. Int. J. Nur. Stud., 30, 197-212

18. Kumar S.,(1990). Cumulative load as a risk factor for back pain. Spine, 15,12,1311-1316

19. Leighton D., and Riley T.,(1995). Epidemiological aspects of back pain: the incidence and prevalence of back pain in nurses compared to the general population. Occup. Med., 45,263-267

20. Ljungberg A.S., Kilbom A., and Hagg G.M.,(1989). Occupational lifting by nursing aides and warehouse workers. Ergonomics, 32 1,57-78

21. Magora A.,(1972). Investigations of the relation between low back pain and occupation III. Physical requirements: sitting, standing and weight lifting. Industrial Medicine 39,11,31-37

22. NHS Estates Health Building Note No. 40. Common Activity Spaces, Vol II, Treatment Areas. Department of Health (1986). HMSO.

23. Pheasant S., and Stubbs D.A.,(1992). Back pain in nurses: epidemiology and risk assessment. App. Erg., 24,4,226-232

24. Seccombe I., and Ball J., (1992). Back Injured Nurses – a profile; a discussion paper for the Royal College of Nursing.

25. Stubbs D.A., Buckle P.W., Rivers P.M., Hudson M.P., and Worringham C.J.,(1983). Back pain in the nursing profession, Part 1 Epidemiology and Pilot Methodology: Ergonomics 26,755-765

26. Stubbs D.A., Buckle P.W., Hudson M.P., Butler P.E., and Rivers P.M.(1985). Nurses uniform: an investigation of mobility. Inter. J. N. Stud. 22,3,217-229.

27. Stubbs D.A., Hudson M.P., Rivers P.M., and Worringham C.J.,(1980). Patient handling and truncal stress in nursing. Proceedings of the Conference on Prevention of Back Pain in Nursing. Northwick Park Hospital, Harrow. BPA, DHSS 14-27

28. The Guide to the Handling of Patients, second edition,(1987). National Back Pain Association in collaboration with the Royal College of Nursing, London.

29. The Guide to the Handling of Patients, first edition,(1981). National Back Pain Association in collaboration with the Royal College of Nursing, London.

30. The Guide to the Handling of Patients, third edition,(1992). National Back Pain Association in collaboration with the Royal College of Nursing, London.

31. Videman T., Nurminen T., Tola S., Kuorinka I., Vanharanta H., and Troup J.D.G.,(1984). Low back pain in nurses and some loading factors at work. Spine, 9,400-404

32. Videman T., Nurminen T., and Troup J.D.G.,(1990). Lumbar spinal pathology in cadaveric material in elation to history of back pain, occupation and physical loading. Spine, 15.8.728-740

BIOMECHANICS OF LOW BACK PAIN

by Michael A. Adams

SUMMARY

The most severe and chronic back pain usually comes from the intervertebral discs.

The apophyseal joints, sacroiliac joints and ligaments are also common sites of pain.

Muscles may give rise to brief attacks of pain.

Discs are most easily damaged by heavy lifting, and the apophyseal joints by twisting

Damage can occur by injury, or by the accumulation of "fatigue" during repetitive loading.

Degenerative changes in spinal tissues may well follow structural damage.

Postural pain may arise from abnormal or chronic loading of undamaged tissues.

Pain-provocation studies suggest that the most common origin of severe and chronic back pain is the posterior part of the intervertebral disc, and the longitudinal ligament which adheres to it. The apophyseal joints and sacro-iliac joints are also painful in substantial minorities of patients.

Pain can be caused by mechanical failure, and the most common mechanisms are as folllows: ligaments of the neural arch can be damaged ("sprained") by forward bending movements; the apophyseal joint surfaces by twisting and backwards bending; the vertebral body by compression; and the disc by awkward bending and compression, or following compressive damage to the vertebral body. In each case, damage can occur during a single application of load, simulating some incident such as a stumble or fall, or by the process of accumulating "fatigue failure" in which the forces remain relatively low but are applied many times. As far as the intervertebral disc is concerned, there is unambiguous evidence that biological (cell-mediated) degeneration follows structural failure, but there is little evidence that degeneration precedes failure.

Pain may possibly arise in the absence of structural failure if high stress concentrations are generated within the intervertebral disc or apophyseal joints. This can occur in lordotic "hollow back" postures, especially if they are held for long periods, and it may possibly occur as a result of excessive or unbalanced muscle activity.

Some people are pre-disposed to back pain on account of psychological factors, or physical factors such as body weight, poor spinal mobility, or easily-fatigued back muscles.

In conclusion, the available evidence suggest that mechanical loading plays a central role in the etiology of most people's low back pain. This applies even if the patient appears psychologically disturbed, or reports no history of trauma, or shows evidence of biological (cell mediated) degenerative changes in spinal tissues.

INTRODUCTION

Back pain is now the most frequent medical cause of absence from work in the United Kingdom. Sometimes, it may be cited as a convenient excuse for taking time off work, but there can be little doubt that many people have real and severe problems.

In certain cases, the problem appears to be mainly psychological. Psychosocial factors are important to the clinician because they affect the likely success or failure of treatment, especially in chronic back pain or when compensation claims are involved. However, psychosocial factors explain only 2 – 3 per cent of new reports of back pain (Ref 15), and in patients who are well motivated at the outset, unhappiness and litigation may simply represent normal human reactions to persisting pain and ineffective treatment.

Identifiable disease processes such as ankylosing spondylitis and rheumatoid arthritis account for only a small minority or patients; as far as the majority is concerned, there is growing evidence that the underlying cause of their back pain is mechanical. It will be shown later that certain types of mechanical loading constitute the greatest known risk factors for back pain.

The purpose of this chapter is to indicate in general terms how mechanical load might lead to low back pain. Specific advice concerning manual handling techniques, and other ergonomic considerations, can be found elsewhere in this book. The information is divided into five main sections. The first tackles the problem of where back pain comes from by considering the relevant anatomy, together with evidence from pain-provocation and pain-blocking studies. The second section reviews the epidemiological evidence which indicates who develops back pain, and in so doing suggests why they do. The third section introduces spinal mechanics and considers how high mechanical loading might cause injury or fatigue ('wear and tear') damage to spinal tissues. "Postural pain" is then introduced as a convenient term to cover mechanical pain which is associated with functional disorders, rather than overt damage or injury. The fifth section describes how living tissues respond biologically to their mechanical environment and to mechanical damage, and suggests how these responses may mask the essentially mechanical original of degenerative changes within them.

THE ANATOMICAL BASIS OF LOW BACK PAIN

The lumbar spine

The spine consists of 26 bones (vertebrae) stacked one on top of the other, as shown in Figure 4.1. Each vertebra has a chunky "vertebral body" which is the main weight bearing structure, and a "neural arch" which is a bony arch protecting the spinal cord. Various "processes" attached to the neural arch act as levers so that muscles can move the spine about.

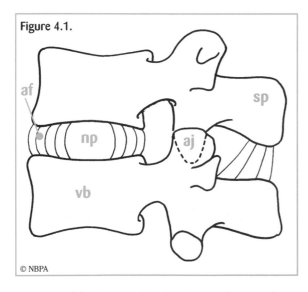

Figure 4.1.

© NBPA

Figure 4.1. (A) Side view of two lumbar vertebrae, posterior on the right. The weight bearing vertebral bodies (vb) are separated by an intervertebral disc which comprises a soft nucleus pulposus (np) surrounded by the tough annulus fibrosus (af). Small apophyseal joints (aj) increase stability. The spinous processes (sp) can be felt by running a finger down someone's back.

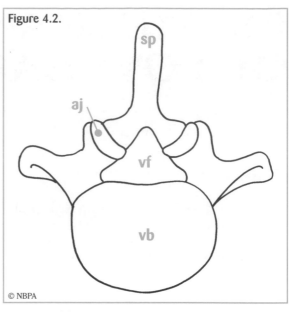

Figure 4.2.

© NBPA

Figure 4.2.(B) Top view of a lumbar vertebra, showing the vertebral foramen (vf) which contains the spinal cord.

Adjacent vertebral bodies are separated by a pad of cartilage called an "intervertebral disc" which consists of a central region of soft hydrated material (the "nucleus pulposus") surrounded by a ring of tough gristly cartilage (the "annulus fibrosus"). Intervertebral discs allow the spine a certain amount of flexibility, and they also play a minor role in shock absorption. Many people have a "slipped disc" (more correctly, a "prolapsed" disc) in which some of the nucleus pulposus is displaced into, or through the annulus fibrosus in such a way that some part of the nucleus or annulus bulges beyond the normal margins of a healthy disc.

Adjacent vertebrae are also linked by ligaments (tough fibrous bands which prevent excessive movement) and by a pair of "apophyseal joints," which are small sliding joints the size of a fingernail. These joints stabilize the spine and protect the discs from excessive movements, specially twisting and bending. In people aged over 40, the apophyseal joints often show signs of osteo-arthritis, such as cartilage loss and marginal osteophytes.

The lumbar spine consists of the five lowest vertebrae and discs. This is a particularly mobile region of the spine, and it is also subjected to the highest forces, so it is not surprising that it is the region most likely to be damaged and painful.

The innervation of spinal tissues

The nerve supply to most spinal structures is uncontroversial and has been summarised recently (Ref 16). However, the innervation of intervertebral discs and longitudinal ligaments has been hotly debated, with negative findings being taken at face value, or attributed to technical failure. According to the widely-accepted account of Bogduk and Twomey (Ref 16) a mixed autonomic and CNS nerve, the sinuvertebral nerve, supplies the posterior and posterolateral annulus fibrosus, and the posterior longitudinal ligament (Figure 4.3). Within healthy discs, free nerve endings of various types have been identified, but only in the outermost few millimetres of the annulus fibrosus. Nerve endings and capillaries can grow in towards the centre of degenerated discs which generally do not exhibit high internal stresses (see below).

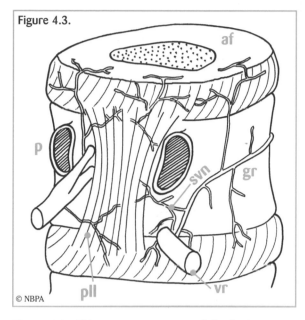

Figure 4.3.

© NBPA

Figure 4.3. Oblique posterior view of the lumbar spine showing the sinuvertebral nerve (svn) which supplies the annulus fibrosus (af) of the intervertebral disc and the posterior longitudinal ligament (pll). The neural arch has been cut away at the pedicles (p). The sinuvertebral nerve is a mixed nerve containing fibres from the grey rami communicantes (gr) and the ventral ramus (vr) of the spinal nerve. (Reproduced from (1) with permission.)

Pain-provocation and pain-blocking studies

A large-scale pain-provocation study was performed recently on 193 conscious patients undergoing surgery for herniated ("slipped") disc or spinal stenosis (Ref 30). Local anaesthesia was applied progressively to the skin, fascia, ligaments, muscles, apophyseal joints, nerve roots, annulus fibrosus and vertebral end-plates. Before each structure was anaesthetised, it was stimulated, either electrically or mechanically. Patients' leg pain could be reproduced only from an inflamed or compressed nerve root, and it was always removed by injecting local anaesthetic beneath the nerve sleeve at the site of compression.

The posterior annulus was 'exquisitely tender' in one third of patients, 'moderately tender' in another third, and insensitive in the rest. Back pain produced from the annulus was similar to that suffered pre-operatively. The posterior longitudinal ligament and vertebral body end-plate were frequently painful, but

it was difficult to stimulate them independently of the annulus. The facet joint capsule produced some sharp, localised pain in approximately 30 per cent of patients, but the ligaments, fascia and muscles were relatively insensitive. Although severe back pain can emanate from the discs (Ref 30,37), there is growing evidence from MRI studies that the majority of abnormal or degenerated discs are not painful at all (Ref 17). It seems that certain types of disc lesion are more likely to be painful than others, and only then if certain other conditions are met, such as chemical irritations or inflammation.

The importance of the apophyseal joints in producing low back pain has been studied by Schwarzer et al. (Ref 36). They injected local anaesthetic into several facet joints in each patient, and reported some pain relief in 47 per cent of patients. However, when the procedure was repeated approximately two weeks later, only 15 per cent of patients reported consistent relief of pain from the same joint on both occasions. The authors concluded that the apophyseal joints are frequently a cause of pain, but questioned the existence of a specific "facet syndrome." The relationship between pain and osteoarthritic changes in the apophyseal joints remains unclear, but the very high incidence of the latter in elderly people suggests that they are frequently asymptomatic.

The sacro-iliac joints have also been investigated using pain-provocation and pain-blocking techniques (Ref 35). Of 43 patients with chronic low back pain below the level of L5-S1, 40 per cent experienced exact reproduction of their pain when the sacro-iliac joints were injected with X-ray contrast medium, and 30 per cent gained relief from their pain when lignocaine was injected.

Muscles and ligaments are probably responsible for many cases of acute back pain which clear up after a few weeks. The role of the muscles in acute and chronic back pain will be considered later.

EPIDEMIOLOGY OF LOW BACK PAIN

The greatest known risk factors for back pain and related disorders are all mechanical. Bending and lifting weights in excess of 11kg (25lb) more than 25 times per days makes a person up to six times as likely to develop a prolapsed disc (Ref 28) and certain awkward manual handling tasks represent an even greater risk for back pain in general (Ref 31). Exposure to vibrations also increases the risk of back pain (Ref 33). It is important to realise, however, that the body can eventually adapt to mechanical loading by becoming stronger (see section 4, below) and that a strong back will be less vulnerable to accidental injury. For this reason, epidemiological surveys probably underestimate the tendency for vigorous manual work to cause short-term fatigue damage to 'unadapted' backs.

The majority of people in high-risk occupations remain unaffected, suggesting that risk factors exist which predispose certain individuals to back problems. Some of these are already known; a long back and a heavy body are associated with increased risk of a herniated disc (Ref 26) and for obvious reasons: these individuals are lifting on longer lever arms, and moving an increased bulk around.

Preliminary, unpublished, results from a large-scale prospective trial conducted in our own laboratory indicate that people with a poor range of movement in the lumbar spine, and those with easily-fatigued back muscles, are also at increased risk of first-time back pain. Poor spinal mobility leads to increased bending stresses acting on the lumbar discs and ligaments (Ref 21), and fatigued back muscles are less able to protect the back from excessive bending during repetitive lifting movements.

Genetic risk factors are suggested by a familial predisposition to disc degeneration (Ref 14) and by the fairly common finding of disc degeneration in both the cervical and lumbar regions of the same individual. Little is known, however, about the nature of the inherited risk factors: they could be biochemical, but equally they could be mechanical characteristics such as small intervertebral discs or short internal levers. Some other non-mechanical risk factors for back pain include smoking, psychological status, and job satisfaction. These factors are generally small, even though they have a high statistical 'significance' in large surveys (Ref 15).

Other influences may be involved in back pain, because all of the risk factors considered above still do not explain most back pain, where 'explain' is used in the statistical sense implying predictive ability. There may be unidentified risk factors waiting to be discovered, or it may be that purely random events and circumstances lead to many people's back pain.

MECHANICAL DAMAGE TO THE LUMBAR SPINE

Mechanical properties of the spine

The apophyseal joints resist forces which act perpendicular to their broad articular surfaces. Thus, they severely limit the range of axial rotation in the lumbar spine (Ref 6) and resist the forward shearing forces on the lower lumbar spine (Ref 20). Little of the spinal compressive force normally falls on the apophyseal joints unless the discs are narrowed by degenerative changes (Ref 5). The apophyseal joints' resistance to compression

comes from the articular surfaces, and from extra-articular impingement of the inferior facet on the lamina below (Ref 24).

Intervertebral ligaments have strengths ranging from about 100N for the posterior longitudinal ligament to about 1kN or more for the apophyseal joint capsular ligaments (Figure 4.4). They resist bending movements of the spine, particularly forward bending.

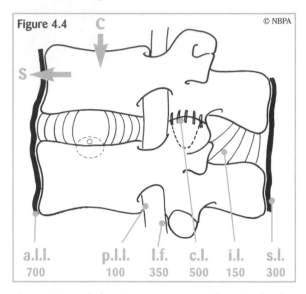

a.l.l.	p.l.l.	l.f.	c.l.	i.l.	s.l.
700	100	350	500	150	300

Figure 4.4 A spinal motion segment as in Figure 3, showing the intervertebral ligaments and their typical tensile strength (in Newtons, where 9.81N = 1kg); a.l.l. = anterior longitudinal ligament; p.l.l. = posterior longitudinal ligament; l.f. = ligamentum flavum; c.l. = capsular ligaments; i.l. = interspinous ligament; s.l. = supraspinous ligament. Compressive forces (C) act down the long axis of the spine, perpendicular to the mid-plane of the discs. The shear force (S) moves a vertebra forwards or backwards relative to the one below. The centre of rotation for forwards or backwards bending normally lies within the region shown by the dotted line.

Tension generated in posterior intervertebral ligaments during flexion acts to compress the intervertebral discs, so that the intra-discal pressure increases by 100 per cent or more in full flexion, even for the same applied compressive force (Ref 11).

Intervertebral discs act like hydraulic 'cushions' between adjacent vertebrae (Figure 4.5). The nucleus pulposus has a high water content and behaves like a pressurised fluid. The inner annulus also behaves like a fluid despite its regular lamellar structure (refs 10-13) but the outer annulus is a fibrous solid which acts as a tensile 'skin' for the rest of the disc, resisting bending and torsional movements. The distribution of compressive stress acting in the proteoglycan matrix of the disc has been measured by pulling a miniature pressure transducer through it (refs 10-13) and typical distributions are shown in Figure 5.

Note that stress concentrations can exist in the middle of the annulus, and that very little compressive stress is measured in the peripheral 3mm (where the nerve endings lie). When a disc is compressed, the pressure in the nucleus causes the vertebral end-plates to bulge into the vertebral bodies and the annulus bulges radially outwards.

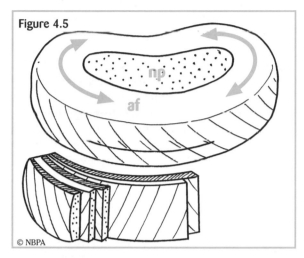

Figure 4.5

Figure 4.5. When an intervertebral disc is compressed, the hydrostatic pressure in the nucleus pulposus (np) is raised, and this creates tensile 'hoop' stresses In the annulus fibrosus (af). (Inset) The annulus consists of concentric lamellae with alternating fibre angles. Note that some lamellae are discontinuous.

Figure 4.6

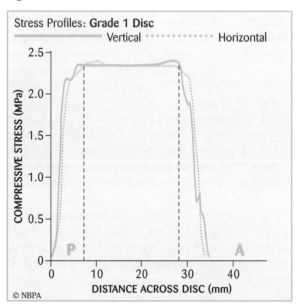

Figure 4.6. Distribution of horizontal and vertical compressive stress along the mid-saggittal plane of a typical non-degenerated 'grade 1' intervertebral disc (**4.6**) and a degenerated disc (**4.7**). Both discs were loaded when the measurements were taken. The central section of each profile, in which stress does not vary with direction or location, indicates a region of hydrostatic pressure. Degenerative changes reduce the size of the hydrostatic region, and increase the size of stress peaks in the annulus, especially the posterior annulus. Adapted from Ref 12.

Figure 4.7

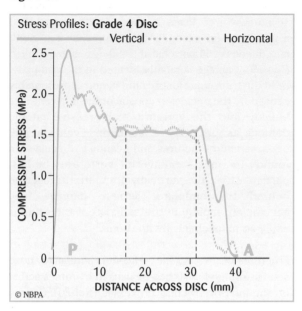

Ageing and degeneration affect the mechanical properties and function of the spine. Age-related changes in discs appear to be due to changes in biochemical composition. With increasing age, the disc's collagens and proteoglycans undergo quantitative and qualitative changes which may be related to nutritional compromise, or the action of degradative enzymes. Similar changes affect other tissues of the body, including the skin.

The most important mechanical consequence of these changes is likely to be the resulting fall in the water content of the nucleus pulposus because this reduces the ability of the nucleus to behave like a pressurised fluid. Nuclear pressure falls, and compressive load is transferred from nucleus to annulus (Ref 12). Overall, the disc bulges and loses height, so that the apophyseal joints resist more compressive load, and the x-sectional area of the intervertebral foramen is reduced. With increasing age and degeneration, all spinal tissues become weaker and less extensible, and spinal mobility decreases.

Structural changes in the discs and vertebrae have a greater effect on spine mechanical function that mere ageing. Slight damage to a vertebral body end-plate, which may not be apparent on x-ray, would allow it to bulge more into the vertebral body, causing a substantial drop in nuclear pressure and doubling the height of stress peaks in the posterior annulus (Ref 13). Other structural changes such as radial fissures in the annulus, posterior disc prolapse, and increased outwards bulging of the outer annulus would have a similar effect.

Injury to the spine

The *vertebral body* is the 'weak link' of the spine and is the first structure to fail in compression.

Its compressive strength depends greatly on the sex, age and body mass of the individual. Failure occurs at much lower loads if these loads are applied repetitively: for example, the compressive strength is reduced by 50 per cent if 5,000 cycles are applied (Ref 19). Damage is mostly located in the end-plate, or in the trabeculae just behind it, and is presumably caused by the nucleus pulposus of the adjacent disc bulging into the vertebra. Compressive fatigue damage is probably a common event in life, because micro-fractures and healing trabeculae are found in most cadaveric vertebral bodies, particularly in the vertically-orientated trabeculae behind the endplate. Fatigue damage may accumulate rapidly in the end-plate if the spine is exposed to mechanical vibrations.

Fractures of the *pars interarticularis* similar to those seen in spondylolysis can be caused by forces acting on the inferior articular processes (Ref 20). Gravity causes the lower lumbar vertebrae to move forwards and down relative to the vertebra below and this bends the inferior facets backwards about the pars interarticularis. Lumbar extension movements also bend the inferior articular processes backwards, whereas lumbar flexion tensions the apophyseal joint ligaments and bends the processes forwards. In this way, alternating forwards and backwards bending movements would create large stress-reversals in the pars interarticularis and may eventually cause fatigue failure within the bone. This may explain why spondylolysis is so common among sportsmen who frequently flex and extend their lumbar spine.

Backwards bending movements generate high stress concentrations in the inferior margins of the *apophyseal joint surfaces*, (Refs 5,24) especially after sustained ("creep") loading which reduced the water content and height of the intervertebral discs (see below). Severe (pathological) disc narrowing greatly increases loading of the articular surfaces, and may cause the tip of the inferior facet to impinge on the lamina below (Ref 24). There is no articular cartilage on the very tip of the inferior facet, so any extra-articular impingement may be painful. Axial rotation of the lumbar spine compresses the apophyseal joints on one side of the body, and excessive movement may damage the cartilage or subchondral bone of these joints. Damage to the apophyseal joint surfaces, either in bending or torsion, may lead eventually to osteoarthritic changes, as in other synovial joints.

The *intervertebral ligaments* which span adjacent neural arches provide most of the spine's resistance to flexion, with the remainder coming from the disc. In hyperflexion, the first structure to sustain damage is the interspinous ligament (Ref 3) so it is not surprising that this ligament is often found damaged in cadaveric spines. Further flexion is required to damage the apophyseal joint capsular ligaments, and still more to injure the disc. If lateral flexion is combined with anterior flexion, then the contra-lateral capsular ligament will be put to an additional stretch and might be damaged before the interspinous ligament. The visco-elastic nature of ligaments and discs increases their resistance to stretching during rapid movements. Conversely, sustained flexion reduces the spine's resistance to bending by 40 per cent in just five minutes (Ref 2), due mainly to "stress relaxation" in the spinal ligaments. Thus, rapid bending movements are more likely to injure the discs and ligaments, and sustained stooping may reduce ligamentous protection of the discs during subsequent activity. The interspinous ligament may be damaged in hyperextension by being squashed between opposing spinous processes (Ref 4). Usually the apophyseal joints or disc would be damaged first, but this depends on individual details of anatomy such as the spacing of the spinous processes. Hyperextension movements bend the inferior articular processes backwards about the pars interarticularis; the facet tip may then damage the posterior margins of the apophyseal joint capsule (Ref 40).

Intervertebral discs are not damaged directly by compressive loading of the spine; compressive failure always affects the adjacent vertebral bodies. Torsional loading normally damages the lumbar apophyseal joints first (Ref 6), but if these are removed, torsion can cause the lamellae of the annulus to separate circumferentially. Hyperflexion injury to an isolated disc, unprotected by the ligaments or apophyseal joints, occurs in the outer posterior annulus. The only loading conditions known to cause discs to prolapse *in vitro* in ways similar to those seen *in vivo* involve a combination of compression, lateral bending and forward bending. Bending stretches and thins the postero-lateral annulus while compression raises the hydrostatic pressure in the nucleus (Figure 4.8a).

In cadaver experiments, prolapse can occur in a single loading cycle if the motion segment is flexed several degrees beyond its normal range of motion, so that the interspinous ligament is over-stretched (Ref 7).

Repetitive application of a moderate compressive force to a fully flexed motion segment causes some non-degenerated discs to prolapse by the gradual formation of a radial fissure which allows soft nucleus pulposus material to migrate into the postero-lateral corners (Ref 8) (Figure 4.8b).

Adding torsion to bending and compression makes prolapse easier. Discs which prolapse most readily are from the lower lumbar spine of cadavers aged under 50 years which show little sign of degeneration

(Ref 7); on the contrary, severely degenerated discs do not prolapse, presumably because the nucleus is too fibrous to exert a hydrostatic pressure on the annulus. Severe backwards bending and compression can cause discs to prolapse anteriorly (Ref 4) but this may be a rare occurrence in life. Pain arising from a prolapsed disc may originate in the disrupted outer annulus fibrosus and the adhering posterior longitudinal ligament. Pain may be exacerbated by the vigorous inflammatory response which occurs in the displaced material.

Structural failure of the disc often involves inwards buckling of the annulus, rather than outwards prolapse of nuclear material. Internal derangements could be caused by previous minor injuries to adjacent vertebral bodies, since such injuries decompress the nucleus pulposus and generate high concentrations of compressive stress in the annulus (Ref 13). Subsequent repetitive loading can cause the inner lamellae to collapse into the nucleus (Figure 4.8c).

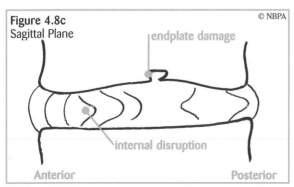

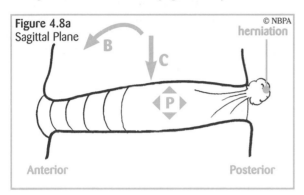

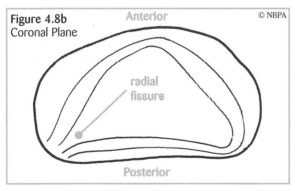

Figure 4.6. Types of structural disruption commonly seen in lumbar intervertebral discs. **(a)** Posterior herniation of nucleus pulposus ('slipped disc') can occur when a disc is

subjected to compression C, at the same time as bending B, which stretches and thins the posterior annulus. **(b)** Radial fissures can grow into the postero-lateral corners of lumbar discs in response to repetitive loading in bending and compression. **(b)** A damaged end-plate depressurises the nucleus and can lead to internal disruption of the annulus.

Spinal loading during manual handling

The above evidence supports the common sense notion that intervertebral discs are most easily damaged by loading in combined bending and compression. During manual handling, the spine is compressed by tensile forces acting in the back muscles as they attempt to raise the upper body and weight into the upright position. The back muscles act very close to the "pivot point" within the discs, so they need to generate high forces to lift even modest weights. Spinal compression can be minimised by lifting slowly, with the weight close to the body (Ref 23). Bending stresses rise rapidly as a person bends forwards as far as they can go and these stresses can be minimised during lifting either by bending both knees and keeping the weight just in front of the feet (Ref 23), or by performing a straddle lift with one foot beside the weight, and the other knee behind it and close to the floor. More detailed advice on lifting is given elsewhere in the book.

POSTURAL PAIN

Posture and stress concentrations in the spine

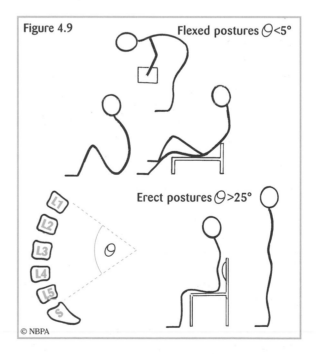

Figure 4.9. The orientation of the lumbar vertebral bodies in the sagittal plane can be defined by the lumbar curvature (θ). This angle increases during erect postures such as upright standing, and decreases, or is reversed, in flexed postures. (Reproduced from (Ref 1) with permission.)

A cadaveric lumbar spine shows a 'natural' lordotic curvature of about 40° in the sagittal plane when cut free from all muscle attachments (Figure 7). In the upright standing posture, this lordosis is increased by about 13-15° whereas upright sitting reduces it by 20-35° (Ref 4). Compared to flat back postures, a lordosis has several disadvantages: it impairs the supply of metabolites to the posterior annulus fibrosus (Ref 9); it reduces the volume of the spinal canal; it increases loading of the apophyseal joint surfaces; and it generates compressive stress concentrations in the posterior annulus fibrosus (Ref 11). These last three effects may explain the dull backache experienced by many following prolonged standing. It seems that the lordotic posture has been advocated in the past because it reduces the hydrostatic pressure in the nucleus pulposus. However, this apparent benefit is lost when the compressive force rises to 3kN (Ref 11), and it occurs at low loads only because the load is transferred from the nucleus pulposus to the posterior annulus fibrosus and apophyseal joints, which are less able to resist it.

The effect of sustained and repetitive loading on spinal mechanics

During the daytime, physical activity drives water from the intervertebral discs and reduces their volume by approximately 20 per cent (Ref 18). Much of the change takes place during the first hour after rising, and changes are reversed during the following night's rest. There is a corresponding diurnal variation in human stature of about 15-25mm. Reducing the volume of the disc late in the day causes it to bulge radially outwards, rather like a 'flat type,' and potentially-painful concentrations of compressive stress appear within the posterior annulus (Ref 10). Diurnal variations within the disc also affect the mechanical properties of the whole spine (Figure 4.8).

Disc height loss in the afternoon leads to increased vertical loading of the apophyseal joints (Ref 5). Conversely, the intervertebral ligaments become slack and resist bending movements less, and the discs are less likely to prolapse (Ref 3). Diurnal changes in spinal mechanics can be readily appreciated by trying to touch your toes just before going to bed, and then tying it again first thing in the morning, when it will be more difficult. Although there are no satisfactory epidemiological studies concerning diurnal variations in the onset of back pain, the available evidence suggest that vigorous bending and lifting movements should be avoided in the first few hours of the day.

Muscle dysfunction and chronic back pain

Back pain may lead to abnormal muscle function, which in turn may lead on to recurrent or chronic

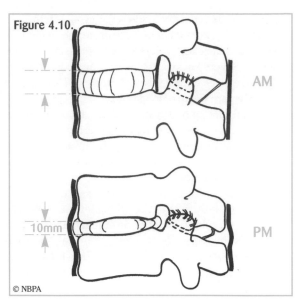

Figure 4.10.

AM

10mm

PM

© NBPA

Figure 4.10. Motion segments in the sagittal plane (anterior on the left) showing the effects of diurnal changes in intervertebral disc height. Late in the day (PM), the dehydrated disc is narrowed, and the apophyseal joints become load-bearing. The ligaments and annulus fibrosus gain some 'slack' and the spine resists bending movements less. (Reproduced from (Ref 1) with permission.)

problems in muscle and underlying tissues. For example, pain may inhibit normal spinal movements, causing muscle atrophy and a reduction in joint mobility. Since the back muscles are required to protect the underlying spine from excessive bending, and since this protection is reduced by poor mobility (Ref 21), the end result of the pain may be an increased risk of bending injuries to the intervertebral discs and ligaments. As a second example, unilateral pain may cause an imbalance in muscle activity leading to asymmetry in spinal posture and movement. As discussed above, small changes in lumbar curvature can lead to high and potentially painful stress concentrations in the intervertebral discs and apophyseal joints. Although plausible, these mechanisms are difficult to prove.

Spinal movements and low back pain

Spinal movement patterns have been used to distinguish between 'normal' and 'back pain' populations. People with back pain tend to move their backs less, and more slowly, presumably because vigorous full-range movements exacerbate their pain. Also, they sometimes show abnormal 'coupling' of movements in different planes (Ref 38). However, there is no evidence that abnormal movement patterns *cause* back pain, and the variability found in normal pain-free people makes it difficult to assign any individual patient to a specific diagnostic group on the basis of spinal movements.

BIOLOGICAL CONSEQUENCES OF MECHANICAL LOADING ('DISEASE' VS INJURY)

Adaptive remodelling

Physical exercise strengthens muscles, whereas disease weakens them. Most of the forces acting on the skeleton come from the musculature, and skeletal tissues adapt to increased or decreased forces by becoming stiffer and stronger, or softer and weaker. The phenomenon is well documented in bone: for example, the racquet arm of professional tennis players contains 30 per cent more bone mineral than the other arm (Ref 27). Elite weight-lifters have dense vertebrae (Ref 25) which are very strong. Manual labourers are more likely to have osteophytes (bony spurs) around the margins of their vertebral bodies, suggesting an adaptive response to increase the load-bearing area of the vertebra and hence reduce compressive stress. Intervertebral discs probably respond in similar fashion, but this is difficult to demonstrate in animal experiments because disc metabolic activity is very low. Thus, adaptive remodelling resulting from vigorous exercise regimes may be masked by the accumulation of fatigue damage within the disc. A small cadaveric study has shown that physically-active people do have stronger discs and vertebrae, but disc strength appears to increase less, or less rapidly, than vertebral strength (Ref 34). This suggests that an abrupt increase in physical workload may lead to disc injuries as disc strength falls behind that of the adjacent vertebrae and muscles.

Most epidemiological studies consider populations of survivors: people who presumably have developed strong backs after many years of hard work. Such studies fail to account for people who injure their backs soon after starting an arduous job, in the period when the discs are still "catching up" with strengthening muscles and bones. This interpretation is supported by the high number of back injuries sustained by young nurses during their first year on the wards (Ref 29), and by the close association between heavy manual work and vertebral osteophytes (Ref 39).

Response to structural failure

Remodelling is a reversible process which appears to be distinct from the progressive degenerative changes which often accompany structural failure within the tissue. (The word 'degenerative' implies long-term deleterious changes mediated by cellular activity.) Ruptured interspinous ligaments deteriorate markedly. Damaged vertebrae heal, but the original shape is not normally regained. Injured intervertebral discs show little sign of true healing, probably because collagen synthesis within the avascular disc is so slow, and

structural changes in the annulus become increasingly common with increasing age. Animal experiments have shown that the discs of rabbits, sheep and pigs degenerate rapidly following scalpel 'injuries' to the annulus (Ref 32). The annulus defect is quickly filled with fibrous tissue, but the fissure progresses in towards the nucleus so that the mechanical integrity of the disc is eventually destroyed. An even more rapid 'degenerative' response to structural damage has been demonstrated on cadaveric material: when discs are induced to prolapse in-vitro by means of high mechanical loading, the displaced nucleus pulposus swells unopposed in surrounding fluid for several hours (Ref 22). Swelling is followed by proteoglycan loss and tissue shrinking during the next 86 hours. In life, therefore, disc prolapse would cause physico-chemical changes in the displaced tissue over a period of several hours which might give an illusion of a slowly-developing condition. This would be followed by long-term structural and biochemical changes in the remaining disc. Similar changes are observed in prolapsed disc material removed at surgery, but they are often assumed, for no apparent reason, to *precede* the disc prolapse.

REFERENCES

1. Adams M.A., (1996). Biomechanics of low back pain. Pain Reviews 3: 15-30.

2. Adams M.A., and Dolan P., (1996). Time dependent changes in the lumbar spine's resistance to bending. Clin Biomech 11: 194-200.

3. Adams M.A., Dolan P., and Hutton W.C., (1987). Diurnal variations in the stresses on the lumbar spine. Spine 12: 130-137.

4. Adams M.A., Dolan P., and Hutton W.C., (1988). The lumbar spine in backward bending. Spine 13: (9) 1019-26.

5. Adams M.A., and Hutton W.C., (1980). The effect of posture on the role of the apophyseal joints in resisting intervertebral compressive force. J. Bone Jt. Surg. 62-B: 358-362.

6. Adams M.A., and Hutton W.C., (1981). The relevance of torsion to the mechanical derangement of the lumbar spine. Spine 6: 241-8.

7. Adams M.A. and Hutton W.C., (1982). Prolapsed intervertebral disc: a hyperflexion injury Spine 7: 184-191.

8. Adams M.A. and Hutton W.C., (1985). Gradual disc prolapse. Spine 10: 524-532.

9. Adams M.A. and Hutton W.C., (1985). The effect of posture on the lumbar spine. J Bone Jt. Surg. 67-B: 625-29.

10. Adams M.A., McMillan D.W., Green T.P., and Dolan P., (1996). Sustained loading generates stress concentrations in lumbar intervertebral discs. Spine 21: 434-8.

11. Adams M.A., McNally D.M., Chinn H., and Dolan P., (1994). Posture and the compressive strength of the lumbar spine. International Society of Biomechanics Award Paper. Clin Biomech 9: 5-14.

12. Adams M.A., McNally D.S., and Dolan P., (1996). Stress distributions inside intervertebral discs: the effects of age and degeneration. Spine Society of Australia Research Award. J Bone Jt. Surg. 78B 965-72.

13. Adams M.A., McNally D.S., Wagstaff J., and Goodship A.E., (1993). Abnormal stress concentrations in lumbar intervertebral discs following damage to the vertebral body: a cause of disc failure. European Spine Society (Acromed) Award paper. Eur. Spine J 1: 214-221.

14. Battie M.C., Videman T., Gibbons L.E., Fisher L.D., Manninen H., and Gill K., (1995). Determinants of lumbar disc degeneration. A study relating lifetime exposures and MRI findings in identical twins. Spine 20: (24) 2601-12.

15. Bigos S.J., Battie M.C., Spengler D.M., and Fisher L.D., et al, (1991). A prospective study of work perceptions and psychosocial factors affecting the report of back injury. Spine 16: 1-6.

16. Bogduk N., and Twomey L.T., (1991). Clinical anatomy of the lumbar spine. Churchill Livingstone, U.K.

17. Boos N., Rieder R., Schade V., Spratt K.F., Semmer N., and Aebi M., (1995). The diagnostic accuracy of MRI, Work perception, and psychosocial factors inidentifying symptomatic disc herniations. Spine 20: 2613-25.

18. Botsford D.J., Esses S.I., and Ogilvie-Harris D.J., (1994). In-vivo diurnal variation in intervertebral disc volume and morphology. Spine 19: 935-940.

19. Brinckmann P., Biggemann M., and Hilweg D., (1988). Fatigue fracture of human lumbar vertebrae. Clin. Biomech. 3 (Supplement 1).

20. Cyron B.M., Hutton W.C., and Troup J.D.G., (1976). Spondylolytic fractures. J Bone Jt. Surg. 58-B: 462-466.

21. Dolan P., and Adams M.A., (1993). Influence of lumbar and hip mobility on the bending stresses acting on the lumbar spine. Clin. Biomech. 8: 185-192.

22. Dolan P., Adams M.A., and Hutton W.C., (1987). The short-term effects of chymopapain on intervertebral discs. J Bone Jt. Surg. 69-B: 422-428.

23. Dolan P., Earley M., and Adams M.A., (1994). Bending and compressive stresses acting on the lumbar spine during lifting activities. J Biomech. 27: 1237-1248.

24. Dunlop R.B., Adams M.A., and Hutton W.C., (1984). Disc space narrowing and the lumbar facet joints. J Bone Jt. Surg. 66-B: 706-710.

25. Granhed H., Jonson R., and Hansson T., (1987). The loads on the lumbar spine during extreme weight lifting. Spine 12: (2) 146-9.

26. Heliovara M., (1987). Body height, obesity and risk of herniated lumbar intervertebral disc. Spine 12: 469-72.

27. Jones H.H., Priest J.D., Hayes W.C., Tichenor C.C., and Nagel D.A., (1977). Humeral hypertrophy in response to exercise. J Bone Jt. Surg. 59-A: 204-8.

28. Kelsey J.L., Githens P.B., White A.A., and Holford T.R., et al, (1984). An epidemiological study of lifting and twisting on the job and risk for acute prolapsed lumbar intervertebral disc. J Orthop. Res. 2: 61-66.

29. Klaber Moffett J.A., Hughes G.I., and Griffiths P., (1993). A longitudinal study of low back pain in student nurses. International Journal of Nursing Studies 30: 197-212.

30. Kuslich S.D., Ulstrom C.L., and Michael C.J., (1991). The tissue origin of low back pain and sciatica. Orthop. Clin. N. Amer. 22: 2 181-7.

31. Marras W.S., Lavender S.A., and Leurgans E.W., et al., (1993) The role of dynamic three-dimensional trunk motion in occupationally-related low back disorders. Spine 18: 617-28.

32. Osti O.L., Vernon-Roberts B., and Fraser R.D. (1990). Annulus tears and intervertebral disc degeneration: an experimental study using an animal model. Spine 15: (8) 762-767.

33. Pope M.H., (1989). Risk indicators in low back pain. Annals of Medicine 21: 387-392.

34. Porter R.W., Adams M.A., and Hutton W.C., (1989). Physical activity and strength of the lumbar spine. Spine 14: (2) 201-3.

35. Schwarzer A.C., Aprill C.N., and Bogduk N., (1995). The sacroiliac joints in chronic low back pain. Spine 20: 31-7.

36. Schwarzer A.C., Aprill C.N., and Derby R., et al. (1994). Clinical features of patients with pain stemming from the lumbar zygapophyseal joints. Spine 19: 1132-37.

37. Schwarzer A.C., Aprill C.N., Derby R., Fortin J., Kine G., and Bogduk N., (1995). The prevalence and clinical features of internal disc disruption in patients with chronic low back pain. Spine 20: 1878-83.

38. Stokes I.A.F., Wilder D.G., Frymoyer J.W., and Pope M.H., (1981). Assessment of patients with low-back pain by biplanar radiographic measurement of intervertebral motion. Spine 6: (3) 233-230.

39. Videman T., Nurminen M., and Troup J.D.G., (1990). Lumbar spinal pathology in cadaveric material in relation to history of back pain, occupation and physical loading. Spine 15: (8) 728-40.

40. Yang K.H., and King A.I., (1984). Mechanism of facet load transmission as a hypothesis for low back pain. Spine 9: 557-565.

Acknowledgements. The work of the author is supported by the Arthritis and Rheumatism Council. Some of the text is adapted from a review paper (1) of the same name in the journal 'Pain Reviews.'

THE BIOMECHANICS OF HUMAN MOVEMENT

by Philippa Leggett

SUMMARY

Efficient movement of the human body involves the application of principles rather than the learning of techniques.

Some of these principles are mechanically based:

- centre of gravity

- leverage

- forces - pressure, tension

- friction.

Some are neurophysiologically based:

- relaxation

- use of the three movement centres - head, shoulder girdle, pelvis

- but all combine in human movement, whether it be movement of :

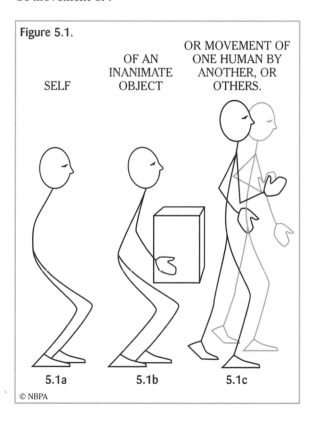

Figure 5.1.

SELF

OF AN INANIMATE OBJECT

OR MOVEMENT OF ONE HUMAN BY ANOTHER, OR OTHERS.

5.1a   5.1b   5.1c

© NBPA

INTRODUCTION

This chapter explains biomechanical principles, with the help of illustrations. The aim is to enable the reader to understand the main forces at work when moving oneself or a load: which movements may be harmful, and which may be better.

Biomechanics is the study of the application of mechanical principles to living tissue, for example, forces and levers.

Biomechanics is usually expressed in numerical terms, but in most of this chapter the principles and their direct application are described without the mathematics. A simple mathematical analysis is outlined at the end of the chapter.

It is common for researchers to analyse movements or lifting actions by working out forces within muscles, pressures within intervertebral discs, and compression forces between vertebrae, on a numerical basis, and so determine the safety of the movement, in accord with the guidelines from the National Institute for Occupational Safety and Health in 1991 (NIOSH 1991).

However, such results should be used with caution, because they involve approximations and simplifications.

most 'safe' limits quoted for force measurements come from cadaver specimens and are consequently only an approximation of the forces that apply in living tissues

the human body is much more than a mechanical structure: the forces applied to living structures also come from psychological, physiological, and chemical sources

measurements taken of a living person are often the measurement of a single activity under controlled and ideal conditions. For example, when analysing a particular type of movement, researchers may choose to ignore rapid acceleration at the start of the move, and to ignore twisting or sideways bending: the human body is too complicated for everything to be measured accurately in all circumstances.

It is beyond the scope of this chapter to explain in detail how the forces are calculated and how approximations are made: the bibliography offers sources for further reading.

However, it is useful to understand the main forces at work in any movement of the body as a guide to working out the most effective way to handle a load or a person.

The capability of the person doing the moving is an important part of the manual handling assessment. People who do not move their own bodies efficiently are not likely to be efficient at moving another.

CENTRE OF GRAVITY

Everything has a centre of gravity which can roughly be approximated to be the centre of the space that the body occupies. This is straightforward with bodies of uniform shape, such as a cube or a cylinder.

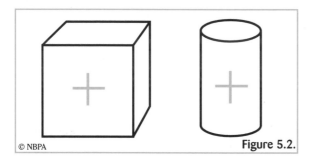

© NBPA   **Figure 5.2.**

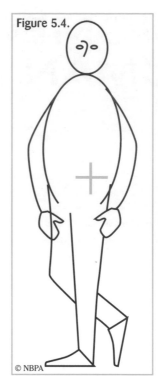

Figure 5.4.

Conveniently, it lies within the pelvis, so standing upright demands little muscular effort. However, people who cannot control their pelvis when standing cannot stand without help.

And in order to walk, the body must be able to shift the pelvis to one side, altering the centre of gravity to allow the non-weight bearing leg to swing forwards (Fig 5.4):

no static pelvic control - cannot stand

no dynamic pelvic control - cannot walk.

The further the centre of gravity is from the centre of the body, the more effort is needed to keep the body stable. As an example, raising the arms above the head causes the centre of gravity to rise, making the body less stable (Fig 5.5).

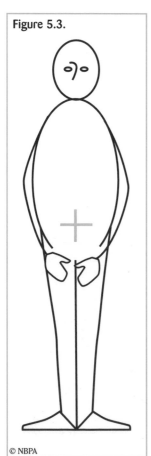

Figure 5.3.

© NBPA

But the human body is not a uniform or regular shape, and alters its dimensions freely. The centre of gravity moves as the body changes position, and may be moving all the time.

When a person is standing upright with the arms by the sides, the centre of gravity coincides with the centre of his physical dimensions (Fig 5.3).

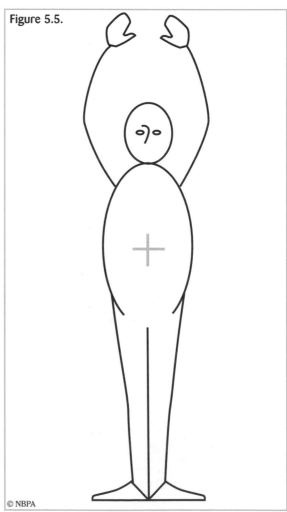

Figure 5.5.

© NBPA

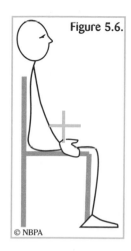
Figure 5.6.

© NBPA

Some movements and changes in position and shape will put the centre of gravity outside the physical body (Fig 5.6), which seems strange, but explains the movement that the body has to make to begin to get out of such positions.

To stand from sitting, moving to the edge of the seat puts the person in a better position as the centre of gravity moves closer in to the body (Fig 5.7a). People who have problems with the muscles of the abdomen, such as elderly frail people, and pregnant women, find this manoeuvre difficult, as to move from sitting, the body must be able to lean forward at the abdomen (Fig 5.7b).

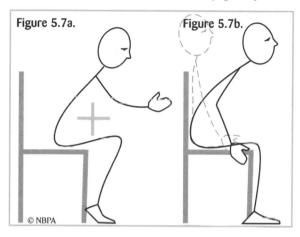
Figure 5.7a. Figure 5.7b.

© NBPA

Kneeling, with the body held high and upright, is a difficult position to move out of. One way is lean backwards first, then, leaning forward, bring one leg up so that the foot is flat on the ground - this brings the pelvis over the supporting foot and the person can then rise (Fig 5.8).

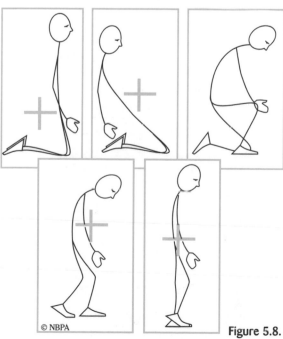
© NBPA
Figure 5.8.

Bodies in bed can present difficulties. Lying flat means that the centre of gravity is in the same place as when the person is standing upright - in the pelvis - so moving the pelvis will turn the body over (Fig 5.9a, 5.9b).

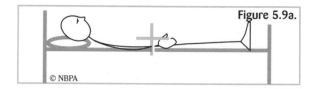
Figure 5.9a.
© NBPA

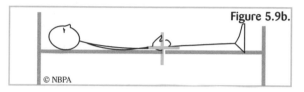
Figure 5.9b.
© NBPA

The centre of gravity of a person sitting upright in bed is far from the body, so it is difficult to handle him without altering his position. This difficulty becomes greater with a slumped person (Fig 5.10a, 5.10b).

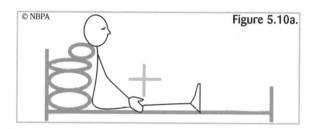
© NBPA
Figure 5.10a.

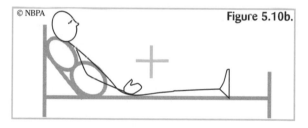
© NBPA
Figure 5.10b.

STABILITY

The line of gravity is the vertical direction down from the centre of gravity. For a body to remain stable, it must retain the line of gravity within its base (Fig 5.11).

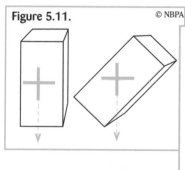
Figure 5.11. © NBPA

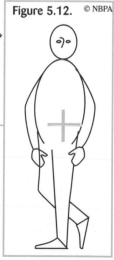
Figure 5.12. © NBPA

When walking normally, a person's centre of gravity moves from side to side, so that the line of gravity always falls along the supporting leg, the foot thus forming the supporting base (Fig 5.12).

The supporting base may be widened:

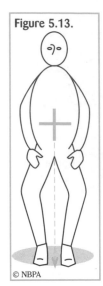

Figure 5.13.

by natural movement of the body – such as standing astride (Fig 5.13)

by changing position - such as crouching (Fig 5.14)

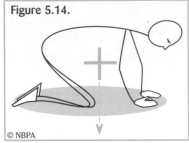

Figure 5.14.

© NBPA   © NBPA

or by artificial means if stability has been lost (Fig 5.15a-c).

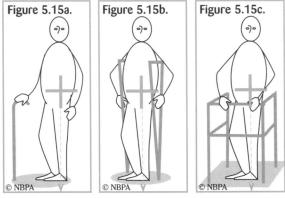

Figure 5.15a.   **Figure 5.15b.**   **Figure 5.15c.**

© NBPA   © NBPA   © NBPA

But stability introduces a problem: the more stable a position, the more difficult it is to move from it.

The positions of sitting, high kneeling, and lying, are much more stable than standing, and especially walking, which provides a small base. This is why divers and speed skaters lean forward: they make themselves unstable to help them move. Ballet dancers are stable for only a few seconds at a time on a tiny base (Fig 5.16a – c).

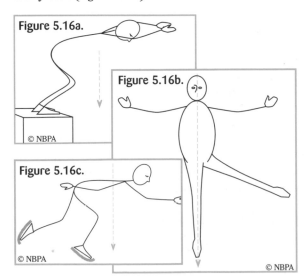

Figure 5.16a.

Figure 5.16b.

© NBPA

Figure 5.16c.

© NBPA   © NBPA

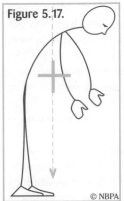

Figure 5.17.

But what happens if instability is created and no movement occurs?

Leaning forward is one of the most common postures adopted by people, either standing or sitting. The centre of gravity moves forward and the line of gravity falls outside the base (Fig 5.17).

© NBPA   The body has become unstable, but why has it not fallen over? As there is no forward movement, the counterbalance opposing the tendency to topple is provided by the effort of internal structures of muscles and ligaments in the back.

The forces exerted by these muscles have to be strong enough to follow the principle involving leverage: the weight of the body is pulling it forwards, the muscles and ligaments are restraining it (Fig 5.18).

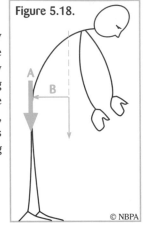

Figure 5.18.

© NBPA

The distances over which these forces are exerted – the lever arms – are of different lengths. The lever arm is the perpendicular distance from the force to the low back. This applies for any direction of force.

The lever arm of the muscles (A in the illustration) is much shorter than the lever arm pulling the body forward (B in the illustration), as the muscles and ligaments are rarely more than a few centimetres away from the skeletal structure they act upon. Consequently, the forces they exert to stop the person toppling are much greater than the force pulling the body through the centre of gravity (Fig 5.19).

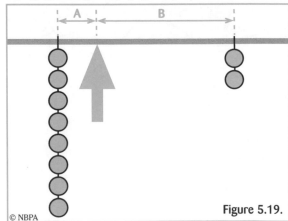

© NBPA   **Figure 5.19.**

It follows that the longer the external lever pulling the body forward, the greater the force the muscles and ligaments must produce to hold the body in this position (Fig 5.20).

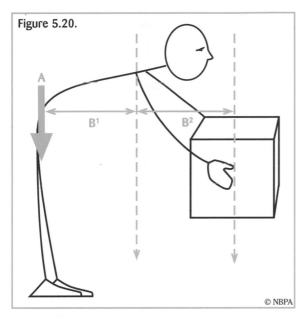

Figure 5.20.

There are two major problems with this:

as muscles contract, the spine is compressed and spinal discs are put under extra pressure (Fig 5.21)

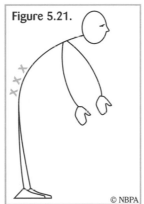

Figure 5.21.

if the position is held for more than two or three seconds, the muscles become fatigued and the body must recruit force from other groups of muscles (Fig 5.22).

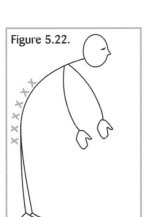

Figure 5.22.

If this position is held, eventually all the major groups of muscles are working furiously to prevent the body falling forward on its nose (Fig 5.23).

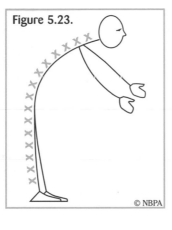

Figure 5.23.

This process is experienced as tension. A person is aware of it, and can observe it in others.

If a person in this position now wants to move something, only the minor muscle groups in the arm are available to provide the necessary effort. However, these muscles are not for strength, but for mobility, and so the intended action has become inefficient (Fig 5.24).

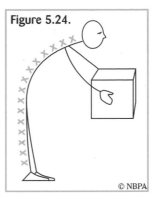

Figure 5.24.

The length of the external lever arm should be reduced where possible. In this example, this is done by bending the knees and spreading the feet so that the base is wider. This brings the line of gravity back into the base, and the body remains stable (Fig 5.25a,b).

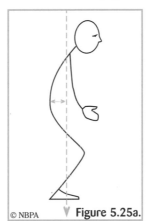

Figure 5.25a.

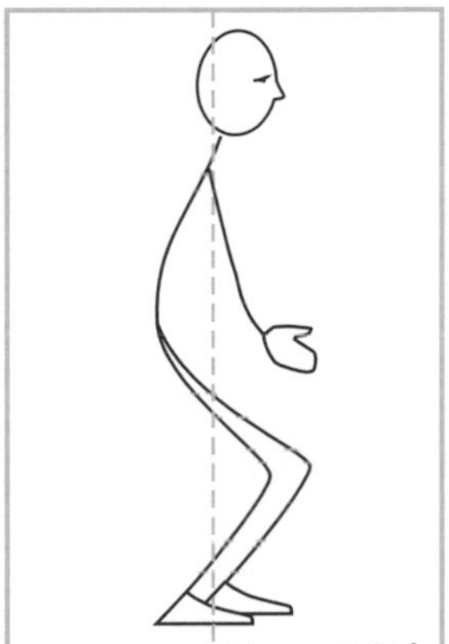

Figure 5.25b.

There is less demand on the muscles and ligaments, there is less tension in the body as a whole, and the major muscle groups are available to counter the effects of gravity, which is what they are designed for, and do as part of a person's normal activity (Fig 5.25c).

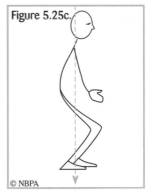

Figure 5.25c.

APPLYING FORCES

It is helpful to consider the human body in two parts:

the 'control centre' – head, thorax and abdomen

the movable attachments of the limbs (Fig 5.26).

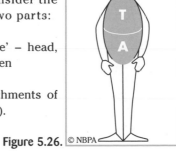

Figure 5.26.

The control centre contains everything necessary for life, and is designed for strength and endurance. Conversely, the limbs are designed mainly for movement and speed rather than for supporting load; they tire quickly when holding weights, or during repetitive movements, particularly when the rest of the body is held still.

The control centre contains the three neuromuscular centres of movement (Vasey & Crozier 1982).

1. the head initiates all body movement

2. the shoulder girdle controls movement of the arms and upper body

3. the pelvis controls movement of the legs and lower body (Fig 5.27).

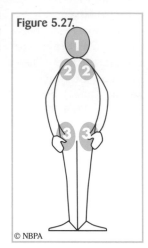

Figure 5.27.

© NBPA

The parts of each limb have more to do with mobility than strength as their distance from the body increases – the more distal the part, the less mass and muscle it has (Fig 5.28).

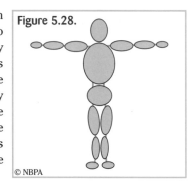

Figure 5.28.

© NBPA

Forces applied at angles

The efficient use of force

A force at an angle acts both vertically and horizontally. Dependent on the angle at which it is applied, the force along one direction will be greater than the other (Fig 5.29).

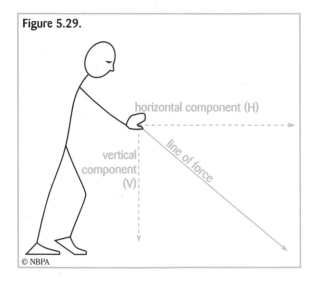

Figure 5.29.

horizontal component (H)

vertical component (V)

line of force

© NBPA

Force applied vertically is evidently a waste of effort if the direction of the force required is horizontal, for example, when pushing a wheelchair (Fig 5.30).

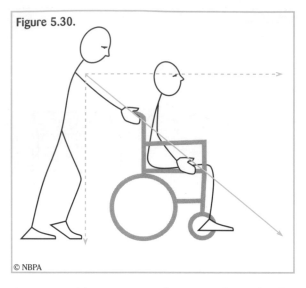

Figure 5.30.

© NBPA

Any vertical force may produce a tendency for the object to rotate, not move in the required direction.

The sensible course is to make the direction of force as close to the horizontal as possible if horizontal movement is required (Fig 5.31a, b & Fig 5.32a, b).

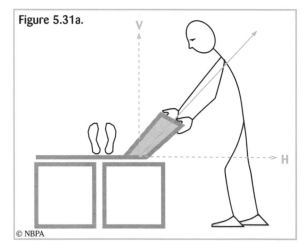

Figure 5.31a.

V

H

© NBPA

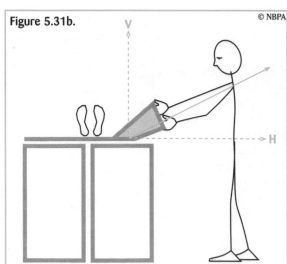

Figure 5.31b.

V

H

© NBPA

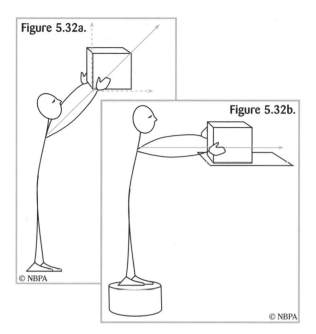

Figure 5.32a.

Figure 5.32b.

© NBPA

To get the force as close as possible to its most efficient direction, the handler must be in the correct posture and/or the height of the equipment must be changed (Fig 5.33).

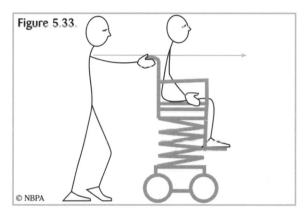

Figure 5.33.

© NBPA

Friction

Every surface material has a friction level, and some materials are designed so that these friction levels contribute to their purpose: a low friction level if movement is required, a high level of friction if movement is unwanted.

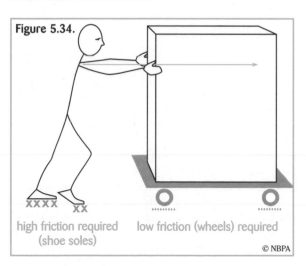

Figure 5.34.

high friction required (shoe soles)   low friction (wheels) required

© NBPA

An obvious example: high friction on the shoe soles of the person pushing an object on wheels with low friction (Fig 5.34).

The use of low friction surfaces is one of the most important principles used in manual handling equipment (Figs 5.35 & 5.36).

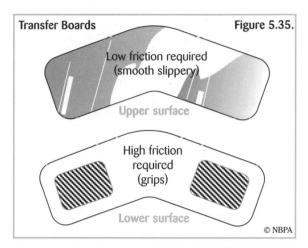

Transfer Boards   Figure 5.35.

Low friction required (smooth slippery)

Upper surface

High friction required (grips)

Lower surface

© NBPA

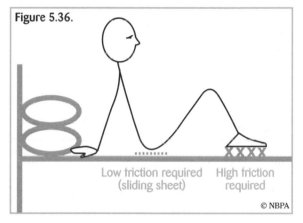

Figure 5.36.

Low friction required (sliding sheet)   High friction required

© NBPA

PRINCIPLES OF HUMAN MOVEMENT

- **ASSESS** the situation. What can be altered ? Must allowances be made for what cannot be altered, such as the existing environment? More manual handling difficulties are resolved by thought and planning than by technique.

- **COMMUNICATE** with others involved about the result of the assessment so that everyone knows what will happen.

- **RELAX.** Avoid tensing the muscles before you starting the movement or it will be inefficient – tension creates unwanted pressure. If the object cannot be moved without tension, it may be too big or too heavy.

- Aim to control the centre of gravity. If a person is to be moved, **CONTROL OF THE MOVEMENT CENTRES** is vital to everyone. Points of contact with another person should be on their trunk wherever possible.

Aim to **REMAIN STABLE**. This probably means moving the feet – the base – to keep up with a moving centre of gravity. Feet too far apart or too deep a knee bend will make the body unstable – this must be avoided.

MAKE THE LEVER ARMS AS SHORT AS POSSIBLE.

Aim to **MOVE SMOOTHLY**. Peaks of effort mean peaks of pressure, which will have to be met by the spinal discs.

AVOID TWISTING OR BENDING SIDEWAYS. Twisting combined with bending forward creates a high degree of spinal compression (Tracy 1995).

LEAD WITH THE HEAD to initiate movement. This applies to everyone involved.

MAKE USE OF FRICTION. The more the friction, the less unwanted movement; the less the friction, the easier it is to produce movement.

DO NOT WASTE EFFORT ON VERTICAL FORCES IF ONLY HORIZONTAL FORCE IS REQUIRED.

USE THE MAJOR MUSCLE GROUPS FOR EFFORT. The minor groups of muscles further away from the trunk are not designed to bear weights.

The more these principles can be applied to any handling situation, the more efficient movement will become. All of these principles can be applied to any handling situation after assessment.

These principles form the basis of efficient movement: the more of them that can be incorporated into a movement, the more efficient that movement will be.

EFFICIENT MOVEMENT IS THE FOUNDATION OF GOOD HANDLING PRACTICE.

Look closely at diagrams or movements when they are demonstrated. How many of these principles are being used? The fewer that can be identified, the more likely is that movement – or illustration – to be poor practice. This is why an assessment must be made first – to discover why some principles cannot be used, such as a lack of space which may make it difficult to shorten the lever arms involved. **THE AIM SHOULD BE TO USE AS MANY PRINCIPLES AS POSSIBLE IN THAT SITUATION TO PROVIDE THE SAFEST COURSE OF ACTION FOR ALL CONCERNED.**

Consider the movements of people who are professional movers, such as athletes and other sportsmen and women, and dancers. They do not end a movement with their head or neck in flexion, and no ballet dancer or figure skater is ever lifted above elbow height without the partner's hands placed firmly around their pelvis or shoulder girdle (Fig 5.37).

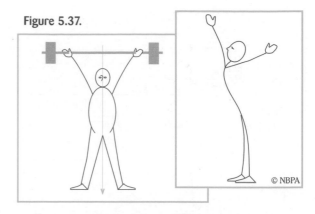

Figure 5.37.

© NBPA

MATHEMATICAL ANALYSIS

It is usual to make biomechanical analyses of human movement on the basis of mathematical calculations. This section gives an outline of these calculations in very simplified form. For more information, refer to the bibliography at the end of this chapter. It should be noted that these calculations are simplistic, and take no account of factors such as acceleration, intraabdominal pressure, or synergetic muscle actions in the calculations given.

Force is calculated in Newtons, found by multiplying mass (weight) by an acceleration:

$$F = ma$$

Gravity is a constant acceleration of 9.81m/s^2 that produces external forces acting on the body.

If the body does not move and is held in a posture, the forces within it are said to be in **equilibrium,** which means that all the forces present in the body must balance each other.

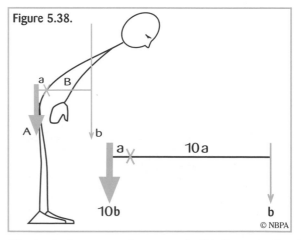

Figure 5.38.

© NBPA

The body is not moving towards the floor, so the external force **b** is being counteracted by a force at **A**. Each force is acting at a perpendicular distance (the lever or moment arm) from the centre of movement, which lies in the lower lumbar spine. If the lever arm of the force **A** is one tenth that of the lever arm **b**, then force **b** must be x10 that of force **A** to equalize the equation (Fig 5.38):

Bb – Aa = 0, so Bb = Aa.

If the force created by this body's weight is about 300N, then the force created by the muscles and ligaments of the lumbar spine is about 3000N (Fig 5.39).

If the body adds another weight of 10kg (about 100N) at the end of another long lever arm, the lever arm at **C** may be 20 times that of **a**, creating a force **Cc** which has to be counterbalanced, as well as **Bb**. The forces within the internal structures of the back must now reach 5000N to hold this body in the same posture (Fig 5.40).

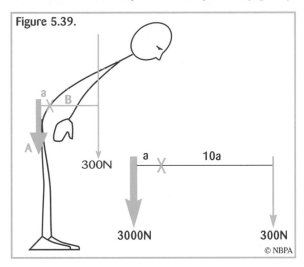

Figure 5.39.

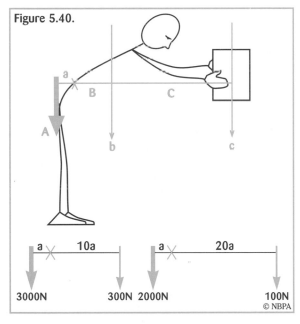

Figure 5.40.

The longer the lever arms from the centre of movement - which may be at any joint in the body – the more force has to be created internally by ligament tension and muscle contraction. In the low back, this muscle contraction produces a compressive force on the spinal discs, and it is the magnitude, speed, and repetition of this compression that can lead to disc damage. (Mc Gill et al 1996).

In these examples, the force has been acting over the lever arm at 90 degrees, but most of the body forces are acting at a different angle, which creates

not one effect but two as the force is calculated in its vertical and horizontal components (vectors).

This is done using constant trigonometric formulae:

The **vertical component** is found by multiplying the overall force magnitude (1000N) by the sine of the angle (30 degrees) which makes

1000 X 0.5 = 500N

The **horizontal component** – which is the one required for movement in (Fig 41) – is found by multiplying the overall force magnitude by the cosine of the same angle:

1000 X 0.86 = 860N

This horizontal force of 860N will produce movement in the required direction – the vertical force is wasted as it will produce unwanted movement.

This arrangement of two force components is reflected in the structure of the spinal disc. The nucleus is structured to resist compressive (or vertical) forces, while the annulus is meant to overcome shearing (or horizontal) forces.

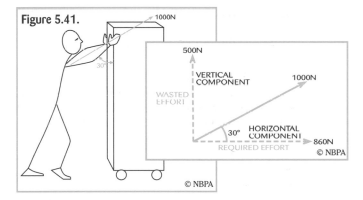

Figure 5.41.

REFERENCES

1. McGill et al. (1996) Ergonomics, 39:9 1107-1119.
2. National Institute for Occupational Safety and Health (1991). A work practices guide for manual lifting. Cincinnati: DHHS (NIOSH) publication no. 81-122.
3. Tracy M.F., (1995). Biomechanical methods in posture analysis, Evaluation of Human Work, Chapter 24, pp 714-748, (ed.) Wilson J.R. and Corlett E.N. Taylor & Francis, London.
4. Vasey J.R., and Crozier L., (1982). A Neuromuscular Approach 1 - 6, Nursing Mirror, April 28 - June 2, 1982.

BIBLIOGRAPHY FOR FURTHER READING
Galley & Forster: Human Movement, Longman, 1982
Pheasant, S: Ergonomics Work & Health, Macmillan, 1991
Macdonald, F A: Mechanics for Movement, Bell & Hyman, 1978
Wirhed, R: Athletic Ability and the Anatomy of Motion, Wolfe Medical, 1991
Williams & Lissner: Biomechanics of Human Motion, Saunders, 1962

THE NEUROMUSCULAR APPROACH TO EFFICIENT HANDLING AND MOVING

by Lesley Crozier and Sheila Cozens

Authors' note: The content of this chapter is not intended to be and should not in any way be considered as sufficient for training purposes.

The system is principle based and does not teach techniques. The process of movement re-education which is involved necessitates attendance on recognised courses for primary, practical, and experiential education, with ongoing assessed practice by suitably qualified personnel. The Neuromuscular Approach has its own established assessment criteria for the application of principles.

The Neuromuscular Approach considers that manual handling skill is dependent upon movement skill. For this reason there are no illustrations of patient handling situations in this chapter. Illustrations may identify a certain posture but do not convey the dynamics of movement, merely indicating an isolated phase within a movement, and cannot show

how the individual got into that position,

for what purpose,

where that movement will continue to,

and perhaps most importantly, how it will continue.

To copy what is seen in a still picture can only encourage a prescriptive or technique-based approach, neither of which is in accordance with the Neuromuscular Approach. The authors consider that body attitudes or hand positions of the figures in illustrations do not translate to movement situations where individual physical characteristics and needs, degrees of tissue adaptation, or current level of fitness of the nurse and patient, have to be considered.

SUMMARY

The Neuromuscular Approach is a dynamic movement system which allows the individual:

to assess his or her movement habits in terms of efficiency and inefficiency

to replace inefficient movement habits with efficient patterns that are reliable and reproducible, applicable not only at work but in all movement situations, to allow and enhance the development of movement skill.

INTRODUCTION

The Neuromuscular Approach to Efficient Handling and Moving is primarily concerned with teaching people to move efficiently, which means moving in a way which produces the least possible fatigue, and strain, and consequently potential and/or actual injury.

The majority of people take their ability to move for granted. The common denominator of all life's activities – daily living, work, recreation and other social pursuits – is MOVEMENT. To perform any manual handling and moving task, an individual has to move: handling and moving **is** human movement –

of ourselves

of objects of all shapes, sizes and weights

of other human beings who have varying and variable needs, dependencies, and so on.

Human movement is essentially reflex, and, therefore, a subconscious activity. Generally, people do not think about how they move, being concerned only with what they want to do.

If a movement does not achieve the desired effect, or if pain or some other difficulty is experienced, then perhaps – but not always – the individual will stop and think. If a movement is effective and achieves the desired outcome, does it matter how the individual moves to achieve that outcome? The Neuromuscular Approach recognises that most individuals develop a habitual pattern of movement which is **inefficient**, and results in tissue adaptation and a predisposition towards injury. This inefficient movement pattern or habit will be the normal reflex response of that individual and it will prevail in all movement activities – including the handling and moving of patients, whether as nurse, carer, or therapist. This pattern will be reinforced by repetition.

THE NEUROMUSCULAR APPROACH

The main aims are:

> to allow the identification and assessment of movement efficiency

> to facilitate the replacement of an inefficient movement pattern with an efficient one.

The Approach is based upon established physiological, physical, anatomical, biomechanical and human movement developmental principles. The application of these principles enables the progressive development of a core pattern of movement which is efficient and reflex, reproducible and reliable. The core pattern is uniquely versatile and applicable to any action, movement, or task, whether occupational, recreational, or social, permitting flexibility in dealing with movement situations.

CONCEPT AND PHILOSOPHY

Humans move in a wide variety of settings and for many and varied reasons: human movement is not concerned **only** with manual handling, and does not occur exclusively in the work place. Nurses move not only when handling patients, but also when carrying out all their other duties, their general activities of daily living, and socially and in recreation. Everyone performs the same basic actions:

> reaching   pushing   pulling
>
> lifting   turning

and **all** these actions involve degrees of risk. One, some or all these actions, in a variety of permutations, form the basis of all physical human activity, whether at work, rest, or play.

The Neuromuscular Approach recognises that:

> most individuals initiate activity in an inefficient, off-balance manner, producing episodes of sustained tissue tension which lead progressively to tissue adaptation – the onset of certain physiological changes – including loss of tissue elasticity. The continuing frequency of the use of this inefficient pattern reinforces the tendency for the pattern to be a habit, and an adaptive, perpetuating cycle is set up within the tissues

and that

> all human movements, if performed repeatedly in an inefficient manner, will result in undue fatigue, strain and potential, if not actual, injury.

Movement skill and efficiency

In any movement, degrees of muscle tension are required for background stability (stability factors) as well as contraction and relaxation of the muscles which perform the movement itself (mobility factors).

In an **efficient** movement there is a precise and subtle blending of these factors to provide a useful, purposeful and co-ordinated movement. A primary requirement for this to prevail is that a movement should be initiated, and the activity continued, with the individual in *dynamic* balance, where the line of gravity of the moving mass – the individual, or the individual plus an added load – remains within the effective, changing base area.

Tissue adaptation

In an **inefficient** movement there is always an excess of background stability tension which is sustained throughout the movement. The tissues rarely if ever recover from these episodes of sustained tension before the next inefficient movement occurs. This leads to fatigue, strain, and consequently potential and/or actual injury (Fig 6.1).

The effect of inefficient movement is that an adaptive cycle is set up within the tissues: figure 6.1

sustained tissue tension

circulatory change ← → cumulative strain

loss of elasticity

predisposition to potential or actual
INJURY

Risk of injury and tissue adaptation

Many people regard 'an injury' as being of acute onset and a specific response to a defined cause. It follows that in practice many people do not necessarily consider themselves to be injured as such, but suffer intermittent or continuing musculoskeletal problems of an insidious and seemingly non-defined nature.

The Neuromuscular Approach suggests that the primary cause of these musculoskeletal symptoms is the physiological effect of inefficient or faulty movement habits. Presenting symptoms are generally indicators of tissue adaptation. Where tissue adaptation is present, individuals are at greater risk of causing further injury to themselves, to co-handlers, and to the patients or loads which they handle.

There are consequently implications for the training and education of individuals who have tissue adaptation. The problems associated with tissue adaptation must be addressed first, before the superimposition of altered movement patterns, so as to avoid exposing the individual to greater risk.

Risk assessment

Formal risk assessment for manual handling tasks is required by the Manual Handling Operations Regulations (1992). However, in every manual handling task, there is also an inherent, less formal process of risk assessment.

Assessment of risk, whether formal or informal, should not focus purely on the heavy, awkward, and unfamiliar task. The Neuromuscular Approach recognises that there is potentially as great a risk in the light, often repeated, and familiar tasks, with which there tends to be less perception of risk.

If any element of manual handling or human movement remains – and this is always the case in the handling of patients – there is always associated risk of injury. The use of mechanical handling devices, such as a standing aid or a hoist, may eliminate some of the risk, but the appliance still has to be pushed, pulled, and turned, and the patient has to be handled by the nurse into the appropriate slings, and so on. Sliding devices for the movement of patients on beds or chairs also involve pushing, pulling, and turning actions.

ESSENTIAL ELEMENTS OF THE NEUROMUSCULAR APPROACH

Conditioning movements

Conditioning movements are integral to and form the essential basis of the Neuromuscular Approach and cannot be divorced from it. Any attempt to portray or teach the Neuromuscular Approach without the inclusion of conditioning movements indicates a lack of understanding of the basic concept and philosophy. After initial tuition their continuance and practice become the responsibility of each individual student of the Approach.

Specific conditioning movements are an essential element in the process of changing movement habits. They constitute slow, gentle stretching movements, each individual working within his or her own limitations to effect change gradually. They are designed to aid the regression of adaptive tissue changes and, besides regaining lost elasticity, which is the capacity of the tissues to deform and reform in response to the forces applied to them, this process progressively increases tissue sensitivity and facilitates the uptake of the core pattern of movement – Patterning Conditioning.

Principles

The Neuromuscular Approach recognises that humans are capable of the five basic actions described in the earlier passage under the heading of Concept and Philosophy. One, some, or all of these actions form, in varying permutations, the basis of all physical human activity whether at work, rest, or play.

All basic actions require equal consideration. If inefficiently performed, all are equally capable of causing injury, whether insidious or acute and, most importantly, following an initial reaching action, all are the same thing - the application of a force.

Any or all of the combinations of these basic actions can be performed using the Neuromuscular Approach's core pattern to achieve an effective application of force, and efficiency, in terms of human movement.

Core pattern of movement

Due to the fact that all basic actions are essentially the same thing - the application of a force - **only one core pattern of movement need be learned**, and applied to all the basic actions. Consequently, the learning of techniques by rote becomes redundant.

The core pattern is applicable to all movement situations in all areas of life and allows the reinforcement and development of an efficient, reflex movement pattern.

The core pattern incorporates established and researched principles:

  physical principles concerning the relationship between the centre and line of gravity and base area

  anatomical and physiological principles related to the bones, joints and muscle tissue structures

  anatomical principles related to movements of the vertebral column

  physiological principles related to muscle and connective tissues

  human movement developmental principles.

Application of these principles allows the appropriate blend of the stability and mobility factors, resulting in the least possible sustained tension where, during both the initiation and the continuation of any movement, the individual is in dynamic balance.

Application of the principles of the Neuromuscular Approach to Efficient Handling and Moving does not mean that every efficient movement will be an effective one – there will always be resistances greater than the ability of the individual to overcome them as when, for example, the load is too heavy, or is unstable.

Using the Approach, the individual makes an internal assessment of his or her capacity to move the load *before the load is moved.* Where necessary, physical or mechanical help is recruited, and the safety of both the handlers and the commodity being handled is preserved.

Modifications can be made to the practical application of the principles according to each unique movement situation.

MOVEMENT EDUCATION CONSIDERATIONS

If efficient movement patterns are to replace inefficient habits, principles of efficient movement must be learned and applied to all aspects of life to allow for the development of efficient, reflex movement skill.

When teaching people to move in a different way, knowledge of the processes involved in the formation of movement habit and adaptive tissue change is essential if they are to be made aware of the potential dangers of such a change: this is true of any movement system.

The Neuromuscular Approach considers that the handling and moving of patients must be viewed within the full context of human movement: manual handling and moving training programmes must provide education in human movement and the means to allow the individual to learn a movement pattern which is efficient and becomes progressively more reflex in terms of being reproducible and reliable and can be applied to any action, movement or task, whether occupational, recreational, or social.

HANDLING OF PATIENTS

The handling of patients variously involves a range of methods, such as:

  verbal and/or manual facilitation of movement

  guidance or assistance of movement

  use of mechanical devices.

Many nurses still consider the primary risk associated with the moving and handling of patients to be lifting, and especially the lifting of the heavy or awkward patient. It seems that this one action – lifting – has been set apart from all other human actions.

The other basic actions – pulling, pushing, reaching, turning – are as frequently, if not more frequently, performed, involve risk, and therefore demand the same consideration. (Note: the Manual Handling Operations Regulations and Guidance (1992) state that manual handling operations means any transporting or supporting of a load, including the lifting, putting down, pushing, pulling, carrying, or moving thereof, by hand or by bodily force.)

There are primary considerations when applying the Neuromuscular Approach principles in any handling situation:

General considerations

The Neuromuscular Approach recognises that current legal requirements, professional codes of practice, and local manual handling policies, must be complied with. Also, adequate assessment and planning of the task must be made before deciding on the action – or nonaction – to be taken.

Specific considerations

The key to movement skill in the Neuromuscular Approach to Efficient Handling and Moving is the application and modification of the core pattern of movement.

From the initiation and throughout all stages of any manoeuvre the handler:

  is in dynamic balance

  engenders forces which are always initiated by movement of the head in a cephalad direction

  does not rely on muscle power or sheer brute force

  induces momentum physiologically, **not** mechanically.

Patient handling situations

If the handler is in dynamic balance, the patient will feel safe and comfortable. This in itself facilitates a positive response from the patient regarding his role in any manoeuvre and any help he can give to the move. If the handler is freed from struggling to maintain her balance and equilibrium, she will be able to control the manoeuvre efficiently and this will give the patient confidence.

The principles within the Neuromuscular Approach to Efficient Handling and Moving and the associated criteria for efficiency of human movement are applicable to all aspects of human movement:

  activities of daily living

patient handling and moving

inanimate loads handling and moving

sport and recreation

the therapeutic handling associated with preventive, re-educative, and rehabilitative therapy.

HISTORICAL NOTE

The title, The Neuromuscular Approach, was devised by John R. Vasey, MCSP DipTP and Lesley Crozier MCSP DipTP and was first documented in 1982* and represented a stage of consolidation and onward development of the work of T. McLurg Anderson, who founded the Institute of Human Kinetics in Glasgow. Anderson's initial concepts and philosophy of human movement continued to evolve through the work of Vasey and others. From the original precepts of some 60 years ago, development by Lesley Crozier and Sheila Cozens, MCSP Lic Ac MBAcC, has continued to uphold the philosophy and has led to the current practice of The Neuromuscular Approach to Human Movement and The Neuromuscular Approach to Efficient Handling and Moving.

FURTHER READING

1 - Crozier L., Cozens S. National Back Exchange Newsletter 1994. Issue no. 6.2 pp .10 11

2 - Vasey J.R., Crozier L. A Move in the Right Direction. Nursing Mirror April 1982

3 - Vasey J.R., Crozier L. Get Into Condition. Nursing Mirror. May 1982

4 - Vasey J.R., Crozier L. At Ease. Nursing Mirror. May 1982

5 - Vasey J.R., Crozier L. Handle with Care. Nursing Mirror. May 1982

6 - Vasey J.R., Crozier L. Easy on the Base. Nursing Mirror. May 1982

7 - Vasey J.R., Crozier L. Safety First. Nursing Mirror. June 1982.

THE MANAGEMENT RESPONSIBILITY

by Moira Tracy and Christine Tarling

SUMMARY

This chapter is intended mainly for directors of organisations, moving and handling coordinators, and back care advisers. It gives guidance about managing handling risk.

A written policy should define people's responsibilities and the arrangements in the organisation for managing patient handling.

People with those responsibilities must have the facilities necessary and the skill to put the policy into effect.

Risk assessments must lead to planning and the allocation of a budget.

The action necessary to reduce risk is indicated.

Employers must periodically review the measures they put in place.

FIVE STEPS

The Health and Safety Executive (Refs 7, 12) has recommended five important steps for success: a policy, staff to put the policy into effect, assessment of risks with appropriate precautions to avoid them, measures of performance, and reviews of performance. In addition, written records should always be kept.

These steps, as they apply to the handling of patients, will help directors to:

attend to priorities first, have a plan, check that what they have done to reduce risks works, and that they do not waste resources

demonstrate that even though they may not yet be complying fully with regulations, they are working energetically towards them. This will help satisfy Health and Safety Executive inspectors as well as staff

in response to civil claims for negligence, show that the organisation has proper systems in place.

In the past, many organisations took action that did not take into account all that was necessary for safer handling. For instance some organisations trained staff to use equipment which was not available in the workplace. Some trained staff to avoid using certain dangerous handling techniques, without instructing managers to enforce this. In claims for negligence, courts ruled against such employers. (see Note A page 70)

In practice the steps need not be taken in the sequence given here. They are essentials that should all be attended to.

The principles outlined here apply to all organisations with staff or volunteers who handle people:

organisations can build on what arrangements they already have

the separate steps all relate to each other

boundaries between each step are not fixed, and changes under any of the headings will have an effect on what happens under all the others.

WRITING A POLICY

A written policy for the safer handling of patients records the system put in place by the employer: a safe system is required in both common law and in criminal law. The policy can be a simple document that forms part of the organisation's health and safety policy.

Not having a written policy would be considered as evidence of poor health and safety management. The need for written policies features in all audit systems and in guidance from the Health and Safety Executive.

Staff need to know what system to work to, and what their rights are. Staff should know and understand the policy, so training may be needed. The policy must:

identify who does what

outline the arrangements for patient handling

be consistent with the organisation's health and safety policy

cover arrangements for staff, patients, visitors, volunteers, relatives, and agency and bank staff at least meet the requirements of the Manual Handling Operations Regulations, 1992

deal with the question of lifting patients manually or with equipment (see Chapter 2)

make clear to staff their duties and their rights (for instance, what they should do if a patient refuses to be lifted by a hoist)

be kept up to date as circumstances change

The policy should not contain anything which is not practical or which managers do not enforce. For example, instructions that there should be no manual lifting cannot be included if there is not enough equipment for staff to use.

The policy can include detailed procedures and plans relevant to patient handling, or these can be written in separate documents.

There is no need for every department to write its own policy, but some may need to write local procedures if these differ from the rest of the organisation's.

All the matters mentioned in this chapter should be covered either in the policy or in supporting documents describing safer handling procedures.

PROCEDURES

Agreements about how safer systems of work are to be achieved need to be made between all providers in the health services, social services, and independent agencies.

Some of the routine processes through which patients pass need to have any risks involved identified, with procedures developed to overcome them. These procedures could cover:

the planned admission of a dependent disabled person into an acute hospital ward

the referral of a dependent patient from one clinical area to another, or from his own home into residential or nursing care

the planned discharge of a dependent patient who uses a hoist into his own home

the safer handling of a very heavy patient (over 176kg or 28 stones) where standard patient handling equipment is not suitable.

Circumstances such as these will involve a multidisciplinary approach by several different teams of staff. Consequently, reaching an agreement and then putting it into effect will require a strong commitment from managers.

Where the moving of a particular patient is known to present risks, procedures are usually developed by the clinical team concerned. A safety audit identifies the problems, and action to reduce the risk must be taken. Some teams develop their procedures as part of their quality awareness programme. It may be appropriate for the quality control manager to ensure that all the procedures are consistent with each other. One team may resolve its patient handling difficulties in a different way from another, and the two methods should be compared to ensure that the risk has been reduced as far as is reasonably practicable.

COMPETENT STAFF

Specific services and people must be provided to put the policy into effect. The precise requirements will depend on all the aspects covered in this chapter, but may include the following:

someone who is in charge of handling issues and advises on everything to do with the handling of patients, such as a back care adviser, or a moving and handling co-ordinator. This person should report directly to a senior manager, such as a board director, who should be responsible for overseeing that the policy is put into effect. Access to competent advice is a requirement of the management of health and safety regulations

occupational health and physiotherapy staff for advice, pre-employment screening, and rehabilitation

a risk manager, health and safety or ergonomics professional

people to give training on handling

people to carry out (or train others to carry out) risk assessments

link staff to promote good practices in wards, departments, and community teams.

Training needs for the people on this list, as well as for all other staff and managers involved in the handling of patients, must be identified. Time and training facilities must be allocated.

Staff members and safety representatives must be consulted and involved in discussing what staff are needed, and what training should be provided.

The first person on the list, the person in charge of handling issues, is probably the key to the success of the policy. Without a competent person concentrating on this, there is usually little progress made.

Where the manual handling is particularly complex, it may be necessary to seek outside help. This may occur in an area where previously no handling equipment was in regular use. Such tasks as turning and positioning patients on an operating table have customarily been done by hand, with perhaps male staff helping to reduce the risk.

Complex tasks of this type are frequently discussed in mutual support sessions such as those provided as a consequence of membership of the National Back Exchange, and at regional meetings of back care advisers and assessors. These meetings take place regularly and give an opportunity for specialists to meet each other to resolve problems. Interprofessional events of this kind are valuable and specialist staff should be encouraged by their managers to attend and contribute.

RISKS AND CONTROLS

Assessment of risks, decisions about necessary controls, and the setting of priorities, lead to immediate action, or planning – and the reduction of risks.

Risk assessment

Chapter 11 describes manual handling risk assessments and discusses three kinds:

1. When working with a patient:

> this is done mentally every time a patient is to be handled. The techniques or equipment to be used with a patient should be noted in the patient care plan if they are not covered by a standard procedure. This is mainly to help communication and consistency between carers. But it is also useful for monitoring, and in case of injury. These purposes should be kept in mind when deciding how much paper work to create for each patient. For nursing people in their homes, facilities are assessed as part of the patient's assessment.

2. For the department or ward:

> this is an annual written assessment of the facilities. It records, for instance, the need for extra equipment, training, or changes around baths or toilets. It must lead to action: local managers should tell senior managers of anything that needs to be done, and introduce improvements within their capabilities.

3. A top level assessment:

> this is the senior managers' judgement of what is needed. Much will depend on the departments' or wards' risk assessments and on the organisation's policy. The outcome is a plan and the allocation of budgets.

Priorities

Managers should identify what needs to be done to control risks so as to comply with the regulations and the organisation's policy. They need to work out costs, and establish priorities. The time within which these needs should be met must be specified.

Managers and directors should keep records of these plans in such a way that they can be used both to review performance, and as evidence in legal proceedings.

Reducing risks

The actions necessary to reduce risks depend on each local situation. The purpose of risk assessments is to identify them.

The main ones to consider are:

> reduce the risk at source where possible. For example, examine each task to see how to avoid the need for hazardous manual handling

> improve the layout, such as space in bathrooms and between beds. The possibility of introducing risks – and consequently how to avoid them – should be considered in the design of new buildings, in consultation with people who know about potential risks. The Department of Health Building Notes (Ref 5) are revised from time to time and give excellent indicators of the space needed in which to use equipment when caring for dependent people

> provide handling equipment and train staff in its use

> training is required at induction, and on regular refresher courses. It is useful to give some of the training in the work place, not just in the classroom

> procedures should allow the work load to be spread through time and between people – for example, patients should not all be bathed on the same day or during the same span of duty

> there must be enough staff to avoid anyone taking risks (Note B)

> fellow workers must be competent (Note C)

uniforms must be suitable for the tasks the wearer has to undertake. The traditional nurse's dress is not suited to most nursing tasks; trousers or a wider, pleated skirt are recommended

carers should keep each other well informed, in writing when necessary, about a patient's needs and the risk of falls

have a procedure for patients whose weight is more than the safe working load of the available hoists

have satisfactory equipment and procedures for emergencies or unusual situations that can be foreseen (see Note D and Chapter 21);

have pre-employment checks to detect staff at risk of back injury (see Note E)

have a procedure for staff reporting back pain (or in the shoulder, hip, or elsewhere) or who have had an injury as a consequence of handling a patient

have a rehabilitation programme for staff who have sick leave because of muscular skeletal injury (see Note F)

liaise with any parties who also care for the patient, such as community nurses or community care assistants, and establish links between hospital and community

improve job satisfaction and reduce stress.

MANAGING EQUIPMENT

Given that the Manual Handling Operations Regulations 1992 require that risks should be reduced by the introduction of appropriate equipment, the evaluation, selection, use and maintenance of equipment must become an important responsibility for a specific person or team.

Access to a resource of products, such as at a disabled living centre, is vital if staff are to evaluate and select appropriate equipment. While there are several publications which evaluate handling equipment, new items become available frequently and no publication will always be up to date. The Department of Health, through its Medical Devices Agency (Ref 4), has funded the evaluation of some equipment and the published results are freely available to staff. Reading these reports will assist staff to make a preliminary choice of equipment appropriate for the handling to be done.

It is useful for managers to have a full inventory made of all the handling equipment that is available to them. Unused hoists in one department may be suitable for use in another. Handling products bought some time ago may now be in cupboards, forgotten. The inventory should be made by an experienced person who knows the range of products available, can identify what is retrieved, and recognise whether equipment has any missing parts.

Equipment used in the community

Equipment for use in a person's home is often designed to criteria different from that used in a clinic, hospital, or nursing home. A bath hoist in a hospital ward may be used ten or more times each day, while in a private home may be used only once a day. A mobile hoist may have to lift only from a low easy chair in a person's home, while a hoist for use in hospital often needs a higher lifting range to reach above the height adjustable bed with a specialist mattress on top. Space is always limited in the domestic home, and any equipment that saves space has advantages. If space cannot be made for appropriate equipment, a manager may have to consider providing services to that patient in a more spacious location, such as in residential or nursing homes.

In the rehabilitation stage of the patient's progress towards discharge from hospital, it is always useful to have in the ward the same type of equipment as that which he will use at home. Not only can the patient gain confidence in using it, but relatives and carers can become accustomed to its use. In certain specialties, such as spinal injuries units, trial weekends at home are often planned before the patient is discharged. Equipment must be available for this so that the patient can be at home without risk.

Since it is common practice for health, local authority and other staff to use equipment in a client's home, managers need to have agreements about how it is to be provided and paid for. The equipment service for the community is generally now funded jointly by health and local authorities' social services departments. This allows staff from both providers to make assessments before prescribing, and to have access to the equipment that they need. The equipment assessor needs to be able to prescribe, and then ensure, that staff and carers are adequately trained in its use with the individual patient. For example, staff employed by the local authority must be able to use hoists paid for by the Health Authority.

When a highly dependent client receives care in his own home from an independent agency, decisions about who provides a hoist or a similar piece of equipment must be made clear. Independent agencies are now the source of most of the nursing or social care given to people in their own home. The local authority social services department is limited in the amount it can spend on its own care services, and must buy from the independent agencies.

Home care service agencies must be registered with the social services department in the same way as residential care homes. They must conform with certain standards and are monitored frequently to make sure the service they provide meets the agreed contracts. Each providing agency has its own management system and must be a good employer. While the social services department contracts unit might insist on health and safety matters being part of the contract, the detail of who provides a manual handling assessment of a client needing a home care service, and who provides the equipment, such as a mobile hoist and slings, must be clarified.

The community occupational therapist in the social services department is the person most likely to make handling assessments and to prescribe what is needed. However, not all occupational therapists are care managers involved in the assessment of need for home care services and the arranging of contracts to meet those needs. A care manager is more likely to be a social worker who may or may not have access to an occupational therapist for advice and assessment of a patient's problems. This care manager may then have to rely on the care agency being able to provide a personal care service to the patient in compliance with the health and safety legislation.

Where a dependent patient is being discharged from hospital to his own home, the community nursing service is often involved with his continuing care. The community nurse can then liaise with colleagues on the ward and establish what handling needs must be met at his home. Occupational therapists and physiotherapists are also involved in the discharge of patients, and in practice the organisation of the home handling equipment is usually done by the most knowledgeable person in the multidisciplinary team.

The home based assessments of patients undertaken by health or community staff often identify the need for handling equipment. If the community loan equipment service does not have a suitable item of equipment available, decisions have to be made. If the risk of injury to a home care worker is high, then without the equipment to lessen that risk, the service cannot be provided. Either the home care service provides care to the patient while in bed, or not at all.

To allow home care staff to lift a patient in and out of bed when the need for a hoist has been identified would be negligent on the part of the employer. Consequently, the availability of a range of equipment is of prime importance. The urgent need for equipment should be dealt with by the community loan equipment service – too often it is left to individual social service teams or community nurse teams to fund and have available an emergency hoist.

There are many problems associated with this type of ad hoc provision. The slings for the hoist are usually not the right design for the patient's needs; the hoist cannot be cleaned satisfactorily between its issues to patients; there is no regular servicing of the hoist and community staff are expected to handle a heavy piece of equipment into and out of a car to deliver and assemble it.

The manager of a community equipment loan service needs to have his own manual handling risk assessment procedures in place and ensure that the storage, delivery and fitting of equipment complies with the Manual Handling Operations Regulations 1992. The delivery of heavy equipment such as hoists and beds requires a tail-lift on a delivery van to ease loading. Consideration must be given as to how equipment is taken up or down stairs.

Equipment instructions

All handling equipment should be delivered with full instructions on its use. These instructions should be written in non-technical language so that all staff can understand them, be well illustrated, and should set out the various situations in which the equipment can, and cannot, be used.

Instructions are often lost, misfiled, or not attached to the equipment. This is a particular problem in the community services where staff work in isolation and without the immediate support of colleagues when faced with problems.

It is helpful to staff to have the manufacturer's instructions on how to use the equipment, as well as personalised instructions for an individual patient, instructions which can form part of the recorded manual handling assessment, and should become part of the care package documents.

Maintenance of equipment

Maintenance can cost a large part of any equipment budget. Mechanical moving equipment such as hoists requires servicing once a year. The current - but under review - British Standard (Ref 1) sets out the annual service procedure and in view of the nature of the equipment used to take the total weight of the patient, regular servicing is important.

TRAINING

All staff must be trained for the jobs they are expected to do. Guidance is given by the Royal College of Nursing (Ref 13), the Chartered Society of Physiotherapists (Refs 2, 3) and the Health and Safety Commission (Ref 10).

In general, all staff must attend a classroom course at induction. Student nurses still tend to have insufficient training and auxiliary nurses may be new to the profession. The duration of courses depends on the level of training that staff have previously received, and on how much change is being introduced. Induction training usually requires a minimum of two days, and the usual recommendation is three to five days (Ref 8) or more. This initial training will be more effective if closely followed by a review day or on the job training.

Regular refresher training is also needed, preferably at least once a year.

Classes must not be too large: for practical sessions a maximum of six students to one instructor is recommended (Ref 3). The instructor should be qualified and experienced to the level set out in the inter-professional curriculum (Ref 11 and Chapter 8).

The classroom course should cover:

  the employer's manual handling policy

  rudiments of spinal mechanics and the causes of back pain

  principles of efficient body movement and posture

  assessing risk and assessing the patient

  how to teach patients to move themselves

  ergonomics - the environment and equipment

  handling aids

  manual handling techniques - but no patient *lifting* techniques

  health, including 'conditioning' or warm-up movements, and awareness of good movement at work and at home

  responsibilities for reporting risks and injuries.

In addition to the classroom work, training and support should continue at the workplace. Some instructors visit wards or help to solve problems with patients. Sometimes, a person such as a link nurse is given the responsibility of making sure staff continue to be reminded of what they were taught, and to report difficulties to the instructor.

Any instructor who observes that someone is unable to reach acceptable levels of competency must inform that person's manager so that a decision can be made about her safety at work.

The 24-hour service given by all care agencies means that training opportunities for staff must be offered within reasonable times suitable for them, as well as fitting in with working rotas. Night staff, bank staff, part time staff are all vulnerable to the possibility of slipping through the training net.

Targets for training need to be coordinated with clinical departments, wards, teams, and agency services. Money needs to be set aside to pay for bank or other staff providing cover for nurses and other care staff on training courses.

Caution needs to be exercised when considering whether to buy the services of an instructor from outside the organisation. Patient handling will continue after the trainer has left. Staff then often feel isolated and let down when left without expert support to work on any problems they identify.

Provision needs to be made also for a training area for manual handling so that equipment handling skills can be learned away from the patient's bedside. This area can become the resource centre for that locality and it may be possible to share facilities between NHS trusts, social services, and local agencies. This close working should ensure that all staff adopt similar attitudes and skills. Apart from a training room with audio visual equipment and necessary furniture, there must be a basic range of equipment so that safer patient handling skills can be taught. This equipment should reflect the range available within the staff work areas, and should also include items less frequently used so that trainees can learn to compare and evaluate equipment themselves.

Training records

Records of training given should be precise, in case they are needed for legal reasons. They should include:

  dates, location, and duration of course

  course contents - equipment demonstrated or practised on, and techniques

  details and copies of written or printed information given to the student for later reference

  warnings given on the course, such as banned lifts

  names of those who attended, with their signatures; name and signature of the instructor.

The instructor should check with the students to learn of any physical condition that might affect a student's ability to take part in the course safely.

Employers should not try to imply that the training makes staff competent and safe, and should not try to make staff sign any disclaimers of responsibility. All that can be expected is to get staff to try and apply their training to the best of their ability.

DOCUMENTARY EVIDENCE

Documentation is becoming increasingly important when defending litigation claims by employees. Managers must keep records that explain what was expected and what took place.

Books and literature

Lawyers frequently ask for details of books and other literature to which staff may have had access to keep professionally up to date.

If there is a library available to staff, questions must be asked about its ability to stock literature to ensure that trainers and staff have access to the latest information on their subject.

Whether or not there is a library, there will be books and journals in the wards or departments, to which staff have access. Managers should decide which documents they need to ensure all staff read.

Qualified staff have a duty to maintain and improve their professional knowledge and competence (Ref 13).

Patient records

Accurate and detailed completion of patient records is vital for the well being of patients and also for the guidance and protection of staff. Facts must be recorded legibly with a black pen and must be suitable for photocopying.

A manual handling assessment form must be completed and included in every dependent patient's care plan. Examples are in Chapter 12. Agreement must be reached on who may complete such a form, and the time limits by when it must be completed and reviewed. It must contain details on how to move the patient, and must be understood by all who care for him.

Staff employment records

Individual records should be kept of each person employed. The records should include her application form for the post she now holds, with her past employment history if she has come from another employer. Records of episodes of sick leave are increasingly important and should contain a note of any action taken as a result of implementing the procedure required by a sickness policy. All other breaks in service, together with the reasons for them, must be recorded. Training records are needed for in-service training and for courses leading to registration and additional professional qualifications. Most professional and registration bodies insist that evidence of continuing education is mandatory for their members to be competent to practice.

Minutes of meetings

Teams of staff may have meetings to discuss matters of common concern relating to their work. These meetings can become a forum where problems and difficulties are identified. This system of open discussion on day to day matters relating to work may encourage an individual team member to raise a matter within a peer group, whereas she may not feel confident enough to discuss it with the team manager. If the team feels that the matter is important, then it is helpful to have it recorded in the minutes so that it can be taken further. All such team meetings should have an agenda with minutes so that problems can be recorded and followed through. Minutes of such meetings must be kept for legal reasons.

Other meetings may be convened for specific subjects. Such a subject might be the implementation of the Manual Handling Operations Regulations 1992. The minutes of such meetings provide valuable insight and evidence on the work identified to be done, and the progress made with introducing new systems.

An expert adviser on manual handling should also keep a record of any discussions with managers where advice was given about the introduction of safer systems of work.

MEASURING PERFORMANCE

A well-known tool for measuring performance is the recording of incidents, (see Note G), which includes accidents and work-related ill health. Having a sore back is not always associated by staff with an accident, and this is why incidents or work-related ill health should be recorded.

As these statistics describe only part of the back pain picture, sickness absence statistics are also needed.

Managers should also note whether specific objectives set at earlier stages have been achieved. This is the time to check how much compliance there has been with the standards set at the policy, planning, and implementation stages. For example, have all the staff due to have training now received it?

Many aspects of compliance with the policy cannot be measured with numbers but can still be evaluated by:

listening to what staff say on refresher training courses

observing their skill and movement

listening to physiotherapists' or link nurses' comments on how nurses handle patients

checking patient care plans and ward-based risk assessments

asking staff their views at meetings.

NOTE A

Enforcing a safe system of work: example of a judgement

In Salvat v Basingstoke and North Hampshire Health Authority, staff nurse Salvat was awarded £13,298 following a back injury incurred in 1983 while transferring a patient from commode to bed with a colleague using a drag lift. There was a hoist on the ward but it was never used except when bathing patients. The nurse had been taught the more suitable through-arm lift, but custom and practice in this hospital was to use the drag lift. The decision was that the health authority had failed to ensure that the lifting was done in a safe manner, either with an approved method of personal lifting, or by use of a hoist. The nurse was not considered to have had any contributory negligence, because "if she had picked up the wrong habits in her training," the judge was not satisfied that she "was adequately or suitably corrected in her employment in this ward."

NOTE B

Providing enough staff: example of a judgement

In Forder v. Norfolk Health Authority, Mrs Forder was awarded £5,000 for an injury sustained in 1975 while lifting a 95kg (15stone) patient up a bed with the assistance of an auxiliary nurse. They used a drag lift, which was the custom and practice in this hospital. Reasons for the decision included: "...it should have been made clear to the nurses in this...ward...that patients of this weight were not to be handled by two nurses alone...it seems...that the defendant allowed an atmosphere to prevail where nurses were encouraged, because of shortage of staff, in the movement of patients without sufficient persons assisting." The judge also commented: On the day in question there were four nurses working on the ward. The plaintiff was in a position where she could have called upon another nurse to assist her if she had thought it appropriate to do so. She did not...but in my view she is not to be blamed for that...despite the fact that she was an experienced nurse. The way the hospital was operated at the time was to create an ethos where nurses thought that their duty required them to perform (this sort of lift) with the assistance of one other nurse.

NOTE C

Fellow workers: example of a judgement

In Page v Enfield and Haringey Health Authority, staff nurse Page was awarded £17,000. The injury occurred in 1977 when a nurse lifting with her failed to lift on the command "lift," with the result that Page took the full weight of the patient.

NOTE D

Emergencies or unusual situations

The regulations require employers to do only what is 'reasonably practicable.' Employers are not obliged to put in measures whose costs greatly exceed the risks. So it may not be legally necessary to spend huge amounts of money on equipment to meet a requirement which is extremely unlikely. In criminal law employers must be able to justify a decision as to why they did not consider a procedure to be reasonably practicable. In civil claims, the burden of proof is lighter. Emergencies are dealt with in Chapter 21.

NOTE E

Pre-employment health check

Chapter 4 describes what is known about the main causes of back injury.

There are few reliable indicators of a person who is at risk, so the emphasis instead should be on reducing risks from the job. Problems can be detected with a new employee more readily during handling training at induction than during a health check. The trainer, the manager, and the occupational health staff consequently need to keep in touch with each other about any problem presented by a new employee during training.

NOTE F

Staff with back pain

Employers should ask their staff to report pain, and should provide advice and treatment from the earliest stage. Any work-related causes should be investigated. Managers, the occupational health staff, physiotherapists, the back care adviser, and any other professionals involved in risk management should keep each other informed about such staff, and about what is being done about the causes of the pain, seeking each other's advice, and possibly making a joint visit to the ward. The role of the occupational health staff is dealt with fully in Chapter 9. Managers, the occupational health staff, and the back care adviser should work together to get the member of staff back to work as soon as possible, albeit with shorter hours at first. This requires careful assessment.

Members of staff will recover faster the sooner they return to some activity, but any assessment of risks in the work they will be called upon to do must take account of their recent experience and the possibility of a relapse if taking up a particular task or tasks too soon. But all jobs should be so safe that there should be no risk even to someone who has not yet regained full fitness.

Under the Disability Discrimination Act (Ref 6), back injured staff seeking a new job or changing jobs can be refused employment only on the basis of a risk assessment that demonstrates that the job does not suit - and cannot be made to suit - the disabled person.

NOTE G

Reporting and investigating incidents and injury

The incident report form should cover near-misses (incidents that could have given rise to injury), as well as injury. The form should include:

the name, date of birth, and address of the injured person

names and addresses of witnesses

the nature of the injury and the part of the body injured

a detailed description of what happened, including the positions people were in and the methods or equipment used

the patient's name, date of birth, weight, and weight-bearing ability, as well as a copy of the manual handling part of the care plan

what systems of work were in place to prevent this type of incident, and what equipment was available

any further precautions to be considered and action taken as a consequence of investigating the incident.

Someone, such as the back care adviser, or the occupational health nurse, should contact the people involved without delay, and investigate the causes. The need for any further action, both to help the injured person and to improve the safety of the job, should be assessed.

This fulfils one aim of incident reporting – to prevent a recurrence. Note also that some accidents should be reported to the Health and Safety Executive (Ref 9). Another purpose of incident reporting is to have a detailed record in case of litigation. The third aim is to gather statistics that will show which are the main types of incidents, such as:

falling patients

non-compliance with policy

no obvious cause,

and to get a measure of their severity by recording what happened as a consequence, such as the extent of sick leave following an injury.

REFERENCES

1. British Standards BS 5827 (1979): Manual Mobile Patient Lifting Devices; BS 5724 (1989) Medical Electrical Equipment.7.

2. Chartered Society of Physiotherapy (1992). Factsheet 9 Patient handling training; Factsheet 9A Manual handling of inanimate loads training.

3. Chartered Society of Physiotherapy (1993). Standards of Physiotherapy Practice for Trainers in Moving and Handling,

4. Department of Health Medical Devices Agency (1997). London

5. Department of Health (1995) Common Activity Spaces. Hospital Building Note no. 40, HMSO, London.

6. Disability Discrimination Act (1995). HMSO - London.

7. Five steps to successful health and safety management. Health and Safety Executive HS(G)65 or the summary booklet IND(G)132L.

8. Health Services Advisory Committee (1992): Guidance on Manual Handling of Loads in the Health Services. Health and Safety Commission.

9. Health and Safety Executive (1995). The Reporting of Injuries, Diseases, and Dangerous Occurrences Regulations.

10. Inter-professional curriculum. A course for back care advisers. (1995).

11. Management of health and safety in the health services – information for directors and managers. Health and Safety Commission (Health Services Advisory Committee). HSE Books.1994.

12. Royal College of Nursing Advisory Panel for Back Pain in Nurses: Patient Handling Standards, May 1996.

13. Code of Professional Conduct for the Nurse, Midwife and Health Visitors, UKCC, June 1992.

THE INTER-PROFESSIONAL CURRICULUM: A COURSE FOR BACKCARE ADVISERS

by Paul Lloyd

This curriculum has been developed in response to the increasing demand from back care advisers appointed by health authorities, and also those employed in the private sector, for a course of instruction which could be taken up by educational institutions.

The curriculum has been drawn up by an expert advisory group drawn from The Royal College of Nursing, The Chartered Society of Physiotherapy, The College of Occupational Therapists, The Ergonomic Society, and The National Back Exchange.

Back Care Advisers are expected to be competent and knowledgeable about handling people in health care or social settings. They are expected to give expert advice on risk assessment, safer working practices, manual handling equipment and its uses, manual handling practices in a variety of situations, manual handling legislation, the prevention and management of musculo-skeletal injuries, and the implementation of educational and training courses for workers at risk of injury.

The curriculum was developed to address all these issues. It is divided into four modules. Each one has a stated aim and learning outcomes. The modules comprise different units of learning, and in total the entire course should involve 135 hours or more of teaching.

The modules:

Health: including occupational health services, epidemiology, biomechanics, and life style.

Ergonomics: ergonomics and task analysis, assessment principles, inanimate loads, design aspects of load handling equipment.

Patient assessment and handling: assessment of patient handling needs, hoists and handling equipment.

Social organisation: legal and professional requirements, problem solving, and implementing change.

This curriculum is under review. A new version will be published in 1997/98.

Information about the syllabus and the setting up of an approved course of training by an educational body may be had from:

Emma Crumpton,
Lecturer in Physiotherapy,
The Faculty of Health and Social Care,
The University of the West of England,
Glenside Campus, Blackberry Hill,
Bristol BS16 1DD.
Tel 0117 975 8416.

THE OCCUPATIONAL HEALTH SERVICE
PART 1 - THE ROLE OF THE OCCUPATIONAL HEALTH SERVICE

by Paul Lloyd

An occupational health service (OHS) collaborates with employers and workers to promote the health and safety of all workers within an organisation.

In the context of patient handling and back injury, the role of the OHS is:

- helping to select staff fit for nursing

- participation in training courses

- monitoring the outcome of training

- assessing and monitoring the working environment

- ensuring that safe systems of work are in place

- investigating and recording accidents, especially back injuries

- producing statistical information related to back injury and its prevention

- undertaking research into back injury prevention, and its management at work

- resettling and monitoring staff in appropriate employment when returning to work after a back injury

- managing and treating back injury at work in liaison with physiotherapists, osteopaths, and chiropractors.

In performing this role the occupational health service works closely with employers and, where they have them, their back care coordinators or trainers, and the health and safety or risk manager or ergonomist, with trades unions, especially their safety representatives, and with other appropriate agencies.

STAFF SELECTION

> ### WARNING
>
> The task is not to select a superman or woman to perform heavy manual handling tasks but rather to redesign the job so that it can be performed by the average healthy man or woman.

Staff selection is based on a health questionnaire which requires truthful answers to be given by the applicant.

The usual question is: "Have you now got, or ever had, any problems with your back?"

If the answer is "No" - further inquiry is not normally necessary where the job has been assessed for risk and safe systems of work are in operation.

But the answer "No" does not necessarily mean that the person is free of any back problems, or that she has a healthy back.

Some conditions may lie dormant for years and may not normally be noticeable. Degenerative changes may also occur without showing symptoms. The person may be unaware of the condition of her spine and the likelihood of trouble ahead. A dormant condition may be triggered by even a minor handling activity.

If the answer is "Yes" - the person should be referred to a qualified occupational health nurse or physician for investigation and assessment. This may take the form of a health or medical examination.

A careful history of any back trouble should be taken and recorded and should include questions about hospital treatment and operations on the back, and the outcome. A visual inspection of the spinal column should be made to note any obvious abnormalities such as loss of lordosis, kyphosis, or spinal curvature, or any limitation in the range of movements.

Depending on the result of this examination, the individual may be referred for a specialist opinion, and depending on the outcome of that, a decision would then be made about future employment. This would normally be:

fit for the proposed work

fit for the work, but with conditions attached

unfit for the work

It then becomes a management responsibility to act accordingly on the basis of these findings.

Safeguards such as a safer handling policy, adequate and competent training, assessment of the outcome of training, and the implementation of safer systems of work in an ergonomically sound environment, should be in place to reduce the risks of a back injury to the lowest possible level.

The Manual Handling Operations Regulations 1992 (Ref 3) should have been fully implemented in health services. There should be no so-called 'heavy work' label attached to nursing. The effect of a safer handling policy will be to reduce the burden of heavy work, although some risks will remain, depending upon the nurse's working environment.

The Disability Discrimination Act (Ref 6) will have an impact on the selection criteria for nurses. This legislation is likely to ensure that the selection of candidates for nursing is conducted on an individual basis which takes full account of the candidate's physical and mental qualities and abilities with regard to their chosen area of work.

There are no nationally agreed selection criteria, and according to an interpretation of the Disability Discrimination Act, there should be no attempt to select on the basis of discriminatory criteria such as height, weight, or disability, even though these may influence the choice of area the nurse is allocated to work in.

Advice on the contribution of an occupational health service in support of the selection of staff is available (Refs 1, 2, 4).

THE BACK INJURED NURSE

When a nurse returns to work following a back injury the occupational health service should be involved from the beginning. Research has shown (Ref 5) that early mobilisation and an early return to work are most beneficial for simple backache if long term problems are to be avoided.

The Royal College of General Practitioners clinical guidelines (Ref 7) challenge the traditional standard of medical management for simple back pain, which relies heavily on rest and analgesic medication. There is no evidence to support the use of rest for simple backache for longer than one to three days.

The aim of managing a nurse with a back injury should be to restore normal function by means of rehabilitation. This should include individually prescribed exercises, hopefully leading to the restoration of the person's full function and the regaining of physical fitness.

There is a need for a fundamental review of policy to ensure that rehabilitation services are available to enable staff to make an early return to work. The occupational health department should liaise with others such as the back care adviser, the risk manager or ergonomist, the physiotherapist, and the injured person's manager, in a programme of action based on the Royal College of General Practioners clinical guidelines (Ref 7).

The occupational health service should also define job and fitness criteria with the employer for every post in the health care setting, whether in an institution or in the community. This would enable the occupational health nurse and the occupational health physician to select or reject candidates for nursing or caring employment, or education for nursing, on a firm basis.

There are no nationally established health criteria for working as a nurse, with the risk that a candidate for nursing, or a nurse, may be refused employment in one place of work for health reasons, and be accepted in another by a different employer.

REFERENCES

1. Health Assessment – Advice to Managers (1995). The Royal College of Nursing, London.

2. Health Assessment – Advice to Occupational Health Nurses (1995). The Royal College of Nursing, London.

3. Manual Handling Operations Regulations (1992). HMSO, London.

4. Occupational Health Services for NHS Staff. National Health Service Executive, HSG(94)51.

5. Report of a Clinical Standards Advisory Group Committee on BACK PAIN (1994). HMSO – London.

6. The Disability Discrimination Act (1995). HMSO, London.

7. Royal College of General Practitioners Clinical Guidlines for the Management of Low Back Pain (1996).

THE OCCUPATIONAL HEALTH SERVICE
PART 2 - A STRATEGY FOR PREVENTION AND TREATMENT OF BACK PAIN IN THE WORKPLACE

by Brian Fletcher

SUMMARY

An occupational health department linked with physiotherapy can provide a service for staff who have back pain.

The physiotherapist would be best placed as a member of the occupational health team. Physiotherapy would support the occupational health team's work in preventing back pain and injury among staff.

The physiotherapist could control a full rehabilitation programme to help staff return to work quickly.

Benefits to the organisation include reduced sickness absence, less need for locums or agency staff, less overtime working, reduced cost of legal charges.

INTRODUCTION

Back injuries are some of the most frequent occupational injuries and the health service has a higher incidence than most other places of work, particularly in nursing (Refs 33,26), see Chapter 3.

Patient handling for the physical work of carrying, supporting, moving or otherwise transferring patients and the disabled remains the commonest source of reported injuries for nurses and other care staff. Musculo-skeletal symptoms such as back ache remain a major problem. The scale of the problem has been identified by a number of workers (Ref 26, 30). This problem must be of concern to the health service for both human and financial reasons.

The focus of this guide, as of the previous three (Ref 28), is the prevention of this problem.

Until comparatively recently, structured functional rehabilitation programmes for injured nurses and other staff, linked to occupational health departments, have been a rarity in the National Health Service. Proposals for such programmes have been made in the past (Refs 30, 12). Previous editions of this guide have referred to special clinics for the rehabilitation of people with musculo-skeletal problems and the suggestion that nurses and carers should act positively to keep themselves fit for work.

There is now some evidence that early management of musculo-skeletal problems may result in speedier resolution of the problems and that prevention strategies in the form of exercise and educational programmes may be successful in reducing the number of problems arising. The Clinical Standards Advisory Group (CSAG) Report (Ref 23) 1994 states that early active rehabilitation is highly effective in preventing long term pain and disability. While it is acknowledged that the onset of back problems is a complex issue, evidence is available to suggest that prevention strategies have a place. One of the conclusions of research in Nottingham (Ref 30) was that staff should have a direct access to physiotherapy clinics through the department of occupational health. This was a consistent request by the staff involved and it is suggested that a physiotherapy service could be linked to and work with the service provided by an ergonomist and a moving and handling advisor. This idea is supported by the CSAG report (Ref 23) which indicates that there is some evidence that the treatment of back pain in the work place can be an effective method of delivering early treatment, preventing chronicity and facilitating an early return to work.

See opposite –
Prevention/Rehabilitation Strategy: Flow chart

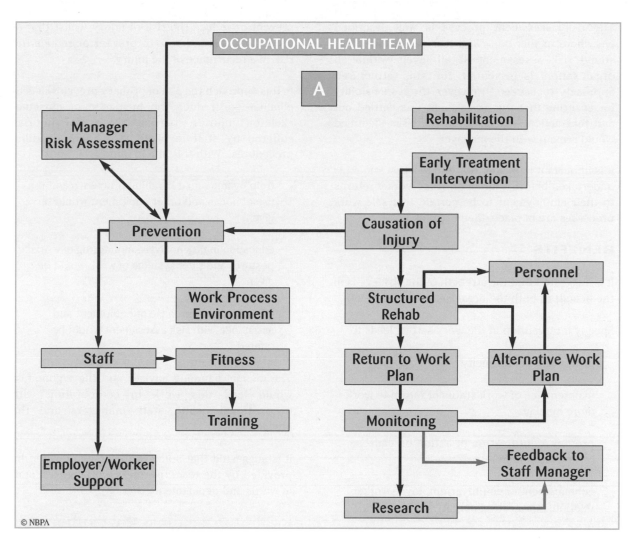

OCCUPATIONAL HEALTH TEAM

In this chapter it is suggested that the whole process as identified in the flow chart should be occupational health based with a personnel link to general management. The occupational health team would be comprised of:

an occupational health physician

an occupational health nurse

an ergonomist

a moving and handling adviser

a physiotherapist

a health and safety risk manager.

Two or more of these functions could be carried out by one individual, for example, the physiotherapist or the ergonomist, but it is important that the physiotherapist should be able to respond promptly to staff who may be referred or self-refer immediately after injury. This is not a new or unique proposal as many industries in the UK and abroad have had similar successful working models of service for some years. However, few have implemented the strategy as a whole although some trusts in the NHS are working towards this model of service.

There are four essential elements to the strategy:

corporate commitment and resources

authority for the team to put the strategy into effect (see flow chart) A

competent and skilled staff

risk assessment process.

Without corporate commitment any scheme will fail. Corporate commitment should include provision of necessary finance for training, equipment, staff and facilities, and the authority given to the physiotherapist to control the return to work of staff who have been injured. Skilled staff are essential but it is important that they work as a team with good working relationships and trust between them and the organisation managers, based on agreed written procedures.

Without this, the structured return to work plan for the injured person, in particular, could be undermined.

The risk assessment process is well described elsewhere in this book and it is self evident that sound risk assessment at all levels within an organisation is essential for this structured approach to succeed. However, the responsibility for ensuring that the assessment was carried out and that action was taken on the risks identified would remain with the manager.

It is important to ensure that the risk assessment is undertaken before a nurse or other worker returns to their employment to be certain that safe work processes are in place. (See Chapter 11.)

BENEFITS

It is suggested that the strength of the strategy is in the benefit to both the organisation and the staff.

Speedy intervention in the work setting leads to:

    prevention of chronicity

    maintenance of work status of return to work more quickly

    prompt identification of action on causes (risk assessment)

    enhancement of employer/employee worker relationships (caring employer)

    reduced stress on staff,

and cost benefits to the organisation include:

    reduced sickness and absence

    reduced need for locums, agency work, overtime

    reduced likelihood of costly itigation

    reduced turnover of staff

    safer working environment

    more effective patient care.

PREVENTION

Prevention programmes in the work setting can be effective if ergonomic interventions are included (Ref 25) and if there is corporate commitment to the process with an emphasis on promoting job satisfaction and reducing job stress. Exercise and relaxation programmes, together with back care education, can be positive contributions.

Prevention programmes may be either primary or secondary. The aim of primary prevention is to prevent or reduce the risk of injury whilst that of secondary prevention is to prevent or reduce the risk of a recurrence of the injury.

In this approach the aim of primary prevention is to eliminate or reduce the incidence of musculo-skeleton injuries, particularly spinal injuries suffered by staff involved in manual handling procedures. With this aim in mind:

    training in manual handling processes and the use of hoists and other equipment would be given

    education in task analysis, monitoring of working postures and safer systems of work would be given

    advice on the purchase of equipment and assistance with risk assessment would be offered.

The manual handling adviser and the ergonomist would lead this work in co-operation with occupational health staff, managers and the physiotherapist.

It is suggested that some of the training would be provided by the team members working with staff in wards and departments (Ref 33).

Role of Preventive Physiotherapy

The specific contribution of the physiotherapist to the prevention programme would be to:

    support the education of staff in back care, the risk assessment process and use of equipment

    give advice on working postures

    provide individual and group exercise programmes

    teach relaxation.

Back care or back school programmes have been incorporated into training for some years (Ref 13) and can include simple bio-mechanics, avoidance of fatigue and identification of correct working postures in everyday activities as well as in working situations. Scheduling of work activity to prevent physical and mental fatigue and identifying the risks of carrying loads, holding static postures, performing repetitive tasks with a flexed and/or rotated spine, and moving in a jerky or unco-ordinated way, are still essential elements of any training programme. Apart from helping prevent or alleviate stress for the individual, the knowledge gained by staff helps them to identify hazardous work environments or processes when carrying out risk assessment.

These essential elements of back care are also incorporated into the Inter-Professional Curriculum: See Chapter 8.

Strength and physical fitness is theoretically an important factor in helping reduce risk or injury though one study (Ref 31) found this to be of limited importance. A combination of factors is probably important; physical fitness in the general sense, neuro muscular coordination and motor skills, flexibility and strengthening of certain muscle groups.

Exercise programmes could be carried out on an individual or group basis and could include stretching exercises to increase and maintain flexibility as part of preparation for more strenuous activity or as an element in pause and refresh sessions for those involved in repetitive tasks or those tasks requiring a static posture. Stretching exercises are the important link in the transition from the sedentary to the active state. Stretching keeps the muscle supple, prepares the body for movement and helps to reduce the strain of the transition from inactivity to vigorous demanding activity.

Bullock (Ref 4) refers to the increase in the number of repetitive tasks requiring a static posture during their performance and the effect of industrial noise or tension, and points out that this has led to the introduction of brief exercise periods during the working day by physiotherapists. Such brief exercise periods, designed by the physiotherapist would:

> provide physical activity not normally done by the person in their work routine

> encourage relaxation either generally or of specific muscle groups

> promote health and physical fitness.

Specific relaxation techniques could be added to exercise periods which individuals could be encouraged to maintain at home and in group sessions at work.

There is a wide range of exercise options: simple stretching exercises (Ref 1), the conditioning exercises used in the Neuromuscular Approach to Efficient Moving and Handling (see Chapter 6), or alternative exercise forms such as Taost Tai Chi or Yoga.

It is appreciated that while encouraging nurses and other staff to exercise is sound in principle, in practice it may not be easy. However, exercise sessions could be carried out in work time as part of a corporate fitness programme.

The introduction of exercises to strengthen specific muscles such as the trunk muscles has been suggested as helping to prevent back pain but there is no real evidence that this is the case (Ref 2). It is likely that dynamic trunk muscle strength and endurance may be more effective in protecting the spinal structures from sudden damaging movements (Ref 22). Such exercises could be included in a general fitness exercise programme.

The Centre for Health Economics discussion paper (Ref 14) refers to a few studies which provide some evidence that workplace interventions can be effective in reducing absenteeism due to back problems and claim to be cost effective,(refs 3, 11, 16, 29).

If it is possible to reduce, even slightly, the impact of sick leave due to back pain prevention programmes such as the one described could be cost effective for NHS trusts.

REHABILITATION

Whatever the level of involvement in a preventive programme, and important as that is, the major role for the physiotherapist in occupational health would be that of treatment of those staff reporting with work related muscular injuries. The thrust of the service would be speedy attention with staff either able to self refer or be referred by the occupational health physician or their general practitioner as soon as possible after the onset of symptoms. A referral directly from the ward or department ought to be possible.

Staff using this clinic would fall loosely into two groups: individuals with acute problems but with no previous history (primary back pain), and those who have previously experienced an episode of back pain (secondary back pain).

PRIMARY BACK PAIN

The facility for early access to assessment and treatment reflects the recommendations in the CSAG report (Ref 23). A procedure for early referral to an occupational health based physiotherapist could be agreed.

A key role in this structured plan would be a physiotherapist specialising in the treatment of musculoskeletal problems who could do a diagnostic triage with appropriate history-taking and a physical examination. If a clear cut nerve root problem or suspected spinal pathology was found, referral to a hospital specialist would be recommended. In most cases where the problem was due to a simple mechanical low back pain, following the examination a non threatening explanation of the problem could be provided by the physiotherapist together with appropriate reassurance that the problem was likely to settle within a few weeks. Treatment would emphasise self care and aim to:

return the individual to normal activities as soon as possible

reduce recurrences.

Manipulation or other pain relieving techniques could be used together with a progressive exercise programme which the individual would be expected to continue working at on her own, with monitoring as necessary (Ref 14). Bed rest would be advised only if essential, and for no more than two or three days. For the organisation, speedy recognition of the cause of the work related injury would enable the ergonomist to advise on measures to eliminate or reduce the hazard.

Good communication between all the health care professionals involved and the supervisors or managers of the individuals, would be essential.

Physiotherapy intervention

The precise intervention would be determined by the problem or problems identified at assessment. A typical problem list could include one or more of: pain, loss of range of movement, loss of function, poor posture, lack of knowledge or awareness, and anxiety. A treatment response might include one or a combination of treatments: mobilisation or manipulation, electro-therapy for symptoms of pain, specific exercises, general exercises or fitness programmes, and correction of posture.

Secondary prevention advice, together with coping strategies to help with self management of problems, would be a major component of any physiotherapy intervention for a patient with back pain.

Included would be advice on:

working postures and work stations

what postures to adopt while working

how to change work stations and activities of daily living to reduce musculoskeletal stress

how to schedule or break up patterns of work

leisure activities to reduce the impact of cumulative stress

self care, health education.

Early activity would always be encouraged and every effort made to keep the individual at work. Exercise regimes are part of any treatment programme and may range from strengthening exercises for spinal and abdominal muscles to a fitness class aimed at reinforcing and encouraging an early return to work. The approaches on exercise range from simple non strenuous routines to intensive programmes of one and a half hours hard exercising, two or three times a week (Ref 17). Another approach (Ref 18) to treating back pain includes the use of passive stretching exercises while at the same time encouraging individuals to take responsibility for their back problem.

Activity has a beneficial effect on muscles, bone, ligament, cartilage, and discs, and experimental studies have shown that healing is enhanced by controlled activity (Ref 19). A controlled study (Ref 9) showed that either remaining active or being given timely information on back care is of benefit. The view expressed by Duane Saunders (Ref 24) amongst others is that most musculoskeletal disorders are an accumulation of the effects of poor posture, faulty body mechanics, and stressful living and working habits. Examples of stressful living are lack of recognition by managers, poor motivation of staff, and pressure to increase work load, and these should be added to the list of causative factors. Treatment programmes can address the physical problems, and allay anxieties and fears, by education and promotion of positive attitudes and belief about back pain.

Negative attitudes and beliefs about low back pain have been said to hinder recovery. One study (Ref 27) shows that such beliefs can be shifted in a positive direction. The intervention used was a psychosocial pamphlet based on the fear-avoidance model of pain. It encouraged a positive outlook, while advocating early return to work. The change in beliefs matched a reduction in the length of short term absence due to back problems, and the number of extended absence episodes also fell substantially. Such an intervention could be introduced as part of the overall treatment intervention. People need to learn that hurt does not necessarily mean harm, but that reduced activity level is likely to lead to chronic disability (refs 7, 32).

Psychosocial management

It is important for all managers and supervisors to appreciate their respective roles not only in the management of staff with back pain, but also in their continuing supportive role for all staff in preventing problems.

Workers should be given attention by their employers (Ref 33). They should know that they are a vital part of the work team and that people depend on them. There is a growing awareness that the relationship of the worker to his or her job and employer plays a pivotal role in determining which workers seek health care intended to deal with their suffering (Ref 8). The CSAG report (Ref 23) identifies the promotion of positive attitudes to activity at work and a need to increase awareness and management of stress and depression. Back pain may restrict physical activity, and work and social activity may both need to be modified in the early stages of treatment. However, it is important that managers recognise this and cooperate with the physiotherapist and occupational health team to make temporary adjustments to the working routine and work process of staff with low back pain. The important issue is to keep the individual at work or ensure a speedy return to work to prevent chronicity. There is rarely any clear clinical basis for advising an individual with simple back pain to stop work or change job (Ref 23).

One of the most important roles of the physiotherapist in industry is the education of people (Ref 5). Education programmes which aim to provide sufficient relevant information to help in the implementation of measures to prevent physical, psychological, or emotional injury or stress could and should be provided to managers, supervisor, and team leaders, as well as workers.

It is recognised that implementing education programmes of this kind is not easy and may require a radical change of attitude and approach by some managers and staff, and yet it fits in well with the principles of the caring employer and the aims of the Staff Charter.

SECONDARY BACK PAIN

The aim of treatment for individuals who have previously experienced back pain would be to alleviate symptoms and to prevent or reduce the frequency of episodes. Treatment approaches used at the primary back pain stage would be applied here, and following an initial assessment those who had developed more serious pathology since the first assessment would be referred back to the doctor or consultant. The aim would be the same: to maintain the work status or encourage a return to work. The pattern of education programmes containing ergonomic advice and advice on pain control would be repeated. The emphasis might be different in some aspects as the individual could be apprehensive about an exercise programme, but the basis would be a progressive exercise regime linked to work activity and again the manager would have an important part to play. Work itself is probably an important factor in reducing chronicity (Ref 20).

A more aggressive rehabilitation programme would be required if chronic pain and disability had become established. A return to work schedule might need to extend over a longer period but whatever the regime implemented, strenuous exercise would be a necessary feature (Refs 17, 10) combined with behavioural therapy (Ref 21).

Rehabilitation programmes could be based on a form of back school, back pain rehabilitation, or a work hardening programme. A back pain assessment and rehabilitation programme for patients with benign mechanical low back pain can demonstrate significant reductions in disability, distress and medical consumption (Ref 7). In this study by Cross et al, two programmes were operated.

One was for individuals who had become disabled and distressed by their pain, and involved the services of a clinical psychologist. The content of the programme included education about the function of the spine, the physical, psychological and social dynamics of back pain experience, pain theory with emphasis on the difference between hurt and harm, and the general benefits of exercise for one hour a day.

The second programme was designed for people who were less disabled and not distressed by back pain. The focus here was preventive rather than therapeutic and included an explanation of spinal anatomy, pain mechanisms, and the benefits of exercise.

The central theme of both programmes was that back pain is not a symptom of severe damage and that exercise and normal activity are likely to result in increased levels of function, or an ability to maintain, levels of function.

The aim of both programmes was to reduce fear of pain and thereby reduce disability. Reduction of pain was not an aim of the programmes.

WORK HARDENING

Work hardening programmes have been defined by the American Occupational Therapy Association (Ref 6) as "an individualised work orientated activity process that involves a client in simulated or actual work tasks. These tasks are structured and graded progressively to increase psychological, physical and emotional tolerance and improve endurance and work feasibility." The effectiveness of such programmes has been reviewed (Ref 15).

An inability to perform certain work related activity could be due to weakness in a particular muscle or muscle group. At the same time tolerance to exercise and activity could be reduced due to a long period of inactivity. A specific progressive task related exercise scheme for the individual concerned could be designed to increase strength, endurance, and aerobic conditioning. Several activities can be included in the one programme to help increase the overall functional level. The programmes described could be introduced in an occupational health setting using the skills of the physiotherapist to lead the programmes and constantly reassess the changed capability of individuals and their ability to cope with the job's demands. Work capacities and skills of individuals could be re-established through rehabilitation, assistance and advice given on modification of the job or work process, or guidance into alternative employment.

RESEARCH

Monitoring of the programme and scrutinising outcomes of intervention are an obvious requirement, but evidence of some aspects of rehabilitation is still not conclusive and it would be essential to collect data on the basis of research projects.

REFERENCES

1. Anderson B., (1981). Stretching. Exercises for every day fitness and for twenty five individual sports. Pelham Books, London.

2. Battie M., (1992). Minimising the impact of back pain: workplace strategies. Seminars in spinal surgery, 4: 20-28

3. Brown K., Sirles A., Hilyer J., and Thomas M., (1992). Cost effectiveness of a back school intervention for municipal empo-loyees. Spine, 17: 1224-1228.

4. Bullock M.I., (1990). Ergonomics, The physiotherapist in the work place. International Perspectives in Physical Therapy, 6.

5. Bullock M.I., (1988). Health education in the work place. In: Isernhagen S., ed., Work Injury – Management and Prevention. Aspen, Rockville: 9-18.

6. Commission on Practice, American Occupational Therapy Association: Work hardening guidelines (1986). Am.J.Occ.Ther. 40: 841-843.

7. Cross C., Rose M., Mickleburgh S., Murphy P., and Grocott D. An audit of a multidisciplinary back pain assessment and rehabilitation service in an acute hospital setting. Back Pain Rehabilitation Programme, Wirral Hospital Trust. Accepted for publication in Musculo-Skeletal Management.

8. Fordyce W.E., et al (1994). Pain in the Workplace: management of disability in nonspecific low back pain, a report of a task force of the International Association for the Study of Pain.

9. Fordyce W.E., Brockway J.A., and Bergman J.A., (1995). Acute back pain, a control group comparison of behavioural vs. traditional management methods. J. Behav. Med., 9: 127-140.

10. Frost H., Fairbank J., Moser J., and Klaber Moffatt J., (1993). A rehabilitation programme for patients with chronic low back pain. European Spine Society 4th Annual Meeting. Bochum.

11. Gundewall B., Liljeqvist M., and Hanssen T., (1993). Primary prevention of back symptoms and absence from work. Spine, 18: 587-594.

12. An unpublished working party report, Healthy Backs for Healthy Workers, Nottingham Health Authority, (1989).

13. Instructor's Syllabus for the Handling and Moving of Patients, 1988. Royal College of Nursing, London.

14. Klaber Moffett J., Richardson G., Sheldon A., Maynard A., (1995). Back Pain, Its Management and Cost to Society. University of York Centre for Health Economics: discussion paper 129.

15. Lechner D.E., (1994). Work hardening and work conditioning interventions: do they affect disability? Phys. Therapy vol.74 no.5.

16. Leiya S., (1993). A cost benefit analysis of a California County's back injury prevention programme. Public Health, 108: 204-211.

17. Maniche C., Lundberg E., Christensen I., et al, (1991). Intensive dynamic back exercises for chronic low back pain: a clinical trial. Pain, 47: 53-63.

18. McKenzie R., (1981). The Lumbar Spine. Spinal Publicationas Ltd., New Zealand.

19. Nachemson A., (1994). Chronic pain – the end of the welfare state? Quality of Life Research, vol. 3, supp.1: 511-517.

20. Nachemson A., (1983). Work for All: for those with low back pain as well. Clinical Orthopaedics, 179: 77-85.

21. Nicholas M., Wilson P., and Goyen J., (1992). Comparison of cognitive behavioural group treatment and an alternative non psychological treatment for low back pain. Pain, 48: 339-347.

22. Nordin M., (1992). Prevention of back pain in industry. In: The Lumbar Spine and Back Pain, Jayson M., ed. Churchill Livingstone, Edinburgh.

23. Report of a Clinical Standards Advisory Group Committee on Back Pain (1994). HMSO, London.

24. Saunders, H. Duane. The Saunders Group, 4250 Norex Drive, Choska, Minnesota, USA.

25. Snook S., (1988). Approaches to the control of back pain in industry, job design, job placement, and education and training. Occupational Medicine. State of the art review, 3, 45-60.

26. Stubbs D.A., Buckle P.W., Hudson M.P., Rivers P.M., and Worringham C.J., (1983). Back Pain in the Nursing Profession. 1, Epidemiology and pilot methodology. Ergonomics, 26: 755-765.

27. Symonds T.L., Burton K., Tillotson M., and Main C., (1995). Absence resulting from low back trouble can be reduced by psycho-social intervention at the work place. Spine, 20: 2738-2745.

28. The Guide to the Handling of Patients (1981, 1987, 1992). National Back Pain Association in collaboration with The Royal College of Nursing.

29. Todd Brown R., Page B., and McMahan P., (1991). Ergonomics in US Railroad Industry. Human Factors Society Bulletin, 34: 1 - 4.

30. Turnbull N., Dornan J., Fletcher B., and Wilson S., (1992). Prevalence of spinal pain among the staff of a district health authority. Occupational Medicine, 42: 143-148.

31. Videman T., Rauhala H., Liinstrom K., Cedercreuty G., Kamppi I., Tolas S., and Troup J D.G., (1989). Patient handling skill, back injuries and back pain: an intervention study in nursing. Spine, 14: 148-156.

32. Waddell G., Somerville D., Henderson I., et al., (1993). A fear avoidance beliefs questionnaire (FABQ) and the role of fear avoidance beliefs in chronic low back pain. Pain, 52: 157-168.

33. Wood D.J., (1987). Design and evaluation of a back injury prevention programme within a geriatric hospital. Spine, 12: 77-82.

MANAGING CHANGE

by Jacqui Hall

SUMMARY

There are several ways to achieve change, but successful change requires a dissatisfaction with the present situation, a vision for the future, and a knowledge of the steps to take, to reduce resistance to the change (Ref 1). Back care advisers need to consider this carefully when introducing change, especially when it involves changing practice.

Developing policies and standards can help in supporting change. Approved codes of practice can also contribute positively in managing change (Refs 3, 19, 20, 21, 22). With support from the Royal College of Nursing and by working on appropriate committees, the back care adviser can find a variety of strategies to overcome resistance to change.

Success as a consequence of management of change, especially with regard to patient handling and moving, is proved in Barbara Lloyd's article (Ref 14).

Such an achievement must give others an incentive to continue to work towards managing change effectively.

INTRODUCTION

Change can be defined as an attempt to alter or make different. It is a major characteristic in all activities of modern society (Ref 5).

This statement may be true of change, but to manage change successfully requires careful consideration of a complexity of factors.

The evolution of the role of a back care adviser has been an example of how difficult and complex it is.

The back care adviser is expected to improve the health of the workforce by reducing the incidence of back injury which is believed to be due to poor or faulty lifting techniques (Ref 15). This is accomplished through advice, training and information, as well as monitoring and supervision of practice.

While the number of posts for back care advisers in health authorities is increasing, there has been little evidence of the requirements for establishing a successful programme for them. Due to the absence of a national strategy, recommendations for setting up effective back care programmes (Ref 15) were hard to find, until the production of Essential Back-up by the National Back Exchange in 1993.

However, implementing the recommendations made by Essential Back-up can provide the effectiveness for successful management of change.

FACTORS INVOLVED IN MANAGING CHANGE

According to Gleicher, in Beckhard and Harris (Ref 1), the factors involved in managing change successfully are:

Dissatisfaction with the present situation,

Vision of a more desirable future,

Steps to take in moving towards that future.

Proof of the success of a management of change, especially with regard to patient handling and moving, is given in an article, *No Lifting – Setting a Nursing Standard* (Lloyd, 1996) Ref 14).

The *dissatisfaction* of having eight staff with back injuries prompted a *vision* of fewer or no staff with back injuries as a consequence of a no lifting standard, and the *steps* taken made this vision a reality.

Therefore, by identifying these key factors involved in managing change the change will be achieved, provided that the resistance and cost is not prohibitive. Egan (Ref 4) suggests another model for change:

assessment of the current scenario

the creation of a preferred scenario

designing a plan that moves the system from the current to the preferred scenario.

The Current Scenario

Find out if a back care advisor is in post, what problems there are in terms of unmet needs, unused resources, unexploited opportunities, and unmet legal requirements.

Preferred Scenario

Determine what the organisation would look like if it were to appoint a back care adviser. The organisation would have to provide patient handling resources, and a suitable training department, linked to an occupational health department, and have a budget to provide handling equipment.

Designing a Plan for Getting There

Devise a plan for moving from the current scenario without a back care adviser, to the preferred scenario, which would be to appoint a back care adviser.

This plan should deal with how results are to be accomplished. The plan would include aspects of audit, risk assessments, ergonomic and patient handling assessments, accident reports, sickness/absence statistics, and supervision and training of staff.

STRATEGIES FOR MANAGING CHANGE

When managing change the change agent will need to select an appropriate strategy for change and recognise its strengths and weaknesses.

Lancaster and Lancaster put forward a variety of strategies for change (Ref 12):

Empirical - Rational

Power - Coercive

Normative - Re-educative

An Eclectic Approach.

The **Empirical - Rational** strategy suggests that it is rational for people to find the outcomes which offer maximum value to the individual when faced with a possibility of risk. Unfortunately, not all people are prepared to face the possibility of risk even for what appears to be a rational suggestion of change.

The **Power - Coercive** strategy assumes a sense of control and recognises that those people with less power will always comply with the orders from the leader.

With the **Normative - Re-educative** approach the emphasis is on the values and attitudes of staff towards the proposed change.

This strategy is based on a bottom-up approach so it can present problems if those in a position of authority feel threatened or suffer from a lack of influence, power and control.

An **Eclectic Approach** considers the other three strategies and forms a combination of strategies rather than isolating one. The change agent can consider what is rational information, whether the back care advisor has a situation for two-way communication, a set of norms for sanctions associated with the change and power to carry out the change.

INFLUENCES ON CHANGE IN HEALTH CARE

Broad influences are seen in health care.

The NHS has seen dramatic changes as a result of Trust status in many areas due to government reforms.

Further changes have ensued due to the reconstruction of financial management in Trusts and fund-holding general practices.

The social provision of services has altered in respect of the assessment and delivery of care due to the NHS and Community Care Act (Ref 16) and technological advances have altered working practices, from the use of personal computers to the introduction of new patient handling and moving devices.

Upton and Brookes (Ref 24) suggest that a political policy change is not totally an isolated decision. It is subject to economic conditions and ever changing technology which influence management decisions. These policy changes have a significant effect on managing change.

Using the back care adviser as a basis for introducing change, the influences can be illustrated as:

POLITICAL –

Due to the Health and Safety at Work Act of 1974 and the Manual Handling Operations Regulations (Ref 6 and Chapter 1) plus other European legislation, it has become necessary to reduce the incidence of back pain and injury in the workplace due to the manual handling of loads.

A back care adviser would be seen to provide programmes to inform the workforce of up-to-date legislation in health and safety and include practical solutions to reduce manual handling of loads, through training and supervision of practice.

ECONOMIC –

The cost of litigation to health authorities due to claims for injuries sustained at work attributed to a lack of manual handling training and/or equipment, is progressively on the increase. Back pain in nursing, in particular, has been seen as very costly (Refs 2, 15).

The National Back Pain Association (Ref 6) quoted 105.38 million certified sickness/absence days due to back pain in 1993/94. The cost to the National Health Service was £480 million each year due to back pain, and the cost to industry in lost production due to back pain is said to be at least £5.1 billion each year (Ref 2).

SOCIAL –

In the social context, the number of people suffering from back pain is excessively high.

The National Back Pain Association frequently produces information based on the statistical evidence of back pain or injury at work.

Often, the cause of their injury was due to handling people (Ref 17).

This in turn can result in many people never returning to full-time employment.

The social implication of being unemployed due to back pain can result in a person becoming demoralised, disabled, and subsequently depressed (Ref 6).

TECHNOLOGICAL TRENDS –

The availability of technology appears to be expanding widely. Not only is it expanding but developments in new technology continue to introduce more and more innovative equipment for personal and organisational use.

Computerised systems and the micro-chip have provided technology that was unheard of 10 – 20 years ago. To reduce manual handling of loads, in particular, the handling of people, new hoisting equipment is being developed which is electrical in many instances and can perform a variety of tasks.

Many of the research and development teams are considering the ergonomic factors and have produced equipment suitable for hospital and home.

Consequently, the individual and his environment are taken into consideration when re-designing the technology required for the task.

The work design attempts to identify those aspects of the job which are particularly hazardous and to redesign them to make them safer (Ref 13).

European directives are encouraging machinery designers and manufactures to meet the European standards in health and safety (Ref 17).

As more emphasis is put on reducing the **manual** handling of loads, new technology is essential to provide alternative approaches to handling people.

CHANGE THEORIES

For the individual or organisation to consider change, it is advisable to determine a model or change theory which suits the situation.

The following three theories of managing change need to meet the requirements for the appropriate pathway to facilitate change. They aim to provide an intervention which can enable the organisation or individual to identify barriers to change and the successful conditions for change to occur.

The origin of classical change theory is credited to Kurt Lewin (Ref 18), who described three steps in the change process:

Figure 10.1.

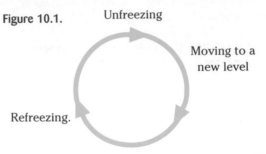

© NBPA

Unfreezing requires a degree of 'thawing them out,' which leads to participants recognising a change is due.

This situation can also generate a problem-solving scenario, which diagnoses the problem and sets about providing possible solutions from a variety of approaches.

Moving to a new level enables those involved to collect sufficient information about the situation to realise the necessity for change. They also need an action plan.

Usually this move to a new level requires the influence of someone who is respected and is knowledgeable about the change proposed. This person also needs to be in a position of power.

The leader is expected to put forward a selection of possible change strategies, which gives the group members an opportunity to take some involvement and responsibility for the change.

Refreezing is a critical stage in the cycle: at this stage continuous reinforcement of the newly acquired behaviour is essential.

Positive feedback, encouragement and constructive criticism are beneficial ways of reinforcing this newly acquired behaviour (Ref 5).

Lewin (Ref 18) also introduced the concept of the force-field analysis model.

Here the driving forces are seen as those that facilitate change, while the restraining forces impede the change.

Put into terms of introducing techniques in patient handling and moving, this force field analysis can be viewed as:-

DRIVING FORCE	RESTRAINING FORCES
Citizens' and Patient's charters	Charter standards being met
Need to provide more training sessions for hospitals and the community.	We've always managed this way
New resources in handling equipment available.	Fear of ignorance of the skill required to use the equipment.
Newly appointed staff with up-to-date methods of handling people	Conflict between staff grades and abilities
Compliance with manual handling regulations	It's never been a problem before.
Legal action for non-compliance with health and safety legislation	Compensation is a management problem – not mine

By using the driving forces thorough selective networks and networking, the restraining/opposing forces could be reduced, enabling the change to be managed effectively and successfully.

Rogers' theory (in Lancaster and Lancaster, Ref 12) has been compared with Lewin's phases of change and has expanded on Lewin's three phases or stages by emphasizing the background of the people involved, the process, and the environment of where the change takes place.

Rogers' five phases in the change cycle are:

awareness, interest, evaluation, trial and adoption.

Lancaster and Lancaster believe that the effectiveness of change is dependent on the participants' keenness and interest in the innovation (the change).

When these five phases are compared to Lewin's three they can be depicted as follows:-

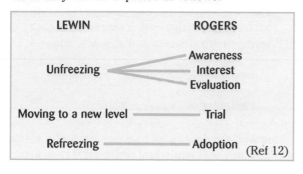

(Ref 12)

Lippitt's theory poses the question – How do we handle change? (Lancaster and Lancaster, Ref 12) He sees the key to change as developing a thorough and well thought out strategy for intervention. He identifies seven phases or stages in the change process as compared with Lewin's three:-

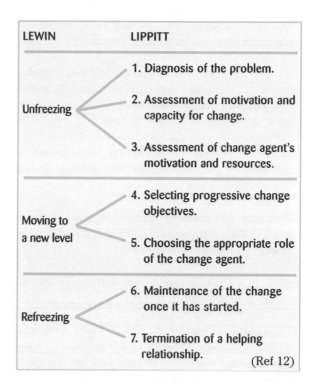

(Ref 12)

Lippitt's stages develop from the step of data collection and problem identification, in stage 1, to assessing carefully the motivation for change. He believes that motivators need to identify factors such as resources, constraints and helpers. There are also the financial considerations and policy control.

During stages 2 and 3 possible solutions to the problems should be identified and pros and cons listed.

The leadership style is all important for the proposed changes to be implemented.

Stage 4 highlights the step-by-step strategy for good planning of managing change. Deadlines are important and a trial period is seen as useful. Thus goals can be re-evaluated as the change process continues.

Stage 5 hinges on the selection of the role of the change agent. It must be recognised by all participants with a common perception of what the change agent is and does. This can then lead to a more successful change.

Stage 6 is the maintenance of the change. Once the change has been established it must not be left to wane. Continual modification and updating of the change can serve to maintain it.

Stage 7 sees the withdrawal of the change agent – although the agent could still be available for consultation. However, the aim is to allow the participants of the change to take responsibility for it.

APPLICATION OF THEORY AND PRACTICE

Managing change also needs to consider the elements of work design and motivation.

Herzberg (Ref 8) distinguished three common forms of job design: job rotation, job enlargement and job enrichment – and then discussed a fourth form, autonomous working groups.

Job enrichment, in particular, contributes to increasing the worker's involvement in the organisation or the job.

Personal achievement and recognition together with feelings of growth and advancement are rewards in themselves (Ref 9).

With this work design in mind there is still the problem of the human factor.

"As a manager, you have a choice. The choice is not between managing change or not managing change but between managing change through people or despite people. In virtually every case, the former is more successful." (Ref 23).

To manage change through people, careful planning is required.

When applying theory to practice, care must be taken when considering a change: consider the following steps:

1, identify external pressures for change, and internal pressures for change.

2, consider the level of change required – is it at individual, group, or organisational level?

3, use a force-field analysis of change to recognise the driving forces and the resisting forces to the change.

4, select strategies that could be used, for example, to:

   unfreeze the change

   effect the change

   refreeze and consolidate the change (Ref 13).

5, select a method to evaluate the change.

6, value the outcomes of the proposed change.

7, praise the involvement of the staff and reward them appropriately. (Ref 11, adapted)

A Critical Pathway for Planning Change (Ref 7)

1, identify need for change

2, persuade stakeholders

3, specify the change

4, plan organisation and people change process

5, create change material

6, implement the change

7, evaluate the change

8, record experience and establish best practice.

Elaine Fazel, describing her experience of managing change (Ref 10), identified the need to change attitudes of having no problems with lifting and handling.

   She persuaded the Wigan and Leigh Health Services NHS Trust that there was a problem with manual handling injuries sustained by staff.

   Through an action plan she established an assessment of handling risks.

   An audit of manual handling activity was made annually.

   Accidents and near misses were recorded and investigated.

   Resources were provided.

   Safest practice for dealing with heavy patients was described in a protocol for staff .

   A questionnaire was sent to all work based assessors to establish patient handling issues.

   In 12 months about £100,000 was spent on equipment for patient handling. Training was given in risk assssment and safer patient handling and equipment use.

   The evaluation of the change in terms of accident reporting and cost in lost hours at work, due to sickness and absence, showed

      1993/94 6,720 hours lost

      1994/95 1,081 hours lost.

This was a reduction of 83.9 per cent. The loss of 6,720 hours was equivalent to £500,000 cash lost. In spending £100,000 on equipment, a relative saving of £400,000 was made, due to a safer patient handling commitment, introduced by a management of very effective change.

REFERENCES

1. Beckhard R, and Harris R (1987). Organisational transitions. London, Addison-Wesley

2. Clinical Standards Advisory Group (1994). Back Pain. HMSO. London.

3. Corlett N, Lloyd PV, Tarling C, Troup JDG, and Wright B, (1992). The Guide to the Handling of Patients, 3rd edition. National Back Pain Association and the Royal College of Nursing. London.

4. Egan G, (1988). Change Agent Skills. B. Managing innovation and change. University Associates, San Diego, USA.

5. Griffiths E, Laxade S, Miller J, (1992). Professional Development in Nursing and Health Care. Managing Change Effectively. Newcastle upon Tyne College of Health Studies. Learning Materials Design. Milton Keynes.

6. National Back Pain Association (1996). Back Facts. NBPA. London.

7. Health Education Authority, (1995) Managing Change Toolbox. A Resource for Local Organising Team Workers to use in Primary Care. HEA. London.

8. Herzberg F, (1968). Cited in Personnel Management: A New Approach, 2nd edition. Torrington D, Hall L, (1991). Prentice Hall International (UK) Ltd. London.

9. Herzberg F (1968) One more time how do you motivate employees? Harvard Business Review vol 46 pp 53 - 62.

10. Fazel E. (1996). ARJO Conference, Darlington.

11. Kotter J.P. and Schlesinger L.A. (1979). cited in Thomson R, (1993). Managing People. The Institute of Management Foundation. Oxford, Butterworth-Heinemann Ltd.

12. Lancaster J, and Lancaster W, (1982). Concepts for Advanced Nursing Practice: The Nurse as a change agent. Mosby -- Year Book Inc. pp 7 - 12.

13. Pheasant S, (1991). Ergonomics, Work and Health (reprinted 1994). Macmillan Press Ltd. London.

14. Lloyd B, (1996). No Lifting – Setting a Nursing Standard. VFM Update, Issue 18, pp 12-13, National Health Service Executive.

15. National Back Exchange (1993). Essential Back-up. Recommendations for setting up effective back care programmes. Middlesex, Scutari Projects Ltd.

16. National Health Service and Community Care Act, 1990. Chap 19. HMSO London.

17. Health and Safety Executive, (1992). Manual Handling Guidance on Regulations. Manual Handling Operations Regulations. HMSO. London.

18. Lewin K, (1951). Field Theory in Social Science. London, Harper and Row.

19. Royal College of Nursing, (1996). Introducing a Safer Patient Handling Policy. London, RCN.

20. Royal College of Nursing, (1996). Code of Practice for Patient Handling. London, RCN.

22. Royal College of Nursing, (1996). Manual Handling Assessments in Hospital and the Community. London, RCN.

21. Royal College of Nursing, (1995). Patient Handling Standards. London, RCN.

23. Thomson R, (1993). Managing People. The Institute of Management Foundation. Oxford, Butterworth-Heinemann Ltd.

24. Upton T, and Brooks B, (1995). Managing Change in the NHS, NAHAT, Kogan Page Ltd. London.

FURTHER READING

Kuorinka I, and Forcier L (1995). Eds, Work Related Musculoskeletal Disorders: A Reference Book for Prevention. Taylor and Francis. London.

RISK ASSESSMENTS: PRINCIPLES AND PREPARATION

by Moira Tracy

This chapter deals with assessing risks from the manual handling of patients in hospitals, nursing and residential care homes and in their own homes in the community.

SUMMARY

Organisations must, by law, carry out manual handling assessments. Assessments are crucial for success in the management of patient handling.

This chapter advises on how to obtain useful results from assessments.

It also covers who should do assessments and the training they require.

Sample assessments are included in Chapter 12.

INTRODUCTION

Legislation requires all employers, including hospital and community trusts, and nursing and residential care homes to carry out manual handling assessments. But in a large organisation, dealing with a variety of situations, there are three questions to ask:

    where to start?

    how to avoid assessments becoming a useless paper exercise?

    how much should be done in writing and what forms could be used?

What follows is practical advice on these questions to people with responsibility for staff's or volunteers' back care. They include

directors, moving and handling coordinators, back care advisers, occupational health advisers and health and safety advisers.

REDUCING THE RISK

The Manual Handling Operations Regulations 1992 (Ref 1) and the EEC Directive (Ref 2) require risk assessments to be made if the employer cannot avoid the need for a manual handling operation which involves a risk of injury. Once assessments are made the employer must take appropriate steps to reduce the risk of injury to the lowest level reasonably practicable.

Reasonably practicable means reducing the risk until the cost of any further precautions – in time, trouble or money – would far outweigh the benefits – see Chapter 1.

A logical method for reducing accidents and ill-health

A professional person planning to start a major training programme or about to buy some handling equipment will probably already have an idea of what is required.

But

    is that picture accurate?
    are efforts really going where they are needed?

Risk assessments will enable you to make decisions based on informed judgement. They will help identify

    what the main risks are,
    where the main needs exist in the organisation.

ASSESSING THE RISK

Assessing risk means first of all being aware of potential problems then determining the extent of concern about a particular problem. For instance

    does it place many staff at risk?

    is it met frequently or rarely?

    is it likely to cause a major injury?

    could it be a task that contributes to cumulative strain each time it is carried out?

But a risk assessment is useless unless it leads to action that reduces risks. These include:

- an immediate decision to change a simple work practice

- purchasing handling equipment and beds

- improving the environment

- agreeing a yearly budget for this action

Assessment increases awareness

Managers and staff both need to be involved in obtaining risk assessments from the areas for which they are responsible. This makes everyone more aware of places where extra vigilance is required. It also emphasises the managers' responsibility to do everything in their power to make work safer.

In some work places, the introduction of risk assessments has improved knowledge and awareness of safety and has prompted a tightening-up of handling policies and the promotion of better practices.

Assessing risk by numbers — or judgement

Some risk assessments are done using a numerical technique. Anything that contributes to a possible risk is given a numerical score. The risk of the task is given a total score, and totals are compared to determine priorities.

The system seems objective and some argue that it gives guidance about when it becomes justifiable to ignore any risks under a certain score.

However, it can also be argued that numerical assessments are neither accurate nor useful.

For instance, where is the risk greater – with an uncooperative patient but lots of space, or with a cooperative patient in a small space?

There is no useful answer to this. There is no practical benefit from trying to decide whether to give a different or larger score for the uncooperative patient or for the small space. The assessor's judgement, looking at the whole setting and taking account of everything that is relevant, will usually be more useful than the application of an arbitrary formula which can account for only a few of the elements that contribute to the risk: informed human beings do a better job than impressive formulae.

Written records

When there has been an accident, or criticism from inspectors, written assessments will demonstrate that a safe system of work is in operation.

If the system is not yet as safe as it should be, well-kept records will show the existence of plans and a budget for improvements. An accident may mean that the assessment was faulty and should be revised, but at least it will help to show that it was made according to the best judgement at the time.

The existence of written policies and procedures which explain how a job is to be done safely may remove the need for a written assessment of that job. A separate assessment would only be needed if the procedure did not control the risk sufficiently, and there was a need to justify the present system and make a note of plans for the future.

The Guidance on Regulations (Ref 1) states: 'in general, the significant findings of the assessment should be recorded and the record kept, readily accessible, as long as it remains relevant. However, the assessment need not be recorded if:

a) it could very easily be repeated and explained at any time because it is simple and obvious: or

b) the manual handling operations are quite straightforward, of low risk, are going to last only a very short time, and the time taken to record them would be disproportionate.'

Written records include patient care plans, and forms such as the ones in Chapter 12.

Managers should also keep a record of their plans, if only in minutes of meetings or copies of correspondence. This should cover the requirements of the regulations as well as produce evidence for any civil court case.

Also, staff should have adequate written information and instruction through patient care plans, and possibly through written policies or procedures. A handling policy or procedure might for instance determine in which cases hoists or lateral transfer aids must be used. But written records are useless if they do not Reflect reality. A written procedure or instructions in a patient care plan are valueless unless they are enforced.

RISKS FROM THREE POINTS OF VIEW

Patients

> The need for a care plan: example of a judgement.
>
> In Munro v. Plymouth Health Authority, a nurse was injured in 1986 while using the Australian lift to lift a very heavy patient up a bed. The patient weighed more than 16 stones, was short, with a rounded figure, and was difficult to handle. Nurse Munro was awarded £172,000, there being no contributory negligence. The judge decided that a hoist should have been used, that it was "reasonably available, that it would have succeeded better than manual handling, that it was necessary for this patient, on this day, that it easily could and should have been used. It should have been specified or stipulated by those in charge of the nursing care plan." He thought that the health authority "needed to put a difficult patient's problem into the hands of a senior person who would specifically herself or himself devise and authenticate a plan for the patient."

The patient care plan must contain clearly stated information on the patient's movement abilities, physical and psychological circumstances, and needs. The plan should include instructions on handling aids, techniques, and the number of staff to be used for various moves. This helps communication between all the carers and is also a record of the system of work in case of injury or for monitoring purposes. (Note A)

In the community, when nurses are visiting patients in their own homes, the patient care plan can be the main assessment and it should take account of the patient's physical circumstances and accommodation, and of the handling aids required.

In hospitals, and in nursing and residential care homes, assessment forms can be made relevant to particular wards or areas. Nurses can tick or circle some items, for instance the type of handling aids used for various tasks. If a ward nearly always uses the same method for some tasks – if patients are usually placed in the bath with a bathing hoist and using the same handling method, for example – then wards could record this as a general procedure, and it need not be written into each care plan.

In addition to reading the care plan, nurses must assess the patient before handling him: if the patient is at this time more dependent than indicated in the care plan, the handling method must be revised to increase the amount of assistance given.

Departments or wards

The assessment of the general situation in a ward or department needs to be done only occasionally. It can be reviewed annually, and amended whenever there are changes.

This assessment should include information such as the space in bathrooms and availability of handling aids, and on the training of staff. An example of a form for such an assessment is included in Chapter 12.

Other areas, such as theatres or clinics, should also make assessments: a guide and a form are given in Chapter 12.

Directors

Many Board decisions implicitly take account of some kind of risk assessment. Decisions on training, uniforms, or budgets for works or new handling aids, should all be based on an evaluation of risks.

Much of the information will be provided by departmental assessments (or, for people being cared for in their own homes, by a survey of the patient-based assessments).

Directors plans should have records of plans for reducing risk.

HOW TO ORGANISE ASSESSMENTS

There are many ways of organising risk assessments and every organisation needs to devise its own system according to the staff it has and its management structure.

The main stages of the process are:

Appoint an assessment coordinator -

Directors in charge of safety should be familiar with what is involved, but a person should be appointed to coordinate the work of introducing assessments.

If there is a back care adviser or moving and handling coordinator, this is an ideal person to be the assessment coordinator: alternatively, it should be someone with an occupational health or health and safety responsibility, or a nurse, physiotherapist, or occupational therapist with an interest in the subject.

The task may require several months of full time work, and the coordinator should be trained to a high level in assessing risks associated with manual handling (see Chapter 8).

Choose the assessors –

In the case of the community trusts, this will be the community sisters or charge nurses visiting people in their own homes.

In hospitals – and in nursing and residential care homes – two different methods have worked well. One is ward managers doing the assessment for their own ward, the other is assessment teams assessing all areas. Each has advantages and disadvantages.

If ward managers do their own assessments, after some training, they are likely to take more responsibility for the practices and to take time to involve their staff in making the assessments. Letting people have this responsibility leads to more follow-up and better practice. But unless awareness among ward managers is high, and they are supported by the coordinator, they may not appreciate risks and may overlook possible improvements. Ward managers may also see the task as a burden that they do not feel competent enough to carry.

If there is a small assessment team, its members will make the assessments with the ward managers. This team could include nurses, physiotherapists, occupational therapists, and works officers. The advantage is that ward managers receive a lot of support from a well-informed team, who may prompt them to think about risks in a new way. The drawback is the possibility that ward staff are not sufficiently involved and do not share responsibility for the assessments. This method also requires considerable time to be allocated for members of the team to be trained as well as to make the assessments.

Planning and preparation

The director in charge of safety, or the assessment coordinator, will have a rough idea of where the main problems are. It would be useful, before starting to make the assessments, to have an outline plan of action and an estimate of the costs of what may be needed for staff training, handling methods, handling aids, and uniforms, for example. The plan can then be explained to assessors during their training.

Another reason to have a rough plan with a cost estimate is that it helps convince assessors and ward managers that the organisation is committed to making improvements.

It is also important to examine any accident or sickness statistics available for the organisation. This is usually not the time to start compiling new statistics as that could delay the risk assessments. This should be done later, when it will help monitor the effectiveness of new measures.

Designing an assessment form: some pitfalls to avoid –

the wording or layout is confusing - everyone has encountered difficult and confusing forms to fill

the form does not prompt managers to reduce risks – but reducing risk is the aim of an assessment, so it should take up a good part of the form

the form does not take everything into account – if it assesses individual lifts only, the larger picture may be missed. A lift on its own may seem quite safe, but it may be one of many, frequently repeated tasks which cause cumulative strain

the form does not encourage managers to use common sense – it must allow ward managers to think for themselves and deal with the main problems. For example, it may distract them from this if it encourages a numerical risk assessment method, or if it asks at every step whether a risk is high, medium or low, or if it asks irrelevant questions.

At this stage, the finance and works managers should be warned of likely outcomes. Assessment coordinators should produce an assessment method and form (examples of forms are given in Chapter 12). Assessment forms should be tested in a few areas before being printed, as a badly designed form may waste a lot of time.

TRAINING ASSESSORS

Ward managers and community staff

The assessment coordinator will need to set up a training programme for ward managers and community staff doing their own assessments.

The training should cover:

    risk factors and assessing risk

    the regulations

    local policies

    practical ways to reduce risk

    how to fill in the assessment form

    the need to involve local staff

    where to get further help

    a demonstration of handling aids.

The duration of the training depends on the existing knowledge of those who will be assessors in future, and on the amount of supervision or support they will have from the assessment coordinator.

Training in small groups, with opportunities for questions, are preferable. Assessors should be offered support from the coordinator if they need it.

If the assessment is to be done by a team visiting the ward, the ward manager should understand what the visit is about and should be motivated to seek improvements. For this reason, ward managers need some training or information before assessments begin.

Assessment teams

If a small team of assessors will visit wards, the assessment coordinator should offer thorough training plus practical experience to be followed by discussion and an examination of their responses. This could take several days. The team will be a group of experts, so their training should be thorough enough to enable them to deal with all the situations they may encounter.

ASSESSMENTS IN HOSPITALS, OR NURSING AND RESIDENTIAL CARE HOMES

The same principles apply to nursing and residential care homes as to hospital wards. Local staff, including physiotherapists and occupational therapists, and any union safety representatives, should be involved. Consultation with them will help to ensure that all the risks are covered, that the best solutions are devised, and that staff feel encouraged to use good practices.

There may be a need to consult a works officer, for instance if changes are needed in a bathroom. If the assessor identifies the need for a hoist, a trial should be organised. The need for trials applies to any handling equipment, including equipment brought to patients in their homes.

Managers should put into effect any changes within their authority and should tell their senior manager of any other needs. Although there should be a written record of this, it is also important at this stage to bring together all managers, and the assessment coordinator to discuss any needs identified by the managers, to solve some of the more straight-forward problems, and for the coordinator to advise and to check that assessments were properly carried out.

Once managers have done what they can, it is up to those at the next level of seniority (for example, clinical nurse managers) to take any further action and to advise the nursing director of anything which still needs to be done. Temporary action to reduce risks should be taken where possible until a senior manager approves the changes.

At this stage, the budget for changes must be agreed, so the manager must be clear about risks and priorities. The assessment coordinator should help in judging these.

Once the nursing director is advised of needs and costs, a plan of action must be drawn up, or the initial plan revised. Other Board members, including the finance director, should be involved at this stage.

It is important that managers should be told what happens to the plans and the progress of the requests they make.

MONITORING AND REVIEWING PROGRESS

Ward-based assessments should be reviewed about once a year, in consultation with staff.

The senior manager and the assessment coordinator should discuss progress, results and any new needs.

The nursing director should assess the effectiveness of the previous year's action and amend plans, policies and budgets accordingly.

Monitoring can be done by –

    analysing incident and sick leave statistics

    watching people work in wards or patients' homes

    consulting staff

    examining a sample of patient care plans

    establishing whether all equipment is being used.

The coordinator can judge if there have been improvements in awareness through discussions with staff and managers, and may learn a lot about what happens in practice from physiotherapists and occupational therapists.

Some hospitals have 'link nurses' or 'resource persons' in each directorate who promote good handling practices: regular reports from them are also a way of monitoring.

REFERENCES:

1. Health and Safety Executive; Manual Handling, Guidance on Regulations , HMSO, 1992.

2. EEC Council Directive: Article 16 (1) of Directive 89/391 (90/269/EEC) 29 May 1990.

This Chapter and examples in Chapter 12 are adapted from the Royal College of Nursing's (April 1996) leaflet, Manual Handling assessments in Hospitals and the Community.

RISK ASSESSMENT: THE PRACTICE

by Danielle Holmes

SUMMARY

This chapter provides an overview of the issues that must be considered when planning to handle a patient in any situation. It establishes the basic principles of the safer handling policy.

INTRODUCTION

All manual handling of patients is dangerous for both the nurse(s) and the patient. Nurses should also be aware that both manual and mechanical handling can be uncomfortable and invasive for the patient.

The best solution is to avoid manual handling altogether. There are a variety of ways that this can be achieved. These range from persuading the patient to move himself to placing the patient in a situation that will avoid the need to handle him. A patient who is in a profiling bed will need significantly less handling than a patient would need in a Kings Fund type bed.

The Manual Handling Operations Regulations (1992) have already been described in Chapter 1. Guidance is provided to help the employer identify handling situations that represent a risk. Numerical guidance is indicated by the figure reproduced below. Where the weight exceeds these figures, a detailed risk assessment is required. It is also suggested that the levels for women should be two thirds of these values (Fig 12.1 & 12.2).

The figures show that the maximum values are 25kg (3st 13lbs) for Men and 16.6kg (2st 8lbs) for women. Both of these values only apply to loads close to the lower body. In any other position the capacities drop significantly. In most situations patient handling falls outside the ideal area close to the lower body, as indicated in the diagram.

TEAM HANDLING

If the load is too heavy for one person, more people may be required to lift the load. It is difficult for several people to share a load safely. This is particularly the case in handling people. In the past when three or four people tried to lift a patient it was quite common for most of the patient's weight

to fall on one lifter injuring her. It is certainly impossible for the load to be shared evenly between four lifters. There is also often too little space for four people to work without falling over each other.

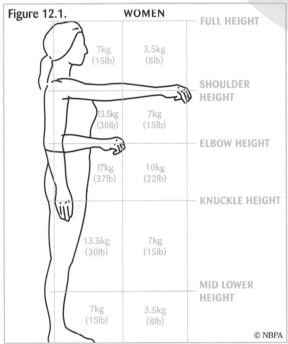

Figure 12.1. WOMEN

FULL HEIGHT — 7kg (15lb) / 3.5kg (8lb)
SHOULDER HEIGHT — 13.5kg (30lb) / 7kg (15lb)
ELBOW HEIGHT — 17kg (37lb) / 10kg (22lb)
KNUCKLE HEIGHT — 13.5kg (30lb) / 7kg (15lb)
MID LOWER HEIGHT — 7kg (15lb) / 3.5kg (8lb)
© NBPA

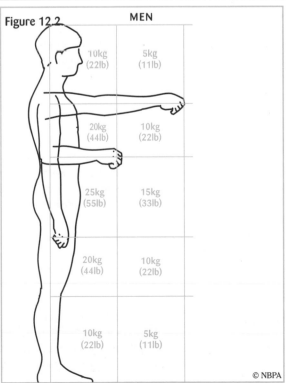

Figure 12.2 MEN

10kg (22lb) / 5kg (11lb)
20kg (44lb) / 10kg (22lb)
25kg (55lb) / 15kg (33lb)
20kg (44lb) / 10kg (22lb)
10kg (22lb) / 5kg (11lb)
© NBPA

The Guidance to the Manual Handling Operations Regulations (1992) address this issue by suggesting capacities for more than one lifter. The Guidance says that two people should not lift more than two thirds of their combined capacity and that three people should only lift half of their combined capacities. The following table shows the effect of these calculations on the weights given for the ideal position close to the lower body:-

	Number of Lifters and their COMBINED capacities		
	One person	Two people	Three people
Men	25kg 3st 13lb	33.3kg 5st 3lb	37.5kg 35st 12lb
Women	16.6kg 2st 8lb	22.2kg 3st 17lb	25kg 3st 13lb

(N.B. These figures are for lifting in the ideal position. Three women lifting close to the floor and at a distance in front of their feet can only lift 5kg! [11lbs]).

The Regulations state that it is the employer's duty to carry out both general and specific assessments. The weight guidelines described above provide a way of identifying manual handling operations that present a risk of injury to the worker. These figures apply to all situations in all types of work including all aspects of the caring professions. When handling inanimate loads such as theatre equipment, medicines, files, etc. it is possible to organise loads and handling situations so that they are within the levels in the guidance. However, very few patients weigh less than the values given in the guidance. Most patients weigh several times these levels. This problem is compounded by the fact that it is hard to lift patients in the ideal position. THEREFORE IT MUST BE ACCEPTED THAT NO PATIENT CAN BE LIFTED MANUALLY.

THE ASSESSMENT OF A MANUAL HANDLING OPERATION

The Manual Handling Operations Regulations (1992) provides a schedule of the factors that must be considered in assessing any manual handling operation. There are five categories to be remembered and acted upon before actually moving the patient or any other load. These are

1. The Task

2. The Load

3. The Environment

4. The Individual's Capability

5. Other Factors

KNOWING THE WEIGHT THE NURSE IS LIFTING

One of the problems of handling and moving is knowing the weight of whatever is being handled. Under the Manual Operations Regulations the employer is required to mark all loads with their weight and centre of gravity.

Under a safer handling policy the weight of the patient is less important than it used to be. Most patients are clearly of a weight that is too heavy to be lifted manually. Equally most patients are clearly not so heavy that they will threaten to break the equipment. However, there will be occasions when it is necessary to know the patient's weight. Unfortunately patients rarely know how much they weigh. At best the patient's own estimate is likely to be too low. The patient tells the nurse what he used to weigh before he started to put on weight and then went "off his feet." This situation is not helped by the fact that patients are hardly ever weighed by the hospital or carers.

Manufacturers are required to label inanimate loads with their weight. However, many objects that nurses have to handle are not marked with their weight. If in doubt about the weight of an object it should be tested, for example by attempting to raise one end.

It can be difficult to assess the amount of force being applied when lifting part of a patient such as a leg. In almost all situations the nurse will know that the patient weighs too much for her to lift all of the patient's body weight. When assisting a patient, the nurse needs to be sure that she does not injure herself by applying too much force.

The weights in the guidance can be compared with the weights of everyday objects. For example a box of five reams of normal copier paper [80gsm] weighs around 12kg (26lbs). Nurses should use objects of known weight so as to familiarise themselves with weights at the levels of the guidance. This will help them to identify situations where they may be lifting too much weight.

The Guidance provides a series of questions to be asked for each factor. The assessment should be recorded under the following headings:-

A description of the Task

The Risks that are identified under the 5 headings above

The measures that are in place to control that risk

Further measures that are required

Review date

Signature of assessor and date of assessment

It is often useful to have different assessment forms for patient handling and for the handling of inanimate loads. Examples of patient assessment forms are shown later in this chapter.

In the following table the factors and questions from Schedule 1 of the Guidance on the Manual Operations Regulations are given with additional notes to assist in assessing handling issues in the health services. Some additional questions that should be asked when assessing patients have been added at the end.

The Task

Define clearly the task to be achieved. Where appropriate, divide it into sub tasks and assess each task separately. Thus deal with the move from the bed to the commode separately from the move from the commode to the wheelchair.

Does the task need to be done? Lifting or sliding a patient out of bed to the commode does not improve mobility. Consider rolling the patient on to a bed pan to reduce the amount of handling needed.

Can the patient be persuaded to move himself? Is the patient capable of moving himself given time and something appropriate to lean on? Could the patient transfer himself if he was provided with a sliding board?

Questions and Notes from the Guidance to the Manual Handling Operations Regulations		Notes
Do they involve	holding or manipulating loads at a distance from trunks?	Almost all patient handling involves taking loads away from the trunk. This is one of the main reasons that nurses must avoid lifting all but the smallest children.
	Unsatisfactory bodily movement or posture, especially:- - twisting the trunk? - stooping?	The task must be designed to avoid twisting with a load. See vv for the walk stance position. Stooping is a common fault in a lot of caring situations. Nurses must avoid stooping even if they are not planning to actually move the patient. The postural stress involved in stooping is damaging.
	- reaching upwards?	Reaching upwards is rarely a problem in patient handling except when something has gone wrong. Nurses must be aware that reaching up is posturally unsound and their ability to take loads in this position is much reduced.
	Excessive Movement of loads especially:- - excessive lifting or lowering distances? - excessive carrying distances?	Lifting or lowering takes the load into the areas where the lifter's capacity to lift safely is much lower. The load must be suitable for the minimum area that it passes through on its journey. Carrying any load over a distance will extend the period of the postural stress and should therefore be avoided.

Questions and Notes from the Guidance to the Manual Handling Operations Regulations		Notes
Do they involve	Excessive pushing or pulling of loads?	Pushing and pulling may be safer than lifting but even these activities are not absolutely safe. See Chapter 5. Some patient handling tasks may involve excessive pushing and pulling forces. For example pushing a wheelchair up a steep slope may involve forces that are too high for safety.
	Risk of sudden movement of loads?	All patients are likely to move in unexpected ways. In all handling situations the nurse must be aware of the risk of a sudden collapse.
	Frequent or prolonged physical effort?	Task allocation where, for example, two nurses are sent round the ward to sit everyone up, should be avoided. Tasks must also be avoided where someone has to hold a patient or part of a patient for extended periods. E.g. holding a patient's leg whilst it is dressed can cause postural stress.
	Insufficient rest of recovery periods?	On busy wards the staffing levels must be high enough for nurses to take rest breaks. Even if nurses are using 'safe' techniques the effort of pushing, pulling and turning may build up cumulative strain.
	A rate of work imposed by process?	This is rarely a problem in patient handling. However, it can occur where there is some task with a deadline such as getting all of the patients in a home ready by nine o'clock so that they can be taken to their day time activities. This risk is more common where there is some form of automated process involving a production line or conveyor belt. There is a risk of this problem arising with some handling of inanimate loads around a hospital.

The Load

Questions and Notes from the Guidance to the Manual Handling Operations Regulations		Notes in respect of the Handling of Patients
Is the load	Heavy?	All but the lightest children will be heavier than the numerical guidelines provided in the guidance. With inanimate loads ensure that they are divided into small enough units so that the loads are within the guidelines.
	Bulky or Unwieldy	The human body is fundamentally an unwieldy load. Some people are especially bulky and unwieldy. Equipment attached to the patient may also increase this problem.

Questions and Notes from the Guidance to the Manual Handling Operations Regulations		Notes in respect of the Handling of Patients
Is the load	Difficult to grasp?	There are no handles or hand holds on people. The only convenient hand hold is the arm pit and we have learned that lifting here is dangerous to nurses and can dislocate the patient's shoulders. If appropriate use a handling belt around the patient to provide hand holds.
	Unstable with contents likely to shift?	All patients are in the nurse's care because they are in some way feeble or ill. The nurse must expect them to move unpredictably. The nurse must always treat all patients as unstable loads and be prepared for them to shift. If she has an expectation that patients will collapse or faint there will be less chance of the nurse being injured.
	Sharp, hot or otherwise potentially damaging?	Some patients will punch or bite the nurse. If this happens whilst nurses are handling a person it can suddenly increase the load or cause the nurse to twist. Consider this risk when choosing a handling technique.

The Environment

Questions and Notes from the Guidance to the Manual Handling Operations Regulations		Notes in respect of the Handling of Patients
Are there	Space constraints preventing good posture?	Beds and chairs etc. always stop the nurse getting into an ideal handling posture. Toilets and bath rooms are often too small to allow safe manual handling. If in any doubt an appropriate mechanical aid must be used. If equipment is not available do not do the task. Furniture that is causing an obstruction but is not required for the task must be moved out of the way. If it cannot be moved it may make the task unsafe, in which case, the task must not be carried out.
	Uneven, slippery or unstable floors?	Beware of spills on polished floors.
	Variations in levels of floors or work surfaces?	Sills and extra steps are a particular risk in the community and in older buildings. In the short term make sure these can be negotiated safely. In the longer term such risks must be removed.
	Extremes of temperature or humidity?	This risk factor is not likely to affect most patient handling situations. However, there may be some situations where it should be considered.
	Conditions causing ventilation problems or gusts of wind?	This risk factor is also unlikely to affect many patient handling situations.
	Poor lighting conditions?	Handling in poor light may confuse the patient or may cause the nurse to miss her footing. This can be a particular problem in the community and on the ward at night.

The Individual's Capability

Questions and Notes from the Guidance to the Manual Handling Operations Regulations		Notes
Does the Job	Require unusual strength, height, etc.?	Nurses and other carers are not selected for their physical strength, nor are they given detailed medical checks of the condition of their spines. Therefore, the task must be designed so that it can be done by the majority of people.
	Create a hazard to those who might reasonably considered to be pregnant or to have a health problem?	There is a risk in any group of female workers that some will be pregnant. Lifting in pregnancy has been identified as a possible cause of miscarriages. If the task is properly designed this risk should be kept to a minimum.
	Require special information or training for its safe performance?	All handling equipment requires special knowledge and training. Ensure that all staff who will carry out the task are familiar with the equipment that will be used.

Other Factors

Questions and Notes from the Guidance to the Manual Handling Operations Regulations		Notes
	Is movement or posture hindered by personal protective equipment or by clothing?	There are several situations in the health care setting where personal protective equipment or clothing can affect the risks of handling patients. For Example – 1. Older style uniforms can inhibit movement. Is there a dress code that ensures that those who handle loads are wearing appropriate easy fitting clothes and flat heeled shoes? 2. Lead aprons are a particular risk factor for Radiographers and for nurses who are assisting them. They can inhibit movement when handling. They significantly increase postural stress. It is very important for people wearing lead aprons to stand or sit with their spines in a natural vertical curve at all times. Beware of having to bend to hold a patient's arm or leg or some other such task.
	Is there a good working atmosphere?	Psychosocial factors including stress, morale, job satisfaction, attitudes to work and attitudes to backache play a part in musculosketal disorders. It is not entirely clear that these factors actually suppress injuries or simply suppress the level of complaints about injuries. Nevertheless, there seem to be fewer injuries if these matters are 'right.'

Additional Questions To Be Considered When Assessing Patients

Are additional procedures to be undertaken while the handing is taking place? e.g. – inserting a bedpan guarding an injured limb doing a dressing	Carrying out two activities at the same time can cause the handler to become unstable and leads to accidents. It must always be avoided. Get another nurse to do the additional task.
What is the condition of the patient?	The condition of the patient may have already influenced several risk factors above. Consider if there is anything further about the patient that will affect the assessment?

CONTROL MEASURES

This section lists possible measures to reduce risk. The items in these lists are applicable to all handling situations. Nurses carrying out assessments should consider their specific relevance to patient handling:-

The Task

Could equipment be better designed for easier use?

Could adjustable equipment and furniture reduce the need for awkward movements or posture?

Can loads be carried for shorter distances even if this means changing the layout of the workplace?

Can heavy items be stored at convenient heights?

Can rest breaks or less tiring spells of work be introduced around the task?

Can the job be re-designed to minimise fixed postures?

Can the job be re-designed to provide more variety?

Can the task be shared or rotated among more staff? (Sharing is only applicable to tasks that are safe. It can be used to avoid damage from repetitive handling. It cannot be used to make unsafe lifts into safe ones.)

The load

Can mechanical equipment such as hoists, trolleys, etc. take some of the strain?

Can the weight be reduced by having smaller containers?

Could handles, wheels or castors help to reduce the load?

Can the task be automated or mechanised?

Can the load be handled by a team instead of by one person? (This will only be a solution in a limited number of cases. Remember that there are severe limits on the effectiveness of several people lifting a single load.)

The environment

Could ramps be installed so that trolleys, hoists, wheelchairs, etc. can be easily moved?

Can heights or work surfaces be harmonised to reduce lifting from one to another?

The worker

Can workers' technique and movement be improved?

Can training be given to change workers' attitudes and perception of risk?

Should workers who are prone to back ache and other ailments be prevented from doing this task?

The organisation

Are there adequate written procedures?

Is there a need for more management reinforcement and supervision?

Is there a need for consultation with other departments, such as supplies?

Can consultation with managers, maintenance staff, or designers facilitate changes?

Can there be more consultation with workers on measures to reduce risk?

Has the management produced a written cost analysis of the risk? See risk control below

SELECTING THE TECHNIQUE

Having considered the factors above the nurse must now decide on one of 4 ways of carrying out the task

1. Let the patient move himself	This may involve some form of support or assistance from the nurse. Ensure that the nurse is not going to be the prop.
2. Use a sliding system	More information on the choice of sliding equipment is contained in the chapter on handling in bed
3. Use a mechanical device	The range of mechanical equipment is described in Chapter 13.
4. Do not do the task	If a safe way of doing the task cannot be found then it must not be done. Review the analysis of the task to see if it can be defined in a different way so that a safe solution can be found. If a safe solution still cannot be found then the task must not be done. An alternative solution must be used until a safe solution can be provided. If necessary the patient may have to remain in bed until appropriate equipment can be obtained.

When it has been decided how to carry out the task the method should be recorded in the patient's care plan and a date set for re-assessment of the task.

CARRYING OUT THE TASK

If more than one nurse is involved decide who will give the command. There must be no doubt which of the nurses is to act as leader. She is responsible for explaining matters to the patient and deciding how to co-ordinate the manoeuvre. (The patient may be asked to give the word of command.) See box below.

Check that the environment is ready

All hazards are removed

Brakes are applied on trolleys, beds and wheelchairs

The height of the bed adjusted

The bed clothing made ready.

Check the individuals' capabilities

Do they know how to handle?

Have they been trained?

Are they fit to handle?

Are they familiar with the equipment?

Are they familiar with the technique?

Are they familiar with the patient?

CO-ORDINATING THE MOVEMENT OF ANY LOAD – COUNT-V-WORDS

It is traditional to co-ordinate lifting with counts such as 1-2-3-lift. The problem with this is that some people lift on the "3" and some lift in the "lift." Thus the lift is not co-ordinated.

It has long been recognised that it is safer to use words such as "ready, Brace, PUSH." The last word can be chosen to suit the action. Words such as SLIDE, PULL and STAND are suitable.

The person co-ordinating the manoeuvre must inform everyone the way in which the move is to be co-ordinated. She must ensure that the command word is known.

EVALUATION AFTER HANDLING THE PATIENT

Once the task has been completed it should be immediately evaluated. This only needs to be an informal process but it should be gone through conscientiously to ensure that handling remains safe.

Consider :-

Has the patient's condition improved?	Is there sufficient improvement to allow the patient to contribute more to the task?	If the answer is yes then the task should be re-assessed.
Has the patient's condition deteriorated?	Is the patient still able to contribute the required effort?	If the answer is no then the task should be re-assessed.
What was the patient's reaction to the technique?	Did the patient resist the move? Did he feel uncomfortable or disorientated in any way?	If problems were experienced the task needs to be re-assessed.
Did all those involved in the task carry out their roles correctly?		If the answer is no then either the person needs to be retrained or the task should be re-assessed.
Did the equipment work correctly?		Report any equipment failures immediately and withdraw the equipment from use.
Did the equipment perform as expected?		If not then the task must be re-assessed or the staff must be retrained in the use of the equipment.

THE DIFFERENCE BETWEEN ASSISTING AND TAKING FULL WEIGHT

Many nurses are injured when they 'assist' a patient to his feet. This happens for two basic reasons.

1. The patient is really incapable of rising from sitting to standing. What the nurse is in fact doing is lifting the patient onto his feet and balancing him in that position.

or

2. For some reason the patient is unable to manage to get to his feet on this occasion and falls back. Nurses instinctively hold such patients up.

BOTH OF THESE CAN AND HAVE INJURED NURSES

The phrase The Patient can stand is often misused. It can and does contribute to injuries to nurses. On some occasions it is used to mean that a patient can get himself to his feet. On other occasions it means that the patient can balance on his feet once he has been lifted there. Staff should be required to use clear statements describing the patient's exact capabilities and exactly how much help he needs.

It is essential that the individual patient is properly and regularly assessed to ensure that he is capable of rising to his feet with a small amount of assistance. Apply the guidance to the Manual Handling Regulations in this situation. The individual lifter should not find herself lifting more than the figures in the guidance. The maximum force is required at the start of an assist from a chair. The weight that can be taken at this point will depend on the exact posture but, as a general guide the nurse should not apply more than 10kg (22lbs) (15kg [33lbs] for male nurses). Familiarise yourself with how much this is by finding inanimate loads of the same weight.

If the patient cannot start to rise this level of assistance is applied, DO NOT TRY TO LIFT HIM.

If the patient suddenly fails to co-operate whilst being assisted to his feet, LOWER HIM BACK INTO HIS CHAIR. Settle the patient back in the chair and find some other way of moving him.

AS SOON AS EITHER OF THESE HAPPEN THE PATIENT MUST BE RE-ASSESSED BEFORE HE IS ASSISTED AGAIN. See Chapter 15

> **WARNING**
>
> **Many lifts and techniques are unsafe.**

CARRYING OUT MANUAL HANDLING ASSESSMENTS

In understanding the process of assessment it is important to see the process of carrying out an assessment as being separate from finding the solution. The assessment is done to identify the risks. When that is complete the solution can be defined. This is then re-assessed and tested to see if it controls the risks that were identified. The solution may not solve all of the risks and may even present new risks of its own. If there are unresolved risks a new solution may be sought or a further assessment may be written to describe the remaining risks.

The regulations require employers to carry out both general and specific assessments of the manual handling operations in the work place.

The general assessment is required to look at:-

the type of work being carried out,

the general characteristics of the loads being handled,

the equipment available

and

the working space.

This assessment should establish the general risks in the work and identify solutions that will meet a range of situations. The regulations recognise that this is sometimes more useful than immediately relying on specific individual assessments. Handling situations found in the work place may be defined as a series of generic assessments.

In some work situations it may be possible to rely on the general or generic assessments. However, in some cases it is necessary to carry out a separate assessment of every lift of every load. This is certainly the case in the health care setting. Every patient's condition is different and therefore every patient presents different risks. Each patient needs to be separately assessed to define the way in which he is to be handled in specific situations.

The following sections discuss the implementation of these assessments in the health services under the headings of **Generic Assessments** and **Individual Care Plans**.

GENERIC ASSESSMENTS

The level of detail required in generic assessments depends upon the area being assessed. The effectiveness of generic assessments in hospital and other fixed locations differs from the effectiveness of assessments in the community.

Generic Assessments in Hospital

When assessing a ward or other fixed place such as a nursing home it is possible to look at the mix of patients, the existing equipment and the physical surroundings. It is possible to arrive at quite detailed conclusions that such and such must be done to make the ward safe. For example, it can be said that with the hoists and space available it is not possible to toilet immobile patients in the toilets and that these people must be toiletted on commodes. The physical changes needed to overcome the limitations can be defined and can be put in hand.

When making an assessment in a ward the nurse can use the generic assessment as a strong basis for the care plan of an individual patient. She can choose from a range of solutions that she is equipped to provide and which the staff know how to implement.

Generic Assessments in the Community

In the community things are different. When carrying out a generic assessment of the community the assessor can consider the different types of situations that have been met. She can consider the changes needed to make those situations safe. However, generic assessments in the community do not make it possible to change rooms nor is it possible to put equipment in place. Such steps can only be taken when a particular person becomes a patient. The actual changes needed can then be identified and carried out. The main value of generic assessments in the community is that they warn management of the normal range of situations that they will have to prepare for in their staff and equipment planning. A generic assessment also serves as guidance to a nurse when assessing the situation in a patient's home.

The nurse carrying out assessments must beware of the limitations of generic assessments. Regardless of the level of detail in the generic assessment the nurse will have to take care to fully assess each patient's needs so that a generic assessment is only applied if it is truly relevant to the patient.

Possible areas for which generic assessments can be carried out include:

transfers from bed to chair, commode, or toilet

patients who have a history of falls

bathing

washing

dressing

undressing

floor coverings, to note risks of hoists on carpets and slippery bathroom floors

difficulties in using hoists: carpets, space

transfers in and out of a vehicle

babies in high-sided cots

the handling of packages and boxes and so on by staff at a health centre.

FORMS FOR INDIVIDUAL CARE PLANS

Assessments of individual's capabilities must be carried out before writing an individual care plan. No specific form has been produced to cover the whole of this process. The process of assessment is complex and depends upon the individual patient and his circumstances. It has not been found useful to reduce this process to a single side of A4.

The results of the individual assessment are to be written up on a care plan. There are three examples The care plan must contain an outline of the patient's condition and abilities. It must then contain instructions on the way in which the patient is to be moved in a variety of everyday situations. The instructions must be provided in a way that can be understood by those who will care for him. Thus, to say that three nurses are needed to toilet a person is not adequate. The plan must say, for example, that two people are required to log roll the patient whilst a third inserts the bed pan. Without these full instructions the nurses would be forgiven for concluding that the three of them were to lift the patient.

As with all assessments the nurse carrying out the individual assessment must have been trained in risk assessment.

FORM 1 Is an example of a generic assessment for a ward in a hospital

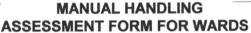

MANUAL HANDLING ASSESSMENT FORM FOR WARDS

WHAT IS THIS FORM FOR?
- Targeted at wards and may not be well-suited to other nursing areas.
- Intended to help ward managers to carry out general manual handling assessments and decide on measures to reduce risk, while keeping a record of their decision-making process.
- Also serves as a Safe System of Work, guiding managers to write down general rules for patient handling.
- Only deals with general handling issues in the ward: detailed assessments of each patient's handling procedure should be recorded in the Patient Care Plan.

TIPS
If some questions cannot easily be answered by a *Yes* or *No* then write down your comments. Add to the form any extra aspects you are concerned about or append a separate page. You will record in this form measures which could further reduce risk. This should include any measures which go beyond your budget or authority, for decision-making at senior management level. You may decide, while filling in this form, that you need to change some of your work practices. To be successful this may need a step-by-step approach, trials and consultation. To allow time for this, make a note of your plan of action and update the form when practices have changed.

ADMINISTRATION DETAILS

WARD: **WEST**
or clinic, area,
surgery etc.

HOSPITAL: **MAIDUP**
or health centre

ASSESSMENT TEAM
Ward Manager: **SISTER HYPOTHETICAL** (name) .... (signature)
Others:

Mrs A lifter Health Care Assistant
Staff Nurse A Repp Safety Representative
Staff Nurse I Link Nurse for Moving and Handling

FOR EXAMPLE
Moving & Handling Co-ordinator
Health and Safety Adviser
Other nursing staff
Safety representatives

DATE: **1st Dec 94**
Date(s) reviewed:

WARD DETAILS

Speciality:	**Geriatric**	☐ MALE
Typical age range of patients:	**Elderly**	☐ FEMALE
		☐ MIXED
Typical number of patients: on a typical shift	**22**	

© NBPA

N.B. When the patient is re-assessed a fresh form must always be used. Corrections to an existing form are a source of errors and confusion.

HANDLING AIDS

EXAMPLES OF HANDLING AIDS

Monkey poles	Sara hoist
Rope ladder	Standaid
Patient hand blocks	Dextra hoist
Turning disk	Ajo side loader
	Carter hoist
	Oxford hoist
Ambulift B (bathing only)
Ambulift C (sling only)
Ambulift D (both sling & seat)
Sliding aid (small/long, sheet/cushion)
Sliding aid (long, rigid) e.g. Patslide

List handling aids used or available in your ward, whether your own or regularly borrowed. If possible use their brand name.

NAME OF HANDLING AID	HOW MANY	IS IT BASED IN YOUR WARD?	OTHERWISE, WHERE IS IT BORROWED FROM?	IN GOOD WORKING CONDITION, WITH ANY ATTACHMENTS IN PLACE?	SUITABLE? (if not, why?)	SLINGS AND OTHER ATTACHMENTS AVAILABLE	CHANGES, REPAIRS OR ADDITIONAL ATTACHMENTS NEEDED	DATE OF LAST SAFETY CHECK (Serial No)
Dextra Hoist	1	yes		Yes need more slings	Yes	1 Extra large sling 1 Large Fabric sling 1 large toilet sling 1 lg. mesh sling for bathing		
Patslide	1	Yes		Yes	Yes	Canvas with extension loops	Additional canvas x 2	
Sara Hoist	1	No	East Ward	Yes			Obtain own SARA for the full time use of this ward	
Patient hand blocks	1 pair	No	South Ward	Yes	Yes		Order a set of hand blocks	
Ambulift Model D	1	Yes	Yes Chair chassis missing	Yes	Yes	1 chair attachment 1 cot hand sling 1 medium patient sling	Remove hand slings Find or order chair chassis 1 small 1 large patient slings	
Small Sliding Sheet	6	Yes	Yes	Yes			Stitching repairs required to 2 sheets	
One Way Slide	1	Yes	Yes	Yes but this is wheelchair size			Order 1 more wheelchairs size plus 2 armchair size and 1 bed	
Transfer boards	0						Order 1 straight one curved transfer boards	

© NBPA

BEDS

List handling aids used or available in your ward, whether your own or regularly borrowed. If possible use their brand name.

MAKE AND TYPE OF BED	HOW MANY	ON THE WARD?	OTHERWISE, WHERE IS IT BORROWED FROM?	IN GOOD WORKING CONDITION, WITH ANY ATTACHMENTS IN PLACE?	SUITABLE? (if not, why?)	ATTACHMENTS AVAILABLE	CHANGES, REPAIRS OR ADDITIONAL ATTACHMENTS NEEDED	SERVICED IN LAST 6 MTH's?
Fixed height beds	3	yes		yes	NO Good for Patient Handling		Replace as soon as possible	N/A
ABC Kings Fund Type beds	12	yes		3 have unspent brakes 2 have broken hydraulics		4 sets of cot sides	Get repairs done 7 days	None
DEF Kings fund type beds	5	yes		yes	This type of bed is not stable if nurses sit on bed to sit patient up		Only use these beds for one-dependent patient's Put on priority list for replacement	Some
ABC Semi Profiling beds	2	yes		Yes	Head section raised manually		Investigate possible fitting of electric motors to lift head and of bed	
Stand-up Beds	0	no	Available from central stores when needed				No need to buy as only needed one or 2 weeks per year	
Turning Beds	0	no	Rented from suppliers when needed				Consider purchase they be cheaper than rental costs	
Profiling beds	0	No					Prepare rolling plan to move to profiling beds	

© NBPA

BATHING

WHAT TYPES OF BATH OR SHOWER ARE IN THE WARD?	HOW MANY	SUITABLY? (if not, why?)
Ordinary Bath	1	Fully ambulant patients only
Parker Bath	1	Use hoist for patients needing assistance
Showers	2	Now Wheelchair access Ambulant Patients only

FOR EXAMPLE
Ordinary bath
Parker bath
Variable height bath
Ordinary shower
Shower cabinet
Shower trolley

SYSTEM OF WORK: List methods used for patients of various degrees of dependency. Which methods are used most frequently; which are used only occasionally?	ARE THERE ANY MANUAL HANDLING PROBLEMS WITH ASSISTING PATIENTS IN OR OUT OF THE BATH OR SHOWER?	ADDITIONAL MEASURES TO CONSIDER FOR THE FUTURE
Half to three quarters of the patients need assistance to get in/out of bath.	There is enough space around both baths	
1. Use ambulift with seat attachment to place semi ambulant patients in the ordinary bath	Access for the Ambulift at the ordinary bath is tricky because only a small slot has been cut out of the casing around the bath	Remove casing around bath until it is re-cut
2. Use ambulift with bathing sling attachment to place non ambulant patients in the ordinary bath	There is some stooping whilst assisting patients to wash.	Reschedule bathing to spread out the work load & reduce prolonged stooping. This will also relieve demand for the Ambulift
3. Or use Dextra place patients in the Parker bath		Submit requisition to replace ordinary bath with hi-low bath
Ambulant patients to use the Parker bath or shower if fully ambulant	Cannot wheel patients into the shower because of step. However patients prefer bath.	Submit requisition for one shower to be changed to allow wheelchair access
If patients need any support or need to be lifted into or out of the bath use appropriate equipment. Do not manually assist such patients	FOR EXAMPLE ✓ Enough room to move freely in a good posture? ✓ Enough room to use a hoist? ✓ Stooping, twisting? ✓ Lifting? ✓ Convenient grab rails etc.? ✓ Floor slippery? ✓ Type of patient? ✓ ref: Health Building Note 40 for correct dimensions of spaces	FOR EXAMPLE • Move or use a hoist, shower trolley, bathing stretcher • Wheel patients into the shower • Cut out casing round bath to improve hoist access • Install a hoist • Take most dependent patients to other ward with better bathroom • Re-schedule bathing to spread out the workload • Install a different type of bath • Move bath away from wall • remove partition walls • Change floor covering

From the above possible measures, write any needs in the summary at the end

© NBPA

TOILETTING

SYSTEM OF WORK: List methods used to assist patients of various degrees of dependency. Which methods are used most frequently; which are used only occasionally?	ARE THERE ANY MANUAL HANDLING PROBLEMS WITH ASSISTING PATIENTS?	ADDITIONAL MEASURES TO CONSIDER FOR THE FUTURE
The smaller toilet is used for patients who do not require manual handling (about 1/4 of the patients).	Not enough grab rails in the toilets Toilet roll holder is in the way in the smaller toilet.	Fit grab rails in all toilets. Use fold away types in larger toilets and move toilet roll holders
The 2 larger toilets are used for more dependent patients with assistance of 1 or 2 nurses	The larger toilets are still smaller than required in Health Building note 40 it is difficult to assist patients as there is not enough room to the sides of the toilets. And wheelchairs cannot be brought into the toilet.	Plan to turn present three toilets into two of the right size
Ambulift or Dextra used with toiletting slings for those who cannot weight bear	Need more toiletting slings to take full advantage of the hoists. N.B. remove hand slings from Ambulift	Submit requisition for Sara hoist for the ward (this will also be valuable in bed to chair transfers)
The Sara is often borrowed for patients who can follow instructions and weight bear	Delays in obtaining the Sara mean it is not always fetched for patients who can benefit from it's use	
If a patient needs more than a few kilos of force to assist use appropriate equipment. Do not attempt to assist if there is not enough space to be alongside the patient	FOR EXAMPLE ✓ Enough room to move freely in a good posture? ✓ Enough room to use a hoist? ✓ Stooping, twisting? ✓ Lifting? ✓ Convenient grab rails etc ? ✓ Commodes adequate? ✓ Floor slippery? ✓ Type of patient?	FOR EXAMPLE • Use a hoist (standing hoist, sling lifter) • Wheel commode over WC • Raised toilet seat • Move WC or move partition wall for more space • Widen doorway • Install or move grab rails • Get door to open outwards • Change floor covering

From the above possible measures, write any needs in the summary at the end

© NBPA

SEATS, WHEELCHAIRS, COMMODES

SYSTEM OF WORK: List methods used to assist patients of various degrees of dependency. Which methods are used most frequently; which are used only occasionally?	ARE THERE ANY MANUAL HANDLING PROBLEMS WITH ASSISTING PATIENTS?	ADDITIONAL MEASURES TO CONSIDER FOR THE FUTURE
Sit to stand/stand to sit - Repositioning in seat - etc.		
At least 1/4 of the patients are non-weight bearing the Dextra, Ambulift or Sara are used to transfer these patients	A quarter of the seats are too low. This reduces independent mobility and causes nurses to stoop.	Plan to replace low seats on a rolling basis
Patients who have only slight loss of mobility are transferred using handling belts and the side transfer.		Requisition for Sara will benefit these transfers
Reposition patients to the back of the chair -		Order sliding boards. These can be used for transfers of patients who cannot stand
1. Using side to side rocking		
2. Use one way glides for patients who slide down the chair frequently		
3. Using hoists for heavy and awkward patients		
If a patient needs more than a few kilos of force to assist use appropriate equipment. Do not attempt to assist if there is not enough space to be alongside the patient	FOR EXAMPLE ✓ Seats too low/too deep ✓ Arms get in the way ✓ Hoist cannot get close ✓ Brakes or wheels defective ✓ Not enough wheelchairs ✓ Floor slippery ✓ Type of patient	FOR EXAMPLE • Use a hoist (standing hoist, sling lifter) • Use a sliding board • Use a turning disk • Sit patient on one-way sliding aid • Sit or kneel by patient rather than stoop • Change type of seat/ used • Get door to open outwards • Label defective items for maintenance

From the above possible measures, write any needs in the summary at the end

© NBPA

BED AND TROLLEY MOVES

SYSTEM OF WORK: List methods used and precautions taken to assist patients of various degrees of dependency. Which methods are used most frequently, which are used only occasionally?	ARE THERE ANY MANUAL HANDLING PROBLEMS WITH ASSISTING PATIENTS?	ADDITIONAL MEASURES TO CONSIDER FOR THE FUTURE
Moving up/down the bed - Move on/off bed pan - - Transfer bed-seat - Transfer bed-trolley	Moving up/down the bed - Move on/off bed pan - - Transfer bed-seat - Transfer bed-trolley - Attending to patients on beds, trolleys or examination couches - Bed-bathing	
Moving up / down bed - about 3 / 4 of patients can move themselves (some using hand blocks or monkey poles.) For others sliding sheet with 2 nurses. Dextra or ambulift is used for patients who are too heavy or too awkward	Three beds are fixed height. These are only to be used for fully ambulant patients who do not need direct nursing care. Do not use these beds for short patients.	Requisition height adjustable beds to replace three fixed height beds. Plan rolling programme to update to profiling beds.
On / off bed pans 3 or 4 patients on every shift require bed pans. 1. Get patient to bridge or use the monkey pole 2. Use log roll 3. Use Dextra or Ambulift		
Use Pat slide for bed to trolley transfers	Do not use the pat slide for heavy patients.	Order Stretcher attachment for Dextra to allow transfers
Transfers bed to seat - see previous page		

If a patient needs more than a few kilos of force to assist use appropriate equipment. Do not attempt to assist if there is not enough space to be alongside the patient	FOR EXAMPLE
	* Enough room to move freely in a good posture?
	* Enough room to use a hoist?
	* Furniture around bed easy to move?
	* Stooping, twisting?
	* Lifting?
	* Straight-lifting hydropneumatic injury patients?
	* Mechanism for height adjustment/controls/defect/rest adequate?
	* Brakes wheels in good working order?
		FOR EXAMPLE
		* Get height-adjustable beds/couches
		* Get profiling beds
		* Put only the most independent patients in fixed-height beds
		* Sit patient on side-way sliding aid
		* Turntable
		* Label defective items for repair or maintenance
		Use handling aids
		  * Hoist
		  * Sliding/Transfer aid
		  * Monkey pole
		  * Rope ladder
		  Patient hand blocks.

From the above possible measures, write any needs in the summary at the end

© NBPA

Other areas of concern

DESCRIBE THE HANDLING AND MOVEMENT ISSUE	ARE THERE ANY MANUAL HANDLING PROBLEMS?	ADDITIONAL MEASURES TO CONSIDER FOR THE FUTURE
Handling of laundry bags (clean linen	Bags are too heavy to be lifted and there is restricted space in the laundry cupboard Staff instructed to take sheets out of bags rather than lift whole bag. (Team brief 20/11/94)	Raise problem with managers to get contract for laundry altered to specify that laundry will be packed in safe parcels.
Removal of Soiled Laundry Dirty laundry is placed in bags supported in a wheeled wire frame	Nurses over fill bags and then have difficulty pulling then out of the frame - Warn nurses to avoid over filling bags	Reduce the size of the laundry bags
FOR EXAMPLE * Uniforms/footwear adequate? * Remaining in awkward postures * Supporting patients' limbs * Handling laundry * Handling food containers * Heavy/awkward objects placed too high, too low, too far * Carrying equipment * Difficulties with other depts/services * Fitness/skill/number of staff		

© NBPA

TRANSFER FROM FLOOR LEVEL

Are falls to the floor frequent? Are patients frequently at floor level? List methods used and precautions taken to reduce risk associated with the falling patient and the fallen patient.	ARE THERE ANY MANUAL HANDLING PROBLEMS WITH ASSISTING PATIENTS?	ADDITIONAL MEASURES TO CONSIDER FOR THE FUTURE
There are 3 to 4 falls on the ward every week. 1. Non dependent patients are taught to get themselves up 2. Dependent patients are lifted using the Dextra hoist All staff have practised movement for breaking the fall of a collapsed patient	Patients being rehabilitated need support. As there is no equipment nurses are walking with patients who are at risk of falling. Nurses follow with wheelchairs whenever possible but there are increased number of occasions when patients have to be lowered to the floor.	Decide on strategy for rehabilitation and obtain walking hoist or hoist with walking harness
FOR EXAMPLE * Avoid situations where the patient is at risk of falling * Check that nurses know technique for dealing with falling patient Use a hoist for fallen patient		

© NBPA

MANAGEMENT CHECKLIST

The following are reminders to managers of systems that should be in place.

Reporting accidents or pain

* An Incident/Accident report form is completed when a member of staff reports pain in the back or limbs or has an accident — ✓ YES ▢ NO   COMMENTS:
* There is evidence that all accident reports have been fully investigated — ✓ YES ▢ NO   COMMENTS:
* Have Occupational Health been notified by phone at the earliest opportunity (daytime hours) — ✓ YES ▢ NO   COMMENTS:
* Were staff advised to consult the Occupational Health Unit when they had a problem with their back or limbs — ▢ YES ✓ NO   COMMENTS: no relevant injuries

Instruction and training

* An up-to-date record is kept of staff attendance at moving & handling courses — ✓ YES ▢ NO   COMMENTS:
* All staff have attended an initial 2-day course — ✓ YES ▢ NO   COMMENTS:
* All staff have attended a refresher course in the past 18 months — ▢ YES ✓ NO   COMMENTS: List of people needing refresher given to Mrs Bass 10/11/94
* All staff, students, temporary staff have been shown how to use the handling aids in the ward — ✓ YES ▢ NO   COMMENTS:
* The Moving & Handling Co-ordinator will be called upon to give additional guidance in the ward if the need arises — ✓ YES ▢ NO   COMMENTS:

Safe system of work

* An initial assessment of each patient's mobility/handling requirements is made during the admission procedure, and updated whenever changes are needed — ✓ YES ▢ NO   COMMENTS:
* Handling methods, staff numbers and equipment to be used are specified in the patient care plan — ▢ YES ✓ NO   COMMENTS: Will write more details then re-evaluate
* Nurses in charge have been made aware of their duty to ensure, so far as is reasonably practicable, that methods specified in the patient care plan are used, recommended moving & handling practices are used, defective equipment is put out of action — ✓ YES ▢ NO   COMMENTS:

Evacuation

* Is there an evacuation plan for the ward? — ✓ YES ▢ NO   COMMENTS:
* Has the plan been approved by the fire officer? — ✓ YES ▢ NO   COMMENTS:
* Has the plan been tested in the last six months? — ▢ YES ✓ NO   COMMENTS: Arrange practice in 1 week
* Is there enough evacuation equipment? — ▢ YES ✓ NO   COMMENTS: Evac Chair needed
* Are structural changes needed for safe evacuation (e.g. ramps in place of steps) — ▢ YES ✓ NO   COMMENTS:

ACTION FOR THE WARD MANAGER

* By the time you have completed this form, you should have initiated some risk-reducing measures which are within your authority
* Some measures will go beyond your budget or authority. List and justify these using the summary sheet following this form. Copy this to your senior manager. It is important to justify any requests as decisions must be made on the basis of risk or benefit versus cost.
* You should review and update this form at least once a year, or whenever there is a change to record.
* Keep this form in the ward as a written record of your manual handling risk assessment.

© NBPA

SUMMARY OF NEEDS AND ACTION PLAN

The following changes will be introduced in the ward's work practices (with target dates for completion). The following equipment, works etc. is needed.

▪ Re-schedule bathing to spread out work load	DEC/JAN
▪ Write more details in patient care plans	DEC/JAN
▪ Dextra Hoist : At least 2 more slings needed (Large and Extra Large) At present larger patients can only be lifted when a sling is borrowed from Ward South. If they need their extra large sling at the same time the patient cannot be moved until the sling is available	JAN/FEB
▪ One large toiletting sling and one mesh bathing sling needed for the Dextra to increase it's usefulness	JAN/FEB
▪ Also lower priority 2 medium and 2 large slings to allow more patients to have their own sling (hygiene)	APRIL
▪ Order own hand blocks so that there is no need to borrow then from another ward	DEC
▪ Order extra canvasses for Pat slide so that there are enough to allow for laundry and soiling.	APRIL
▪ Order one way glides 1 Wheelchair. 2 Armchair and 1 bed sizes	FEB
▪ Order 1 straight 1 curved transfer boards	DEC
▪ Organise stitching repairs to two small sliding sheets	NOW
▪ Casing around bath to be removed until it can be re-set - necessary to reduce strain manoeuvring hoist	NOW
▪ Submit requisition to replace ordinary bath with hi-lo bath	APRIL
▪ Arrange for one shower to be made accessible for wheelchairs	JUNE
▪ Sara Hoist being borrowed from Ward East is very useful for handling several patients. The ward needs it's own Sara hoist. This would be used at least 100 times per week and would also free up the Dextra for other tasks. Requisition a Sara hoist	APRIL
▪ Order slings for Ambulift hoist and find or order chair chassis	FEB
▪ Move toilet roll holders to ease access in toilets	DEC
▪ Provide Grab rails in all toilets (N. B. in larger toilets these must fold back for access with hoists etc.)	DEC
▪ Plan to rebuild toilets as two toilets in accordance with Health Building Note 40	1 YEAR
▪ Replace low chairs by higher chairs	1 YEAR
▪ Replace 3 fixed height beds by height adjustable beds	JUNE
▪ Repair broken Hydraulics on beds	NOW
▪ Repair broken brakes on beds	NOW
▪ Investigate Electric head lift for Semi-Profiling beds + purchase of stand up bed	MARCH
▪ Programme of replacing all beds with electric profiling beds	3 YEARS
▪ Negotiate with laundry to reduce size of linen packages	DEC
▪ Reduce size of laundry bags	DEC
▪ Order stretcher attachment for Dextra	APRIL
▪ Establish strategy for Rehabilitation including equipment needed	MARCH
▪ Order Evac Chair	

Continue on additional pages if necessary

▪ Re-evaluate in February then every 3 month

Remember to justify any needs on the basis of risk levels, cost, and benefits that should be gained. For example:
* Why is the change needed?
* How would it improve the present situation?
* How many staff/patients would it help?
* How frequently would it be used?
* Would it bring other benefits (e.g. independence to patient, quality of care)?
* Have you consulted anyone on the technical feasibility? Had a trial?

© NBPA

There are three examples of Care Plans

FORM 3 Patient Care Plan: Moving and Handling Section (hospitals, residential homes)

Patient Care Plan: Moving & Handling Section

| Patient's name | JOE PATIENT | Named Nurse | A. M. BUSY | If patient is totally independent, tick here and ignore the rest |

Body Build

Obese	✓	Tall
Above average		Medium	✓
Average		Short
Below average

Problems with comprehension, behaviour, co-operation (identify)

NONE

| Weight (if known) | 15 St |

Handling constraints, e.g. disability, weakness, pain, skin lesions, infusions (identif)

Painful right hip Patient requires minimal Assistance

Admitted for investigation of painful hip

| Risk of falls |
| High | | Low | ✓ |

Into bath or shower   Not applicable.

HANDLING AID		WHICH BATH	SUPERVISION	INDEPENDENT
Ambulift	✓	Parker	People 1 2 1
Dextra		Var height
Shower chair		Standard	✓	Additional Information
		Any	Use sliding aid with towel to transfer to ambulift

Transfers (including to/from: bed, wheelchair, commode, toilet)

HOIST		ASSISTANCE	INSTRUCTION	SUPERVISION	INDEPENDENT
Ambulift		People 1 2 1	Additional Information
Dextra		Side	✓
Carter/Oxford		Combined		Uses sliding board
Sara / Standaid

Toiletting

HOIST		ASSISTANCE	INSTRUCTION	SUPERVISION	INDEPENDENT
Ambulift		People 1 2 3 1	Additional Information
Dextra		Side	✓
Carter/Oxford		Combined		Uses sliding board
Sara / Standaid

Walking

NO WALKING	✓	ASSISTANCE	INSTRUCTION	SUPERVISION	INDEPENDENT
		People 1 2	Distance walked/ Additional Information
		Walking aid

Move up/down bed

HOIST		HANDLING AIDS	INSTRUCTION	✓	SUPERVISION	INDEPENDENT	✓
		Sliding aid (fabric)	✓	Additional Information
		Rope ladder		Warn pt that fabric slide is very slippery
		Hand blocks	✓

Sit up over side of bed

| ROPE LADDER | ✓ | SLIDING AID (fabric) | INSTRUCTION | SUPERVISION | INDEPENDENT | ✓ |

Move on/off bed pan

| HOIST | | ROLL PATIENT | PATIENT BRIDGE | MONKEY POLE | NOT USED | ✓ |

Transfer to/from trolley (or bed etc)

| SLIDING AID (rigid) e.g. Pat | | SLIDING AID (fabric) e.g. Easyslide | INSTRUCTION | SUPERVISION | INDEPENDENT |

Other instructions

Review after consultant's ward round 4/3/95

(Use a different box each time the assessment is reviewed)

| Date(s) assessed: | 1/3/95 | Assessor's signature: | A. M. Bussy | Proposed review dates | 4/3/95 |

© NBPA

FORM 4 Patient Care Plan in the Community: Moving & Handling Section

Patient Care Plan in the Community: Moving & Handling Section

| Patient's name | Miss A Lot | District Nurse | Sister A Ready |

BODY BUILD

Obese		Tall
Above average	✓	Medium
Average	✓	Short	✓
Below average

Problems with comprehension, behaviour, co-operation (identify)

NONE

| Weight (if known) | 8 st |

Handling constraints, e.g. disability, weakness, pain, skin lesions, infusions (identify)

Multiple Sclerosis - Unable to weight bear

Lower limbs tend to go into spasms. upper limbs lack co-ordination. Can support trunk

RISK OF FALLS

| High | ✓ | Low |

TASKS	METHOD TO BE USED	DESCRIBE ANY REMAINING PROBLEMS LIST ANY OTHER MEASURES NEEDED
Transfer Bed to Wheelchair	Keep Patient in bed at present	There is a high risk of falls & injuries to Carers if the patient is moved
Transfer to toilet	Use bed pan (Roll onto bed pan)	APPLY URGENTLY FOR HOIST & WHEELED SANICHAIR (environment for these is OK)
Move up / down bed	Sliding aid (fabric) with two carers Roll onto Towel under shoulders. Sit up using towel (kneel on bed next to pt use "sit down" to sit her up Then rock to position sliding sheet Use palm to palm thumb grip to move up the bed	Stooping at low bed is risk for nurses putting on hoist sling and moving patient in bed is unsafe with low bed. ORDER HEIGHT ADJUSTABLE PROFILING BED
Bathing	At present. bed bath	Take care to avoid stooping at bed. Kneel whenever possible Wash in bathroom on Sanichair ASAP ORDER ADAPTATION OF SHOWER

Examples of Methods/Control Measures

Organisation	Furniture
• Number of staff needed?	• Reposition/remove
• Patient stays in bed	

Equipment
• Variable height bed   • Patient hand blocks
• Hoists   • Rope ladders
• Slings, belt   • Turntable
• Bath aids   • Sliding aids
• Wheeled sami-chair   • Stair lift
• Monkey poles

Examples of tasks
• sitting/standing
• toiletting
• bathing
• transfer to/from bed
• movement in bed
• sustained postures
• walking
• in/out of car

Examples of Problems/Risk Factors

Task	Carers
• Is it necessary?	• Fitness for the task ,freshness or fatigue?
• Can it be avoided?	• Experience with patient? with handling team?
• Involves stretching, stooping, twisting, sustained load?	• Skill: handling, using equipment?
• Rest/recovery time?	

Patient
• Weight, disability, falls etc.

Environment
• Space to manoeuvre, to use hoist?   • Flooring uneven? OK for hoist?
• Access to bed, bath, WC, passageways?   • Furniture: movable? height? condition?
• Steps, stairs?   • Bed: double? low?

(Use a different box each time the assessment is reviewed)

Date(s) assessed:	28/2/94
Assessor's signature:	
Proposed review dates:	31/12/94

© NBPA

FORM 5 Patient Care Plan: Moving and Handling Section (hospitals, residential homes)

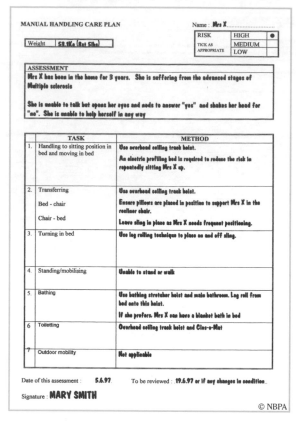

MANUAL HANDLING CARE PLAN   Name: Mrs X.........

| Weight | 53.1Kg (8st 5lbs) |

RISK	HIGH	●
TICK AS APPROPRIATE	MEDIUM	
	LOW	

ASSESSMENT

Mrs X has been in the home for 3 years. She is suffering from the advanced stages of Multiple sclerosis

She is unable to talk but opens her eyes and nods to answer "yes" and shakes her head for "no". She is unable to help herself in any way

	TASK	METHOD
1.	Handling to sitting position in bed and moving in bed	Use overhead ceiling track hoist. An electric profiling bed is required to reduce the risk in repeatedly sitting Mrs X up.
2.	Transferring Bed - chair Chair - bed	Use overhead ceiling track hoist. Ensure pillows are placed in position to support Mrs X in the recliner chair. Leave sling in place as Mrs X needs frequent positioning.
3.	Turning in bed	Use log rolling technique to place on and off sling.
4.	Standing/mobilising	Unable to stand or walk
5.	Bathing	Use bathing stretcher hoist and main bathroom. Log roll from bed onto this hoist. If she prefers, Mrs X can have a blanket bath in bed
6	Toiletting	Overhead ceiling track hoist and Clos-o-Mat
7	Outdoor mobility	Not applicable

Date of this assessment :   5.6.97.   To be reviewed : 19.6.97 or if any changes in condition.

Signature : MARY SMITH

© NBPA

These examples may be adapted to suit reader's needs. There is no obligation to follow any given format. Note that the control measures shown in the examples are not applicable to general situations, they relate only to the patient's for whom the assessments were made.

WARNING - FORMS WITH CHECK BOXES

Forms with check boxes are easy to fill in but they do create their own risks. It is possible to tick the boxes and fail to provide the detailed information that is needed to explain what has to be done.

Assessors must remember that the purpose of the form is to inform others about what needs to be done. They must not assume that those reading the form have the same level of knowledge.

Managers must take steps to ensure that those carrying out assessments complete the additional information sections of such forms.

CONTROLLING RISKS UNTIL CHANGES ARE MADE

If the solution cannot be put into place immediately the manager must consider interim steps to control the risk. The level of risk depends on the patient and the environment. In many cases the situation is such that there is a delay before the necessary steps can be implemented to establish a safe system of work. For example, a patient in the community may need a height adjustable bed. The manager must commit to provide such beds within an appropriately short time. It ought to be possible to provide a normal bed within 24 hours. Meanwhile, steps must be taken to reduce the risks to staff. Examples of the action that must be taken until the bed is provided are:-

- carers should kneel on the bed or floor to reduce stooping

- provide a hoist or a sliding board for transfers to and from bed

- provide a fabric sliding aid or a hoist for moves up and down bed

- provide a fabric sliding aid for turning in bed

- provide a one-way sliding aid to stop patient sliding down in bed

- keep the patient in bed until equipment is available

- provide extra staff

- provide low stools for carers

Managers must be aware of the many people who may be put at risk in the handling of an individual patient. Those at risk include all carers, family, nurses, physiotherapists, chiropodists, etc.

WHEN A SAFE SOLUTION CANNOT BE FOUND

There will be rare occasions where no safe solution can be found. In such cases the first solution is to nurse the patient in bed or an arm chair until the problem can be resolved. If no action is to be taken to remove an identified risk, and staff are to continue to carry out the task, then the managers must produce a written costed justification of their actions.

The cost justification must show that the costs of taking action to remove the risk were out of proportion to the risk.

This must be done if the employer is to have any hope of defending any claim as a result of running the risk. The cost case must be in writing before any accidents occur (see Chapter 1).

COMMUNICATIONS WITH PATIENTS AND RELATIVES

Assessments in the community are likely to lead to recommendations to move furniture or introduce handling equipment. A particular problem can be the need to replace a double bed with separate beds so that the patient can be properly cared for in a hospital bed. Changes will need to be discussed with relatives and family. If any resistance is encountered, nurse managers must be informed. Managers must take action to eliminate or reduce the risk. If the patient or the family do not agree to the necessary changes, the nurse manager must change the level of service to ensure that staff are not put at risk. For example, it may be necessary to nurse a patient in bed if he refuses to have a hoist. If the patient also refuses to have a height adjustable bed it will be necessary to withdraw service.

Discussion of these subjects can be greatly assisted by the provision of pre-printed booklets that explain the equipment and how it works. The booklet should make it clear that equipment **will** be used if necessary.

Similar problems can be encountered on the ward or in the nursing home. Again, a booklet can be a useful way of reinforcing the need for change.

In the last analysis it is a sign of incompetence for the nurses to continue to offer care without using equipment that has been specified. The nurse is deliberately putting her self or her staff at risk.

ACKNOWLEDGEMENTS

This chapter includes some contributions by Moira Tracy. Moira provided the basis of most of the forms that are shown as examples. Brian Fletcher and Ruth Okunono contributed sections for the community. Thanks are also given to other members of the RCN Back Pain Panel. Contributions from the following institutions are gratefully acknowledged:

1. The Victoria Infirmary NHS Trust, Glasgow

2. Nottingham Community Health NHS Trust

3. Community and Priority Services Unit, Lanarkshire Health Board

4. North Tyneside Healthcare NHS Trust

5. Commicare NHS Trust, Blackburn, Hyndburn and Ribble Valley Health Care NHS Trust

6. Community and Mental Health Services NHS Trust, Glasgow

The section on general manual handling assessments was adapted from Institute for Occupational Ergonomics 'Safer Handling of Loads at Work - A practical Ergonomic Guide' by R BIRNBAUM, A COCKCROFT, B RICHARDSON, N CORLET'T, University of Nottingham, NG7 2RD; 1991.

Bibliography - see overleaf.

BIBLIOGRAPHY

EEC Council Directive:	29 May 1990	Article 16(1) of Directive 89/391/EEC (90/269/EEC)	EC
H.S.E	1992	Management of Health & Safety at Work Regulations – Approved Code of Practice	HMSO
H.S.E	1992	Personal Protective Equipment at work Regulations 1192 – Guidance on Regulations	HMSO
H.S.E	1992	Provision in use of work equipment regulations – Guidance on regulations 1992	HMSO
H.S.E	1992	Manual Handling Operations Regulations 1992 – Guidance on Regulations	HMSO
H.S.E	1992	Workplace Health & Safety Welfare Regulations	HMSO
H.S.E	1993	Residential Care homes	H.S.E.
H.S.E	1994	New & Expectant Mothers at Work – A Guide for Employers	H.S.E.
H.S.E	1995	A Guide to The Reporting of Injuries, Diseases & Dangerous Occurrences Regulations 1995 (RIDDOR)	H.S.E.
H.S.E	1994	Manual Handling – Solutions You Can Handle	H.S.E.
H.S.E	1994	A Pain in your Workplace – Ergonomic problems & solutions	H.S.E.
H.S.E	1991	Successful Health & Safety Management	H.S.E.
H.S.E	1993	The Costs of Accidents at Work	H.S.E.
Health Building Note 40 (new update version now in 4 volumes)	1995	Common Activities spaces	Department of Health & Social Security
HSAC	1992	Guidance on Manual Handling of Loads in the Health Services updated version imminent	H.S.C.
HSAC	1993	Getting to Grips with Handling Problems, Worked Examples, Assessment in Reduction of Risk in the Health Services	H.S.C.
RCN	1996	Manual Handling Assessments in Hospitals and the Community – An RCN Guide	RCN

THE GUIDE TO
THE HANDLING OF PATIENTS

Part Two:

Safer Handling in Practice

TYPES AND FEATURES OF MANUAL HANDLING AND MECHANICAL LIFTING EQUIPMENT

by Julie O'Keefe

INTRODUCTION

This chapter looks at the wide range of hoists and small handling equipment that is now available. The market for this equipment has expanded greatly since the introduction of the Manual Handling Operations Regulations (MHOR 1992). With such an array to choose from it is often difficult to establish what is best for an individual or for several people in an institution such as a ward or residential home.

This chapter aims to:

>   provide detailed advice on the purpose of moving, handling and lifting equipment

>   discuss what needs to be considered when choosing equipment

>   consider the advantages and disadvantages of using different items of equipment

>   consider different situations in which the equipment can be used.

The ultimate aim of using this equipment is to:

>   facilitate independence

>   provide a safe means of moving and transferring a person from one place to another

>   maintain the dignity of the person it is being used for

>   minimise potential hazards that can lead to injury.

Types of equipment are discussed in detail. However, reference to individual products with supplier details may be obtained from the Disabled Living Foundation.

USING AND LOOKING AFTER MANUAL HANDLING AND MECHANICAL LIFTING EQUIPMENT

Training

All staff require thorough training in the use of any equipment they will be using with patients in their care. They should have the opportunity to learn about and try out the equipment before using it to move and handle a person. They should have the opportunity to practise on other colleagues and then be supervised whilst using it for the first time with a disabled or ill person.

It is the responsibility of the manager to ensure that all staff have adequate, up to date training and regular refresher sessions on how to move and handle people safely. All new staff should attend training sessions or be trained by experienced staff where the equipment will be used, and be given time allocated to practise with the equipment.

It is the responsibility of all members of staff to inform their manager if they feel they need more training and practice before feeling confident to use the equipment. Training records should be kept, and these should include details of dates and the content of training courses. Managers should ensure that staff are brought up to date at least once a year.

Training should include teaching staff the importance of documenting what method of moving and handling a person is to be used by the team as well as the exact type of equipment, for example, the name of the hoist and the size of the sling. This helps the whole team to provide co-ordinated care and reduce the risk of injury to themselves and their patient.

Maintenance

The manager is responsible for ensuring that all the equipment used in a hospital or other clinical setting is maintained regularly and that it is kept in good working order. In a person's home, the disabled person or carer, or a visiting health care worker, will need to ensure this is done.

It is useful to appoint one person who will be responsible for seeing that all equipment, particularly mechanical equipment such as hoists, is maintained and regularly inspected for wear and tear. Other routine tasks that are essential such as charging powered hoists, and inspecting the castors to make sure they are running efficiently, should be done regularly: a routine ensures that these tasks are not overlooked. A written record should be kept with the equipment so that it is easy to see when it was last inspected.

If someone using any equipment becomes aware of a fault that is potentially dangerous, or a patient or carer is injured or dies, the details should be reported to the Adverse Incidence Centre (AIC) see useful organisations at the end of this chapter. The AIC will investigate the report and take action. This may be to issue a Device Bulletin, Safety Notice or Hazard Warning. These are circulated to relevant agencies including health service supplies departments, social services, and health and safety officials.

Servicing

British Standard 5827:1979 specification for mobile, manually operated patient lifting devices recommends that hoists should be tested at intervals of not more than 12 months. Many hospital departments have their hoists serviced on contract by the hoist manufacturers.

Care should be taken to plan for regular servicing of a hoist in a patient's home. Responsibility for servicing should be established when the equipment is installed. Problems can occur if the money for the hoist has come from several sources. Although this standard does not officially apply to hoists which are not mobile, it is advisable that these also are serviced every year.

Replacement

Equipment has a limited life – some companies recommend that a hoist is replaced after ten years.

Insurance

When people have bought equipment privately, or have been loaned equipment from statutory or non-statutory agencies, they should consider insuring them. It may be worth including the more expensive items of disability equipment on existing household insurance policies. It is advisable to consult a variety of insurance brokers since many of the companies offer preferential rates to people with disabilities.

Hospitals and residential homes will usually have adequate insurance cover. The premiums can be lower if a regular service contract is arranged with the manufacturer.

MOBILE SLING HOISTS

Mobile sling hoists eliminate the need for manual lifting. They do not give a person independence, but they reduce the physical effort and strain on the carer. They are used to move a person, for example, from bed to wheelchair to bath. Mobile hoists should not be used to transport people over long distances. An overhead tracking hoist or specific wheeled equipment, such as sanichair, should be used instead.

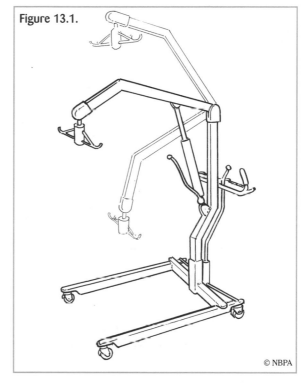

Figure 13.1.

© NBPA

Points to consider when choosing a mobile sling hoist.

Height of chassis –

> a low chassis keeps clearance height to a minimum to get the hoist underneath furniture, such as divan beds or reclining armchairs with filled in bases.

Width of chassis and leg width control lever –

> the front of the chassis can be widened by a hand operated lever, by kicking out the legs using a foot, by foot pedals, or by electrical power. Some hoists have a chassis which widens in parallel at the front and back. Always ensure that the hoist will pass through narrow doorways.

Length of chassis –

a long chassis makes the hoist more difficult to manoeuvre. Note that a longer boom length requires a longer chassis to provide stability during the lift.

Shape of chassis –

the majority of models are U-shaped, others are C-shaped. A C-shaped chassis can be an advantage when lifting someone as the boom and spreader bar are brought in from one side. Many people prefer this as it does not give them the impression that the spreader bar will touch their face while the sling is being fitted. Also, a person can be transferred from a chair into a nearby bed without turning the hoist, by pulling it backwards once the person is comfortable in the sling, and then towards and under the bed.

Boom length –

a longer boom is useful for a taller or bigger person as it provides more leg room. The knees do not have to be on either side of it – instead, both knees can be placed to one side. This can make it easier to position the patient and reduces the risk of knocking the knees.

Rotating spreader bar –

if the boom is angled upwards to form a peak (peaked boom) it usually allows the spreader bar to rotate through 360 degrees. This increases the likelihood of manoeuvring the person into the correct position. Peaked booms bring the person nearer to the mast as the boom rises. Consequently it may be necessary to rotate him so that his knees do not knock against the mast; padded bars are especially important if the boom is peaked since the spreader bar will come close to the patient's face as the boom descends.

Tilting spreader bar –

these are Y or wishbone shaped, with three sling attachment points instead of two. A positioning handle, located at the mast end of the spreader bar, can be used to tilt or angle patients while in the sling, to sit him more upright for positioning on a chair or toilet, or in a reclined position for transferring to a bed.

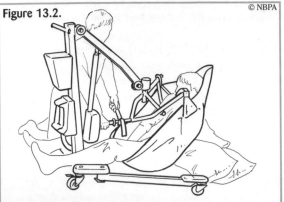

Figure 13.2.

© NBPA

Points of suspension on spreader bar –

the more points of suspension for the sling on the spreader bar, the more comfortable the person will feel. Consequently people may prefer Y shaped spreader bars. Four points of attachment are available on some models.

Lifting height –

this indicates the lowest and highest height of the spreader bar, but should be used as a guide only. The lifting height will depend on the size of the person and the size and style of the sling. If a hoist is to lift someone to a high surface, such as a treatment couch or a bed on raised blocks, it should be tried out with various slings and different sized individuals.

Lifting from the floor –

most models will lift from the floor someone who has fallen over. Some require extension hangers that clip to the spreader bar, and some companies recommend a sling that is one size larger than would usually be used.

Brakes –

brakes are fitted on almost all models of hoist. They are not normally applied unless the hoist is being used on a slope, or if the patient's legs are likely to go into extensor spasm, causing the hoist to move. It is often better to leave the brakes off when using the hoist on a flat surface as the hoist will then move towards the person when the weight is taken, rather than move away, and this reduces the risk of injury. Also, when lifting from the floor or lifting with a hoist which has a peaked boom, if the spreader bar gets too near to the person's face, the hoist can be pushed away quickly using a foot. Brakes should be easy to operate.

Castors and wheels –

small front castors and wheels keep clearance height to a minimum so that the hoist can be positioned underneath furniture, such as divan beds. Larger rear castors and wheels offer less rolling resistance and are easier to push around on certain floor surfaces, especially carpet. They also give the person a smoother ride.

Diameter of turning circle –

the diameter is often difficult to calculate, and sometimes it depends on the position of the fifth wheel which acts as a pivot. Hoists should be turned only as a last resort, as this manoeuvre is likely to result in the carer having to twist or turn her spine, which may cause injury. It is preferable to rearrange any obstructions in the working area so that the carer need only pull the hoist backwards. Then, if possible the patient should be transferred to the equipment on which he can be moved from place to place.

Steering Mechanism –

a fifth wheel is sometimes situated at one side of the chassis, or centrally under the mast. It helps the carer guide the hoist in a straight line and is a pivot on which the hoist can be turned on its own axis. Some models have a metal device that is flipped over the rear castors or wheels to lock them parallel to one another so that the hoist can travel backwards and forwards in a straight line.

Capacity –

the hoist should be of the correct capacity for the weight of the person to be lifted. Heavy duty hoists have a capacity of 190kgs (30 stones) or more.

Dismantling –

most hoists must be dismantled to be transported, taken to a patient's home in a car, for example. However, the component parts often exceed the weight guidance in the Manual Handling Operations Regulations 1992. A small number of hoists can be folded, and they are useful where space is limited and storage is a problem.

Weight –

the heavier the hoist, the more difficult it is to push around, especially with a person in it.

Mobile sling hoists can be operated using either a winding handle, hydraulic pump, or battery.

Mobile sling hoists: with a winding handle –

Advantages:

they tend to be cheaper than powered hoists

they do not require charging

the speed of ascent and descent can be controlled easily and accurately

descent or ascent is easy to stop at the required height.

Disadvantages:

the person in one has no control over the lifting action

some winding handles are positioned on top of the mast and wind in a horizontal plane, and carers may have to adopt a poor posture to do this, particularly if they are short in stature. Winding handles at a fixed height on the mast wind in a vertical plane and are less likely to cause this problem

if the carer stands directly in front of the handle which is positioned in the vertical plane, and winds it, there will be increasing stress on the wrist and elbow joints. It is preferable to stand to one side while winding

using a winding handle to lift a heavy person is more strenuous for the carer than using a pump action or battery powered hoist.

Mobile sling hoists: operated by a hydraulic pump –

Advantages:

the pump handle usually rotates so that the carer can operate the hoist from either side, reducing the need to adopt a twisted posture

using a pump action to lift a heavy person is less strenuous for the carer than a winding mechanism.

Disadvantages:

the person in the sling has no control over the lifting action

the speed of ascent and descent cannot always be controlled accurately

although a pump action is less strenuous for the carer than a winding mechanism, it can be tiring if the carer is doing several manoeuvres in a short time or is using several hoists with different people, in the community during the course of the day, or on the ward

the pump handle is often positioned too low for the carer to be comfortable while standing. Sitting on a chair or bed may be more comfortable when pumping

lifting a heavy person with a hydraulic pump is more strenuous for the carer than using a battery powered hoist

hydraulic hoists tend to be jerky in their movements when the patient is being lifted

the handle is a distance from the patient. It is difficult to calm or reassure the patient while operating the hoist. The carer cannot push on the patient's knees for final positioning without excessive stretching and twisting

these types of hoist often need two nurses to move a patient.

Mobile sling hoists: battery operated –

Points to consider when choosing this hoist:

controls – if the controls are on a wandering lead the patient can control the ascent and descent

lifts per charge – it is useful to know, on average, how many lifts the hoist will make without recharging. The figure may vary between manufacturers as there are no standard criteria for testing this. This calculation should not be used instead of a low battery indicator as the power used for each lift will vary according to the weight of the person being lifted, the height of the lift, and so on

removable batteries – batteries that can be removed and recharged away from the hoist may be useful if there is no power point near the hoist. However, they can be a disadvantage in a hospital or home where detachable components can be mislaid

low battery indicator – this indicates when the battery is running out of power. It may be either audible or visual or both. This is often useful in wards or homes where there is a chance that recharging may be forgotten or where irregular use leads to confusion over the amount of charge left in the battery

spare battery – some hoists are supplied with more than one battery as standard, and can consequently be used twenty four hours a day, as required by night staff

emergency stop button – if the patient using the hoist is controlling it, and becomes frightened or starts to have a fit, the carer can stop it immediately with an emergency stop button without using the handset. The button must not be in a place where it can be pressed unintentionally

emergency manual lowering device – if the carer needs to stop the hoist quickly midway through the lift, the person in it would need to be lowered quickly. If the handset can be used this should not cause a problem, but if it is broken or the power fails, a manual emergency lowering device is essential.

Advantages:

the carer expends only minimal energy

if the controls are on a wandering lead the patient can control the lift and have a degree of independence

if the carer is controlling the lift, she can stand close to it and reassure or help the patient as

the mast and boom are not in the way

if the person in it is controlling the lift the carer's hands are free – to guide the legs, for example

the task may be done by one carer only instead of two

batteries located in the base are unlikely to obstruct the patient's legs as he is being lifted and lowered

batteries located on the mast usually have a charging point at the same level so that the carer does not have to stoop.

Disadvantages:

the speed of ascent and descent cannot be varied

batteries must be recharged regularly

they cost more than mobile hoists with a pump or winding mechanism

batteries located in the base will usually have a low level charging point as well. This means the carer may have to stoop to connect the charger

batteries located on the mast may cause an obstruction – patients may catch their legs during ascent and descent

batteries that detach from the hoist may be mislaid in a ward or home

powered hoists are generally heavier to push than manual hoists because of the additional weight of the motors and batteries.

MOBILE SEAT HOISTS

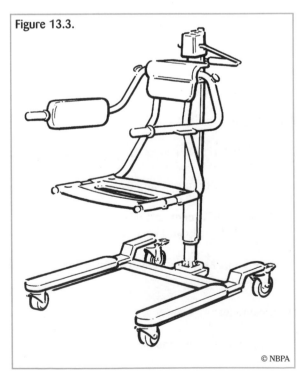
Figure 13.3.

© NBPA

When choosing this hoist the general points in the section above dealing with mobile sling hoists should be considered.

Mobile seat hoists enable a carer to lift and transfer a person in a seat as opposed to a sling. Seats give less support than slings, so the patient has to be given help to balance. He can face forwards or sideways.

Mobile seat hoists can have several optional extras including:

a commode pan so that the hoist can be used as a commode

leg rests that allow a person to extend his legs while being transferred. The angle of his legs can be varied using different length straps

weighing scales so that the person can be weighed while seated on the chair without having to be transferred to scales. These scales are available for all types of hoist

a detachable sub-chassis that forms a mobile chair which can be used as a sanichair, reducing the number of transfers the patient and carer have to make.

MOBILE STRETCHER HOISTS

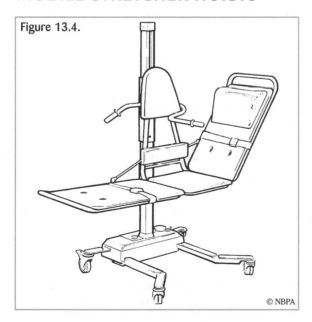
Figure 13.4.

© NBPA

When choosing a mobile stretcher hoist the general points in the section on mobile sling hoists should all be considered.

Mobile hoists with a stretcher attachment have a longer chassis than seat hoists and this makes them more difficult to manoeuvre. They enable the carer to lift and transfer someone in a semi-reclined or supine position: to move a person, for example, from a portering trolley to a treatment couch.

TOILETING/STANDING HOISTS

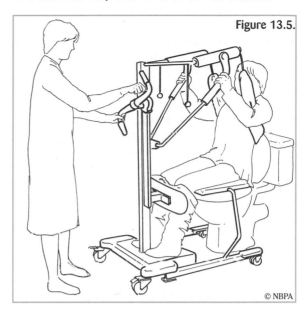
Figure 13.5.

© NBPA

Toileting/standing hoists can be manually operated or battery operated, and the features discussed in Mobile Sling Hoists, above, should be considered when one is being chosen.

Toileting/standing hoists can be used alone or as part of a dual purpose hoist that has an interchangeable boom and spreader bar, so that it can also be used as a standard mobile sling hoist. To convert it from a standard sling hoist to a standing/toileting hoist, the spreader bar is slid out from the boom and replaced with an alternative one. This consists of two fixed bars that project upwards at an angle. A narrow loop sling is attached with hooks at either side. Some models have handgrips below these hooks. A knee pad is inserted at the base of the mast and a footboard is attached to the rear of the chassis.

With a toileting/standing hoist a carer can transfer a person from sitting to standing and if necessary move him while standing. This is useful for transferring a person to the toilet as one carer can then remove clothing and wipe that person's bottom or change a continence pad, or wash the lower half. Additionally it gives a patient some independence while needing help to stand but not in need of complete support from a supportive sling such as a hammock or divided leg.

The commonly used sling for this manoeuvre is a narrow padded band sling which is positioned around the lower back and underneath the arms, halfway down the patient's back and not under the axilla. However, some manufacturers make slings with restraining straps to go around the front of the patient's body. These are useful if a patient unexpectedly lifts up his arms. The knee pad allows him to brace his knees once he is standing. The carer should make sure that the patient has enough strength in his upper body to be lifted from this position.

This sling should only be used with someone who can take some weight through the legs, although this is not always essential. The sling is not suitable for all, and special care should be taken with anyone who is confused or who may move awkwardly and slip through, or with someone who has weak or painful shoulder joints, for example from hemiplegia or arthritis, as there is a risk that the shoulder joint could sublux.

A patient must be assessed by a competent person to establish whether or not this type of sling is suitable for him. A check should always be made with the patient's occupational therapist or physiotherapist if there is any doubt.

A person who is being transferred may prefer to be supported in a sitting position rather than standing. A seat support can be inserted into the chassis base and this helps to redistribute weight from the back and arms and increases the person's comfort. However, hoists should not be used as a method of transport over long distances. A ceiling mounted hoist or specially designed wheeled equipment, such as a wheelchair or sanichair, which have wheels larger than the castors of a hoist, should be used instead as they are much easier for the carer to push and manoeuvre.

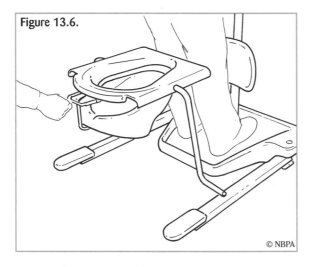

Figure 13.6.

© NBPA

Things to consider when choosing a dual purpose toileting/standing hoist:

> the ease with which the spreader bars can be exchanged

> the weight of the spreader bars

> the size and the bulk of the spreader bars

> where the spare spreader bar will be stored.

Note that the replacement spreader bar may need to be lifted above waist level to be fitted, although if the hoist boom is lowered, the spreader bar can often be handled at a safer height.

Walking hoists –

Some hoists have the option of a walking harness which can be used during rehabilitation if the patient is unsteady on his feet. These allow the patient to face away from the hoist when wearing the sling, so that the hoist can provide support from above and behind. This type of hoist is also useful for supporting someone while he is being put into a standing frame. Other types of walking hoists provide support with a spade shaped seat and a horseshow shaped arm rest with handgrips.

POWERED OVERHEAD HOISTS

Overhead hoists eliminate the need for manual lifting. In some situations the patient can be independent and control the lift if the controls are on a wandering flex and the patient can put the sling on and off. If the hoist is operated by the carer, minimal effort is needed.

Points to consider when choosing overhead hoists:

Manual tracking systems –

> movement along the length of track (traverse) can be manually operated. Manual operation is more strenuous for the carer who must pull the person, supported in a sling, across the track. This is usually done with a pulley. These systems are becoming less common because of a risk of injury to the carer.

Powered tracking systems –

movement along the track is powered by one of these methods, using a hand held control:

1 Mains power with a visible cable that extends from a point on the track to the hoist motor. As the motor traverses along the track the cable moves along with it. Generally, these are suitable for moving distances of up to three metres.

2 Mains power with the cable concealed within the track

3 Mains power with a built in power conductor along the track and no visible or concealed cable.

4 Battery power with a charging point located on the track. The hoist motor should be returned to this point after travel to ensure that the battery is recharged and the hoist remains operational. Note that the patient can travel for longer distances using these concealed power sources.

5 A battery back up system with some mains powered models means a person can still be transferred if there is a power failure.

Rotating spreader bar –

all spreader bars rotate through 360 degrees, giving more opportunity to manoeuvre the person into the correct position. Padded bars are important as the bar is often brought in close to the patient's face.

Points of suspension on spreader bar –

the more points of suspension for the sling on the spreader bar the less scrunched up the person will feel. Consequently, some may find Y shaped spreader bars more comfortable.

Tilting spreader bar –

these are Y or wishbone shaped, with three sling attachment points instead of two. A positioning handle can be used to tilt or angle the person in the sling, to sit upright to be put on a chair or toilet, or in a more reclined position to be transferred to a bed.

Lifting range –

this is the height that the hoist is able to lift in one manoeuvre. The lifting tape can be extended, for example, if used in a room with high ceilings. However, the actual height through which the hoist can lift cannot be extended.

Lifting from the floor –

most models will lift a person from the floor. However, some require extension hangers that clip on to the spreader bar; some companies recommend using a sling that is one size larger than the person would usually use.

Emergency lowering system –

a manual wind down facility or a battery powered device should be available so that the person can be lowered in an emergency, such as during a mains power failure. Systems of this kind are for lowering only.

Controls –

a splash proof handset enables the hoist to be used safely in a bathroom. However, the handset should not be fully submerged in water. Manufacturers may be able to supply waterproof controls at extra cost. Air pneumatic controls are an alternative to waterproof. Infra red controls are available and work like a remote television control, having no wanderlead connected to the hoist.

Capacity –

always check what an individual weighs to ensure that the correct capacity hoist is used.

Heavy duty hoists are available with a capacity of 191kgs (30 stones) or over.

Types of powered overhead hoists include, ceiling track hoists, gantry hoists, X–Y tracking, free standing and wall fixed:

Ceiling Track hoists

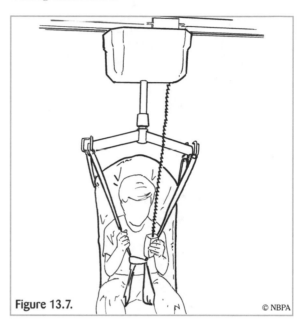

Figure 13.7.   © NBPA

Points to consider when choosing a ceiling track hoist:

Layout and design –

the layout, design and position of furniture in the person's home or on a ward: do these allow a straight track to be used? Could the patient transfer from bed to wheelchair, to bath and toilet without turning a corner? If not, can the room be rearranged in some way?

Incorporating turns –

ceiling tracking can incorporate angle and turns. Angled tracks can often make major adaptations, such as putting a bath in a new place, unnecessary.

Turntables –

ceiling tracks can incorporate a turntable device. The carer can then turn the person by hand so that travel can continue along the track in another direction.

Portable units –

a hoist light enough to be moved by hand may be useful. These hoists can be detached from one track and used on others in different places, for example over the bath, over the bed, and over the toilet. These can be useful in hospitals and residential homes.

Advantages

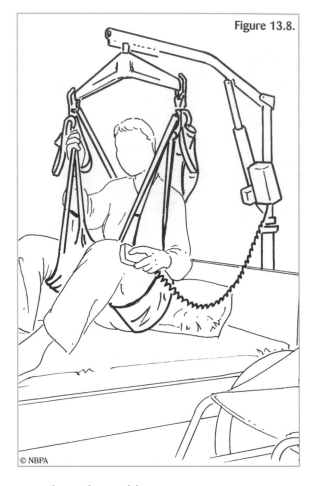

Figure 13.8.

© NBPA

reduces the need for storage space

the person in it can retain some independence if able to control the lift

a patient can transfer without help if able to negotiate the slings

there is less risk of injury to the carer than with a mobile hoist

they are safer than mobile hoists when transporting a patient over longer distances.

Disadvantages

they are permanent fixtures which may require structural alterations to be made to the property before installation

the pick up and set down points are limited to the line of the track

angled tracks are more expensive than straight tracks

a turntable limits an individual's independence because help is needed to change direction

they are more expensive than mobile hoists.

GANTRY HOISTS

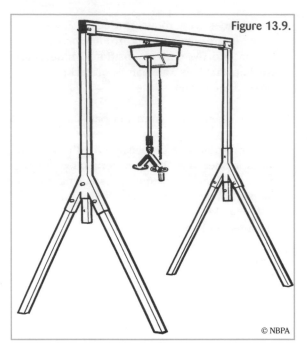

Figure 13.9.

© NBPA

The hoist motor is located on a floor standing gantry A frame.

Advantages

useful as a short term, non permanent solution or where a ceiling fixed hoist is unsuitable, such as when a patient is terminally ill or in temporary accommodation

can be positioned almost anywhere, for example, over the bed to enable a bed to wheelchair transfer to be made

can be moved from one location to another

the person in it can retain some independence if able to control the lift

a patient can transfer without help if able to negotiate the slings

there is less risk of injury to the carer than with a mobile hoist.

Disadvantages

heavy and awkward to move unless on castors or wheels

people do not always feel stable during transfers, but some gantries can be fixed to the wall on one side to increase stability

the pick up and set down points are restricted to the path of the gantry

they are more expensive than mobile hoists.

Wall fixed overhead hoists

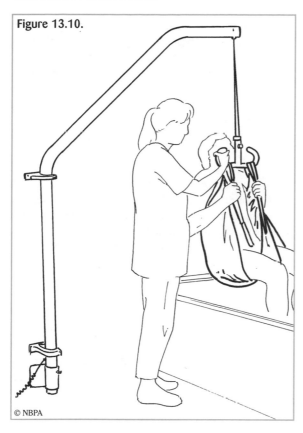

Figure 13.10.

© NBPA

Wall fixed hoists have an arm that can be swung through 90 degrees to enable, for example, a transfer from bed to wheelchair to be made.

Advantages

swinging frames can be fixed in various locations in a ward or home, allowing a portable hoist to be attached

they are useful for transferring people short distances, for example from bed to chair or wheelchair

they can be used in confined spaces where a mobile hoist cannot go

a hand held control on a wandering flex gives the patient the independence of controlling the lift.

Disadvantages

more expensive than mobile hoists

they are permanent fixtures

their use is limited as only a short transfer can be made.

Free standing overhead hoists

Overhead free standing hoists consist of a floor standing cantilever gantry.

Advantages

free standing hoists are easily removable and are useful as a short term solution, for example, for a patient with a terminal illness or one who does not want a permanent hoist

useful for transferring people short distances, for example from bed to chair or wheelchair

can be used in confined spaces where a mobile hoist cannot go.

Disadvantages

their use is limited as only a short transfer can be made

patients do not always feel stable during transfers

they are more expensive than mobile hoists.

X-Y Tracking Hoists

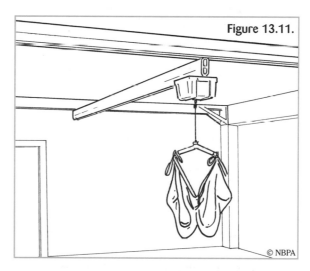

Figure 13.11.

© NBPA

Two parallel tracks are positioned on either side of the room and a moving section of track runs between them enabling a person to be picked up or set down almost anywhere. This is ideal in wards, physiotherapy rooms, and sensory rooms.

Advantages

the pick up and set down points are not restricted to one path of track

no storage problems

the person in one can retain some independence if able to control the lift

a patient can make a transfer independently if he can negotiate the slings

there is less risk of injury to the carer than with a mobile hoist they are a safer than mobile hoists for transporting someone over longer distances

they are less complex to instal than ceiling hoists as they are fixed to the wall or pillar.

Disadvantages

they are permanent fixtures which may require structural alterations to be made before installation

there is extra cost but it is offset by the increased convenience and avoidance of any need to move the installation if the room is changed.

SLINGS AND SUPPORT SYSTEMS

Selecting the correct sling for an individual to wear is crucial for the patient's comfort, function, independence and willingness to use the hoist. Often, people have difficulty accepting the need to use a hoist because the sling has been chosen incorrectly, and does not provide enough support, is too small, or causes pressure and discomfort. Failure to use the hoist may put the patient and carers at risk of injury.

Clothing has to be removed, for example, for toileting, before most slings are put on. This is often unacceptable to patients as it is not dignified.

The choice of sling depends on:

the amount of support a person needs

the tasks to be undertaken

the comfort of the patient when being lifted

the abilities of the patient to help when being lifted

the ability of the carer.

Points to consider when choosing slings:

Sling markings –

BS 5827 1979 Mobile, Manually Operated Patient-lifting Devices, specifies that each sling shall be clearly marked with the manufacturer's name and address, the model number or name of the hoist for which the sling is designed, the safe working load of the sling, the size, and the washing and drying instructions.

Number of slings –

two slings should always be provided for the patient and two complete sets of slings should be ordered for institutional use: when one is being cleaned, another is available for use.

Compatibility –

some manufacturers stipulate that only their slings can be used on their hoists because of liability if there is an accident. However, some companies allow their slings to be used on other companies' hoists. In these cases, it is advisable to obtain written permission from the hoist and sling company manufacturers.

Size –

all manufacturers supply a range of sizes, but corresponding sizes will vary from one company to another. As it is essential to use a sling of the correct size, frequent reassessment is essential, particularly if the person is likely to gain or lose weight. Some manufacturers colour code their slings for size.

Fabric –

different sling fabrics are available including synthetic, which is durable, easy to wash and dry, and fairly easy to place in position. However, it may cause sweating when sat on for a long time. Mesh is preferable for bathing transfers as it allows the water to drain through and dries quickly after use. Sheepskin lined and quilted slings are more comfortable to use, particularly for someone who is sitting on them for a long time, but they are not designed for pressure relief.

Amount of fabric –

the more fabric there is in a sling, the more support it will offer and the larger the area over which the person's weight will be spread. Hence, hammock slings, which have more fabric, cause less pressure and are consequently usually more comfortable than band slings. This is particularly important for people who are susceptible to pain.

Loops or chains –

these are attached to the sling and they hook on to the spreader bar. They should be used to position a person in the sling and not to try to increase or decrease the size of the sling. It may take several attempts to position the patient successfully and comfortably. Once this has been done, marking the loops or chains that have been used will avoid wasted time in the future. Chains look more institutional than loops and may not be acceptable to everyone.

Points of suspension –

the more points of suspension for the sling on the spreader bar the less enclosed or scrunched up the patient will feel. This is an important consideration for people who are susceptible to pain. Hoists with more than two points of suspension are common.

Putting slings on –

A good posture must be maintained while putting slings on.

If possible, the bed or treatment couch should be pumped up to a comfortable working height (usually waist height).

When the leg or foot rests are left on the wheelchair, commode or arm chair it is easier to position the slings underneath the thighs if the person's legs are supported.

It is incorrect to stand and bend over to lift the legs up. The carer should squat in front of the patient and rest the patient's foot on her thigh so there is enough room under the patient's thigh to manoeuvre the sling.

Band slings

These are usually two pieces of fabric in a small and narrow rectangular shape.

Following a Department of Health hazard notice, it is not recomended to use two band slings with any patients.

Hammock slings

These are usually a rectangular piece of fabric and may be with or without a commode aperture.

Advantages

this sling provides support and comfort for the patient as the body weight is supported over a large area of fabric, and pressure areas are unlikely to form

it can be used to lift a person from the floor

the patient does not need to cooperate.

Disadvantages

hammock slings are difficult to put on and take off when the person is seated and it is usually easier to roll someone on to the sling when he is lying down

patients often have to remain sitting on this sort of sling, so the type of fabric is important as increases in temperature and a crumpled sling will increase their discomfort and the risk of pressure sores, particularly important for people who have a loss of the sense of touch

this sling is usually available with or without a commode aperture and provides little or no access for washing

patients cannot put the sling on independently

if the sling is fitted incorrectly and the patient goes into an extensor spasm, it is possible that he could slide out

if this sling is used for toileting the person's clothes will need to be removed before hoisting and he will have to go back to the bed to get dressed again.

Divided leg slings

A divided leg sling is a U shaped piece of fabric with or without head support.

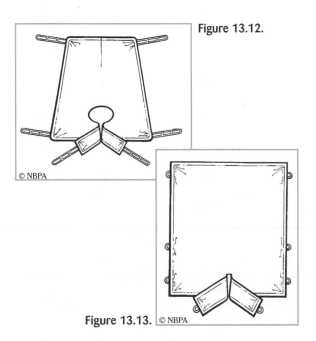

Figure 13.12.

© NBPA

Figure 13.13. © NBPA

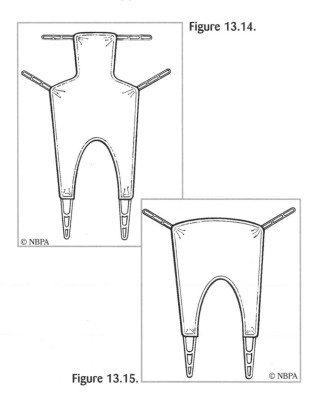

Figure 13.14.

© NBPA

Figure 13.15.

© NBPA

Advantages

they are available with or without a commode aperture. They provide good support as long as they are positioned correctly, with the commode aperture lined up and the leg bands under the patient's mid thigh

they are generally comfortable as the person's body weight is distributed over a fairly large area. However, pressure on the thighs may become uncomfortable

this sling is easily put on while the patient is sitting or lying

it can lift from the floor

the patient does not have to cooperate

The leg bands may be used in a variety of ways. Three examples:

A leg band under each leg and crossed over in the middle keeps the person's legs together and is dignified, although it restricts access for toileting and washing. With care the sling will not crumple under the thighs to cause discomfort and pressure. Some makers have a system of loops which holds the leg pieces together, so that the person's legs are held in adduction without having to cross the loops over. With the leg bands in this position and the correct sized sling, it is virtually impossible for someone to fall out.

A leg band under each leg but not crossed in the middle keeps the legs apart and is not dignified. However, it gives good access for toileting and washing.

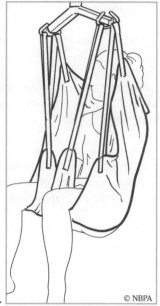

Figure 13.18. © NBPA

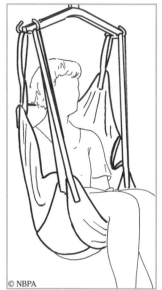

Both leg bands under both legs keep the legs together. Care is necessary using this method with a patient who has a neurological condition as he may slide out if he goes into extensor spasm.

© NBPA **Figure 13.19.**

Disadvantages

the need to remove clothes for toileting before hoisting may mean the patient must first be transferred to a bed

with both leg bands under both legs the patient may slide out of the sling if he goes into extensor spasm

the leg pieces can feel uncomfortable

support is not adequate if the leg pieces are too narrow or if they are not positioned correctly under the patient's mid thigh.

Toileting/access/independence slings

These are combination slings that provide split leg support, upper back support, and a thoracic or waist strap.

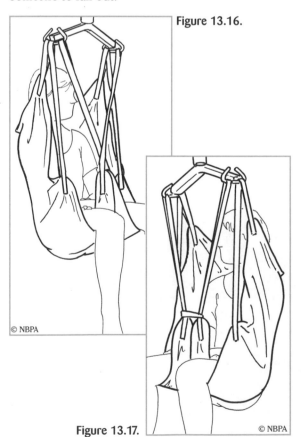

Figure 13.16.

Figure 13.17. © NBPA

Figure 13.20.

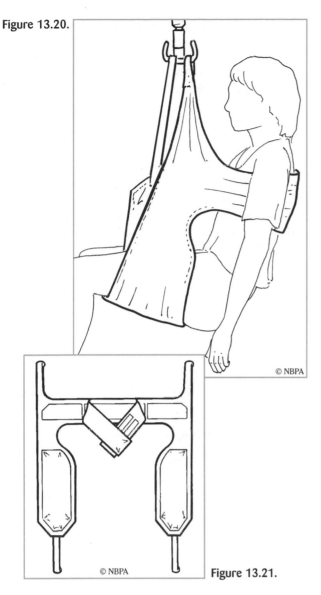

© NBPA

© NBPA   Figure 13.21.

Advantages

this sling can be put on in most positions, sitting, lying on the floor, and so on

the patient may be able to put it on without help

toileting and washing is straightforward.

Disadvantages

it does not provide enough support for everyone: people with reduced or no muscle tone may slip through the sling

although it is available with head support, most patients who do not have head control will rarely have the necessary trunk control to use it

the thoracic/waist band may feel restricting although it does not have to be done up tightly

the patient must cooperate if he is not to slip through the sling as he could raise his arms above the head.

Walking harness/dressing sling/standing harness

These slings are used mainly with an overhead track hoist to assist with walking, standing or dressing. They support the trunk area of the body. They can be adjusted with Velcro straps.

Figure 13.22.

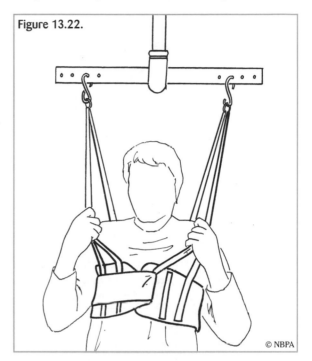

© NBPA

They can also be used with a mobile hoist to help someone stand up from a chair, especially a chair with a deep seat. The standing harness is often used for rehabilitation by physiotherapists for walking practice or for maintenance of good health, as with kidney drainage.

Amputee slings

Figure 13.23.

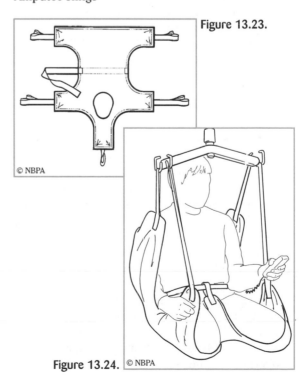

© NBPA

Figure 13.24. © NBPA

Although many manufacturers sell specially designed amputee slings, a one piece or hammock sling used on a conventional spreader bar may serve just as well. However, the sling may need to be supplied with extra long straps or chains at the front edge if the person is to sit upright.

Stretcher slings

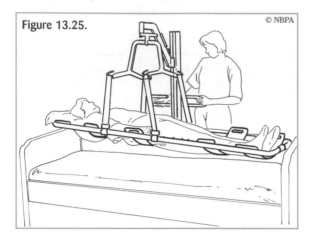

Figure 13.25.   © NBPA

These are used to transport a person lying supine. Some stretcher slings are made of fabric, others are solid. If they are to be used during an x-ray, they should be x-ray translucent. The solid stretchers are usually made of several components and this makes it easier to transfer the patient: the two halves of the frame are placed around the patient lying on the bed, or floor, and then joined together. The supporting slats are then slid under the patient's body at regular intervals and clipped into place.

Made to measure slings

The majority of manufacturers will adapt or produce slings to meet an individual's specific needs. However, a sling will often take up to eight weeks to make and can be too expensive. In addition, there is no guarantee that it will solve the problem as there is no way of trying it before it is made. It is best to be sure there is no ready made sling which is suitable before ordering a special even if it means trying many different styles and sizes.

SMALL HANDLING EQUIPMENT

Small handling equipment enables a person to be transferred from one place to another, for example, from wheelchair to bed or wheelchair to commode, with or without assistance. When a carer is assisting someone and using small handling equipment the carer will usually have to take some, if not all of the person's weight.

Guidance on patient handling must be followed to avoid injury.

Most types of handling equipment require the full cooperation of the person being moved for it to be done safely. If the carer believes that the patient will be deliberately uncooperative – or inadvertently uncooperative because, for example, he does not understand what is happening – other equipment such as a mobile hoist should be used.

Small Transfer Boards

Small transfer boards are used to slide a patient from one level surface to another, for example, from bed to wheelchair or wheelchair to commode. They are usually tapered at either end to assist the transfer. A person moving himself must shuffle his bottom and use his arms and legs to move sideways. If necessary, a carer can help the person to do this.

Where possible, the patient should be encouraged to use his arms and legs to lift himself across to avoid rubbing on the transfer board, which can lead to skin marking and pressure.

This is particularly important for people with reduced or lost sense of touch, for instance, with a spinal injury.

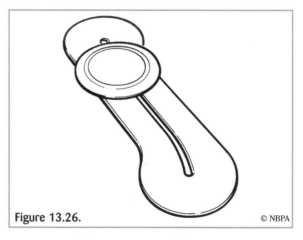

Figure 13.26.   © NBPA

Transfer boards with low friction sliding material and moveable sliding sections are helpful as the friction occurs between the board and the material or the moveable section, and not the person's skin.

Advantages

the boards are cheap, portable and relatively easy to use

they are available in various widths, lengths and curves

a curved board is especially useful on chairs as it makes it possible to transfer people around fixed armrests. It is also useful in cars, as the open car door often interferes with the use of a straight board, and a curved board allows the person to transfer more easily to the middle of the car seat.

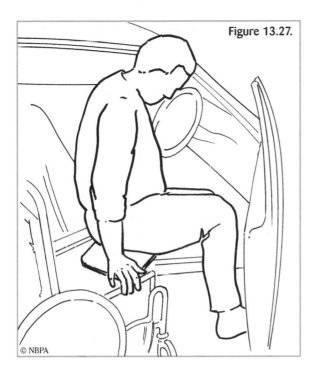

Figure 13.27.

Disadvantages

two level surfaces are advisable for an easy transfer.

the person to be moved must have some degree of sitting balance

the edge of the board can sometimes cut into the patient's skin, particularly if he has a reduced or lost sense of touch

many of these boards have no handles so that some people may find them difficult to pick up and position correctly

they can be too heavy for some people

fingers may be trapped under the ends of the board

a carer giving help must take care not to twist during the transfer.

Supine transfer boards

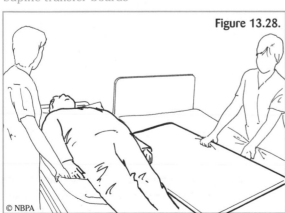

Figure 13.28.

A supine transfer board is a solid, large board with a slippery surface which is used to transfer a person in a supine position from one level surface to another, such as from a trolley to an operating table or from a bed to a stretcher. It is sometimes used in conjunction with a sliding sheet (see following section).

Advantages

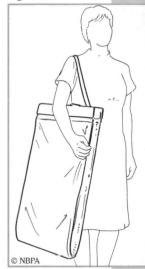

Figure 13.29.

there is no need for manual lifting

the board is easier to store than the fabric version as it can be hung on the wall or stored under a trolley. Some solid models may fold

it is easier to clean than the fabric version which needs frequent laundering

some have built in handholds

some are radiolucent and can be used in X-ray or MRI departments.

Disadvantages

when a person is transferred from one surface to another, the two levels should preferably be the same or similar height, although it is possible to transfer from a higher surface to a lower

the board is less comfortable than the fabric version

not all models can be sterilised, so some may be unsuitable for use in such places as operating theatres.

Sliding sheets and netting

Large sliding sheets and netting are used to slide a person lying supine from one level surface to another, for example from bed to stretcher, or from trolley to operating table. One or two carers can then guide the person in the required direction by pulling the sheet. Some models have hand loops sewn into the fabric for the carers to grasp.

This sheet can be used to slide under a person who has fallen in a tight or awkward space and who needs to be moved to where he can be hoisted.

Low friction fabric rollers

Low friction fabric rollers enable independent or assisted movement to be made:

in one direction only – a person lying on one can slide up the bed but is prevented from slipping down again

in more than one direction across a level surface, from trolley to examination couch and back, for example, or up and down the bed.

A low friction material roller is similar to a cross section of a sleeping bag which is open at both ends. It is padded, and the inner surface is made of a slippery material.

Small low friction fabric rollers (large cushion size) can be used:

independently – a person with good sitting balance and sufficient arm or leg strength may be able to slide from one surface to another or up and down the bed. He should use arms and legs to push or pull. The roller may need to be placed in position by the carer

with partial help – the roller can be used to slide a person who can push with one arm and one leg while the carer supports the weaker side with a shoulder or through arm technique. It can also be used like a small transfer board to slide a person from bed to wheelchair, from wheelchair to sanichair, and so on

The roller can also be used to turn a person in bed as his bottom can be moved from side to side, and the multi-glides are designed to move in any direction so can rotate a body through 90 degrees to help a person get in or out of bed.

Advantages

the low friction fabric roller is versatile and easy to use

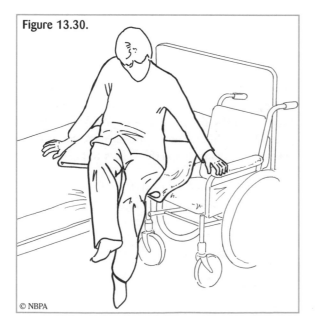

Figure 13.30.

© NBPA

there is no need for manual lifting as the person is slid from one place to another

a person can be rolled on to it easily or, if sitting, the roller can be tucked a short way under his bottom to move him up the bed

low friction rollers with handles allow the carer to secure a firm grip, reducing the risk of injury.

Disadvantages

this roller may not be suitable for someone with pressure sores or a dressing on his bottom as the movement may cause pain, even though the skin does not slide across the surface

the roller should not be used to move heavy people because of the effort needed

some are made of fabric which cannot be wiped clean easily. Precautions must be taken to avoid cross infection if the roller is to be used for more than one person. Ideally, all patients should have their own. Some rollers are made of a waterproof material that can be wiped clean, and others have waterproof covers, but some of these tear easily.

The roller or the covers must be laundered frequently. Consequently, in the community each patient should have two, and a busy ward or residential home should have an adequate supply. Some can be sterilised in the autoclave.

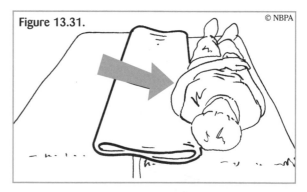

Figure 13.31.

© NBPA

Full length low friction fabric rollers are available in various widths, and are mainly for use in hospitals to transfer people lying down to a trolley or stretcher, or to roll a patient over in bed.

Advantages

there is no need for manual lifting

the fabric roller is more comfortable to use than the board versions

it can be left under a patient in bed, ready to use when the person has to turn. A high friction insert can stop the person sliding down when sitting.

Disadvantages

when a person is transferred from one surface to another, the two levels need to be the same or similar height

the fabric roller is not as easy to store as the board versions as it is more difficult to put it under a trolley or hang on a wall

the cover is not always washable. Some can go through an autoclave and some have disposable covers.

Turning discs

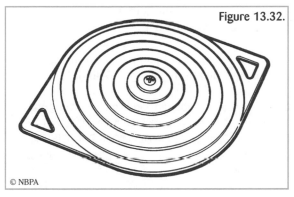

Figure 13.32.

© NBPA

A turning disc is made up of two discs that rotate against one another. There are two types. Some are moulded plastic with a slip resistant surface, on which a person places his feet to move through 90 degrees and make a swivel or pivot transfer. It can be used by someone on his own, or with help from a carer.

The other type of disc is made of two flexible fabric discs with a slip resistant outer surface for standing on, and a slipperey, low friction inner surface. It can be used to move someone's feet in the same way as the solid discs, and can also be used for placing under a person's bottom on a bed or in a chair to help him swivel round. Because they fold up they are easy to carry around.

Advantages

as the transfer is made, the person is swivelled round and his feet do not have to be turned or adjusted

if the person cannot move his legs or feet, but has enough upper body strength to make the transfer, the feet can be placed on the disc and it will automatically swivel round as they move around. This should minimise the risk of the feet being hurt or caught during the transfer

discs with a small handle are easier to move although the handle increases the size of the disc.

Disadvantages

the larger the disc, the greater the risk that it will get in the way of the carer's feet. Small diameter discs are less common, but do not present this risk

for smooth operation the person's weight must be at the centre of the disc, and if he can take weight through one leg only, then that foot should be placed at the centre of the disc so that the disc will rotate. The best position for the foot should be marked so that everyone knows where it is

most discs are subject to friction. Some of the solid discs have ball bearings in their swivel mechanism and should be chosen and used with care as they are difficult to control, especially with light weight patients

turning discs should not be used to turn heavier people, as their weight will preventthe discs turning. However, a carer should not give manual assistance to a heavy person.

Transfer handling belts

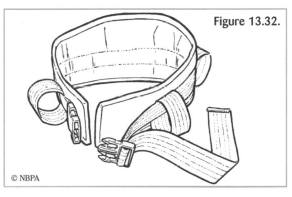

Figure 13.32.

© NBPA

Transfer handling belts are worn by the patient to provide the carer with a safe, secure handle to graps during transfers or while helping the patient with a sliding transfer, using a transfer board, or during walking practice. These belts avoid the need for the carer to grasp the person's clothing. The belt is usually adjustable in length to fit different people and is fastened around the waist with a clasp or buckle. Some are available with integral looped handholds which may be positioned width or lengthways, and these give the carer a secure grip. Padded versions may be more comfortable for some patients.

Handling belts enable the carer to:

have a secure grip

bring the person closer, thus bringing his centre of gravity near to the carer

work in a more upright position.

Advantages

provide a good grip

they are cheap

some people prefer a belt to a sling as it is more secure

if there are handles attached to the belt, it is probably more comfortable for the person using it

a wide, padded belt is comfortable to wear

it can be carried easily, either in a pocket or as part of a uniform

a velcro fastening is quicker and easier to fasten than a buckle, but the hooks can get caught on the patient's clothing, tend not to be so adjustable, and can deteriorate rapidly if not carefully laundered

car seat belt type fastenings are easy to put on.

Disadvantages

the Royal College of Nursing Code of Practice 1996, and the guidance in the Manual Handling Operations Regulations 1992, mean that using a belt around a patient to lift from sitting to standing is no longer acceptable

a belt does not enable a carer to give help from the best position: the patient's weight is more easily moved from his bottom than from the waist

narrow, unpadded belts can dig into the person's waist.

EQUIPMENT FOR MOVING A PATIENT AROUND

Wheelchairs

It is advisable to move patients from place to place by using specially designed transport equipment. The size and position of the wheels on equipment has a greater influence on the ease with which it can be pushed than its weight; large wheels are easier to push than small castors. It is consequently eaiser to move a patient in a wheelchair or sanichair than in a mobile hoist. Other useful wheelchair features include:

flip up foot plates and foot rests

swing away or removable leg rests

swing away or removable arm rests

an elevating seat.

If a carer finds it difficult to push someone in a wheelchair, it is possible to add a powered drive unit which either replaces a front castor or attaches as a fifth central wheel between the rear wheels. This wheel is powered by a battery and is controlled by the carer or by wheelchair user with a joystick. Although the unit is designed to provide assistance over difficult ground or for travelling long distances, the motor and its battery are usually quite heavy and consequently make the wheelchair harder than it would otherwise be to push when it is not switched on.

Patient trolleys

The AT2000 trollery has an extendable transfer surface which unwinds and retracats under the patient, enabling lateral transfers to be made on and off beds and couches at the push of a button. It eliminates all manual handling in the transfer of a patient weighing up to 209kgs (458lbs).

Comprehensive, unbiased and up to date product information can be obtained from the Disabled Living Foundation. Disabled Living Foundation Data-Off-Line and the DLF Hamilton Index contain full details of thousands of products used to move, handle and lift people. Handling people – Equipment, Advice and Information (1994), is a comprehensive resource that covers the legal perspective, ergonomics, different moving and handling environments, access, and transport, as well as product information and supply and provision criteria.

BEDS: HOW TO MOVE PEOPLE IN BED

by Danielle Holmes

SUMMARY

There are many ways of moving patients in bed. There are more than sufficient types of equipment and techniques available to mean that nurses do not have to lift patients who are in bed. However, the first step is to ensure that the patient is in the right bed and has the right mattress. Getting these right can in themselves reduce the patient handling load on the carers.

INTRODUCTION

The first consideration when looking at a patient's handling needs in bed must be "Is the patient in the right type of bed?" The relatively small cost of what are often called 'specialist' beds is rapidly repaid in the improvement in the patient's care and reduced amount of direct nursing effort needed. Putting the patient in the right bed can pay for itself. For example, if patients are in beds that turn them automatically, the number of nurses needed might be reduced. The incidence of pressure sores will certainly be reduced and there will be a real saving in the cost of caring for these wholly avoidable injuries.

The second consideration is to ensure that the patient is on the right mattress. The proportion of patients with reduced or no mobility seems to be increasing. If these patients are to be protected from pressure sores they must be nursed on mattresses that reduce the pressures.

Thirdly the nurse should consider the ancillary devices that are needed to complete the handling task. The employer must ensure that a full range of devices is available.

Fourthly the appropriate handling technique must be selected. This selection should take into account all of the factors listed in Chapter 12 in the assessment of the handling tasks.

Finally the environment must be safe for the handling task to be performed. There must be enough space for the nurses and the equipment to move properly. If there is not enough space there is a risk that someone will be injured reaching to hold the patient or trying to turn a piece of equipment in too small a space (Ref 1).

TYPES OF BED

Most hospitals now use a bed that is known as The King's Fund Bed. This is a height adjustable bed with the a back rest built into the head board. This bed is vastly better than the old fixed height beds that it replaced. Nevertheless, when this bed is used for patients with limited mobility there is a considerable amount of manual handling that has to be done by the nurses. Patients are continually being lifted up to the back rest for meals and drinks and then away from the back rest so that they can lie down. All of this manual handling is time consuming, dangerous for the nurses and dangerous for the patients.

The King's Fund type of bed is not now purchased in other European countries. A number of manufacturers only produce this type of bed because some British hospitals are still specifying it in their purchase orders.

The original King's Fund bed ought to be now considered as only being suitable for patients who are virtually fully ambulant. This type of patient is becoming increasingly rare in hospitals today. Even areas such as ENT have a large proportion of elderly and infirm patients who have other problems that limit their mobility. The original type of Kings Fund beds should not now be purchased by hospitals unless they need it for patients who are fully mobile.

Many hospitals are now buying a bed with a section that raises the head end of the mattress instead of having the older back rest support in the head board. This bed is being called a Kings Fund bed but it might be more properly known as a semi profiling bed. This is better for handling but it is not as effective as a full four section profiling bed.

With effect from April 1998 there will be a European standard for a four section profiling hospital bed (Ref 2). This will, like the King's Fund standard, be a purchasing specification. It will not be compulsory to make or purchase beds to this standard. Purchasers may choose to specify that beds should be made to this standard or to other standards. Most, if not all, UK manufacturers have stated that they will be making beds to the European standard.

N.B. The European standard should not be confused with the CE mark. The CE mark is a manufacturing standard. All medical equipment sold in the UK from June 1998 will have to bear the CE mark. Assuming that the manufacturers comply with the appropriate regulations they will be able to sell Kings Fund beds with a CE mark. This does not mean that such beds are safe for manual handling.

General issues in the selection of beds

All patients must be nursed on variable height beds. It is essential to be able to bring the patient to the right height for each activity. Different heights are needed for giving nursing care; making the bed; getting the patient out of bed, etc. The bed manufacturers specify the heights that their beds can be used at. If the range of heights excludes some staff they will either have to stop staff nursing patients in the beds or be provided with a bed that can be used safely.

Handle operated, variable height mechanisms cause the nurse to stoop with a twisted spine. If the bed is occupied, the effort required in this dangerous position is considerable. Electrically operated beds should be selected when purchasing.

Hydraulic jacks are notorious for breakdowns and can be uncomfortable for the patient. Unless the hydraulics have been properly maintained the movement can be jerky. This is uncomfortable for all patients and is quite disorientating to the confused patient. Electrically operated systems are much smoother and are now quiet enough for the ward environment.

Braking systems can cause back strain either through failure when a patient is being moved or because the levers are difficult to reach or operate. Ensure that brakes are efficient and easy to operate. Avoid beds with brakes operated only on one side of the bed. Make sure that the brakes operate on all four wheels.

Ensure that the bed and hoists are compatible

Check that the chassis of the bed does not interfere with the legs of the hoist. This check must be carried out with the bed in both highest and lowest positions as well as in the middle. Many beds have a chassis or frame to which the wheel and the rest of the mechanism are attached. In some designs, part of the mechanism comes below the chassis at some stages of the cycle. Check that this will not be a problem when using the hoist.

Check that the hoist lifts high enough to lift the patient off the bed. There can be a particular problem lifting large patients off the bed when a pressure relief mattress or over lay is being used.

Make sure that the chosen bed and hoist will work together with the mattresses that are to be used.

The bed must be able to take the weight of the patient. Most beds in the UK are designed to take up to 176kg (28 stones). Any large hospital or community can expect to have some patients who weigh more than this. Therefore it is foreseeable that they will need a few beds that have higher capacities. See below.

Local equipment policies should include a specification for purchase of beds in order to avoid as many of these pitfalls as possible.

Variable Posture or Profiling Beds

These beds consist of three or four platforms that are linked together to form the bed surface. They can be brought into a profiled shape. Most of these beds are operated by electricity and can be controlled by a hand control. The patient can use the control to adjust his own position in bed.

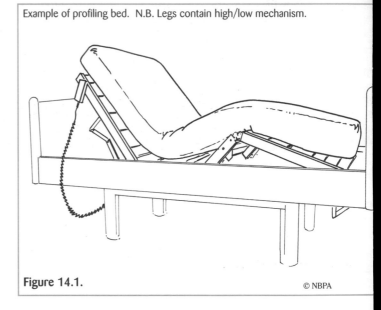

Example of profiling bed. N.B. Legs contain high/low mechanism.

Figure 14.1.   © NBPA

A patient in such a bed can be sat up in bed and laid down without any need for handling. This has many benefits:-

The patient can be moved whenever necessary to ensure that he is not stuck in one place. This can be an important part of avoiding the onset of pressure sores.

If the patient is conscious he can move the position of the bed himself without the need to call a nurse. This is particularly valuable where a patient is being cared for at home and often has to be sat up and laid down at times to suit the nursing arrangements. With a profiling bed the patient can regain a measure of independence and, incidentally, may be able to manage with fewer visits from carers.

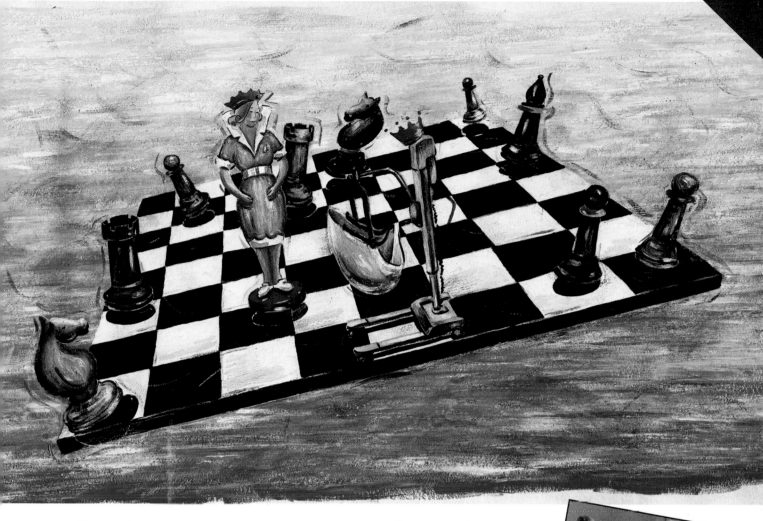
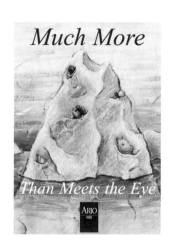
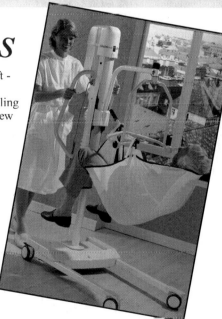
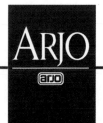

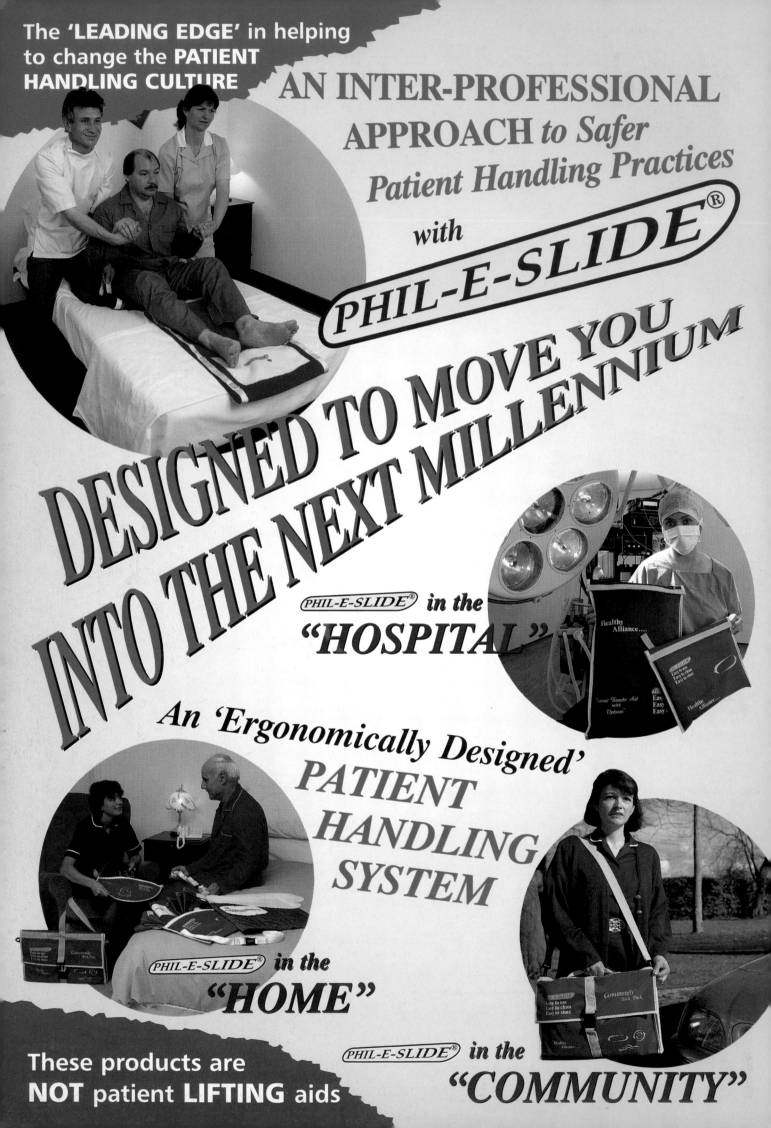

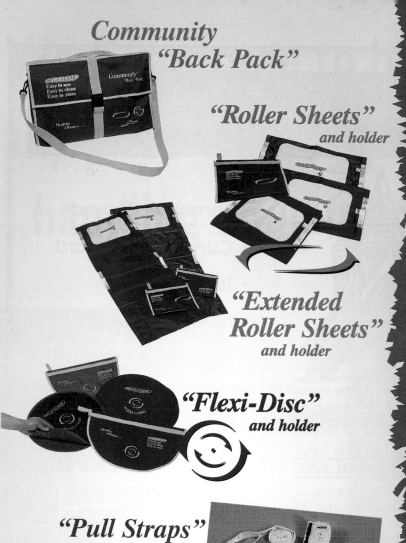
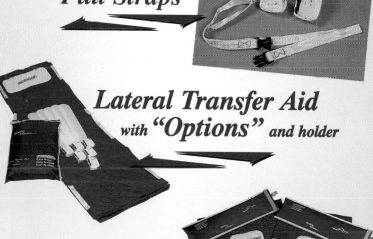
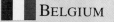 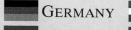
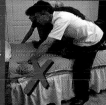
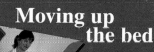
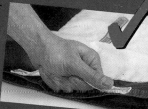

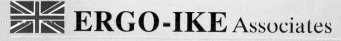

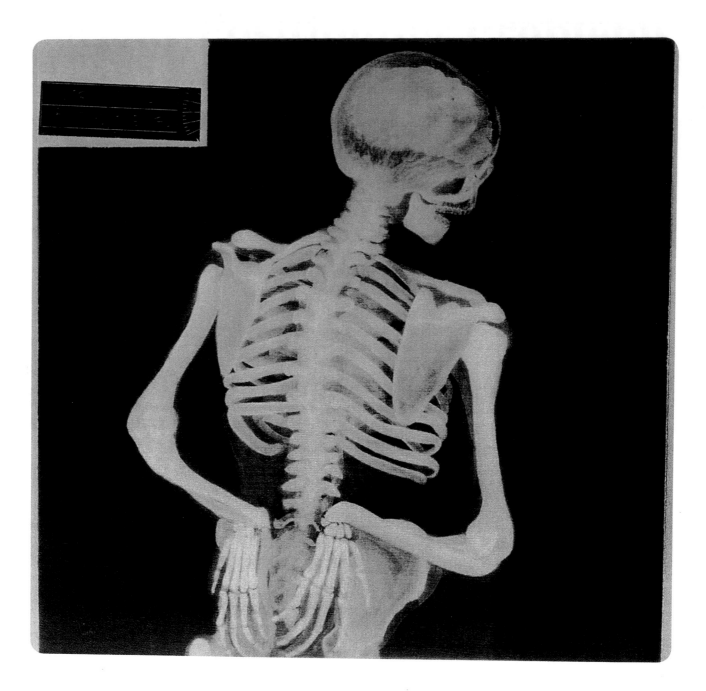

"I want to help my patients without becoming one."

Back pain doesn't kill, it tortures.

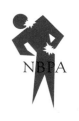

National Back Pain Association, 16 Elmtree Road, Teddington, Middlesex TW11 8ST

Even patients who are incapable of moving themselves can be moved by one nurse.

There is a reduction in nursing costs. Fewer nurses are required for the routine tasks of moving patients in bed. There is a reduction in manual handling and therefore a reduction in days lost with back pain. There is also the longer term benefit of a reduction in losses due to compensation paid to injured nurses.

The costs of moving to this type of bed can be more than offset by the benefits.

These beds are available in all metal designs for hospital use and in designs with wooden finishes to make them more suitable for nursing home and domestic situations.

It is recommended that a purchasing policy is commenced so that over a period of years existing beds will be replaced with variable posture beds in all areas where nurses have to handle dependant patients.

Special Beds

In addition to the above, there is a wide range of beds designed for special purposes, such as following severe injuries or prostration and where pressure sores occur or are likely to occur.

The Air Fluidised Bed

The mattress section of this bed consists of very small beads that are fluidised by a controllable stream of warm air being pumped through them. When the airflow is switched off the support surface solidifies. The fluidised bed provides a surface that spreads the weight of the patient as evenly as possible across the whole area of the patient's body. This reduces tissue interface pressures dramatically.

Any liquid waste that falls into the bed passes through the beads and is collected in a container at the base of the bed. This process takes fluid away from the skin reducing the risks of maceration.

This bed is both heavy and large. It can be hired leased or purchased.

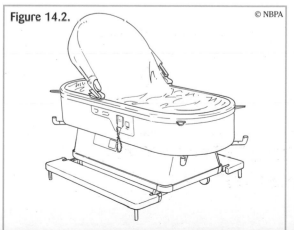

Figure 14.2. © NBPA

This bed is appropriate for patients who will remain in the bed for an extended period to recover from their injuries. It is suitable for patients with severe injuries including burns. It is also suitable for patients who are suffering from severe pressure sores, thermo regulation, flap and graft surgery and for those patients who need pain relief.

The air fluidised bed is not suitable for patients who will get out of bed on a frequent basis.

A hoist is essential to get patients in and out of this bed if the patient is unable to help himself. An overhead hoist is best. This can be fixed to the ceiling or on a gantry. If it is necessary to use a mobile hoist, ensure that the legs will go underneath the bed and that it will lift high enough to get the patient over the top of the bed.

The older models of the air fluidised bed were heavy and large. Newer models have many improvements but the bed remains large. The beds have built in steps or a platform for nurses to stand on. On the older beds the back rest had to be lifted manually. This lift is unsafe as the strain on the nurses back can be quite large and it is hard to avoid twisting. Some new models now have an electric back rest to ensure that the nurse does not have to lift the patient manually. If the patient is to be sat up this feature must be obtained.

The air fluidised beds can cause back strain in nurses if they are treated like conventional beds. It is essential that staff should be instructed in their use by the supplier when they are installed.

Turning Beds

There are many of these on the market and they should always be provided when heavy and highly dependent patients are nursed. Types include electrically or manually operated turning frames. Turning frames with net mattresses and net suspension beds. Turning beds are extremely beneficial for nursing patients with major trauma, extensive burns and pressure sores.

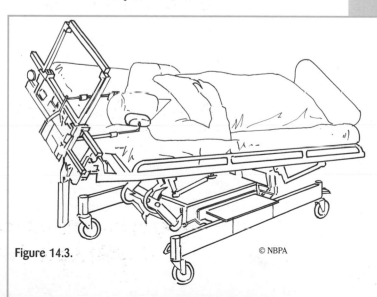

Figure 14.3. © NBPA

Electrically operated turning and tilting beds are often supplied in Intensive Care and Orthopeadic Units. These beds are often particularly wide and nurses should be aware of the need to lean over to reach the patient. Sliding sheets should be used to move the patient whenever possible. Care should also be taken in these units to organise equipment so that patient-handling is not obstructed.

One of the major advantages of these beds is that they can be programmed to operate continuously or at fixed intervals. There is no risk of the nurses failing to make a turn because they are too busy elsewhere. The use of one of these beds reduces the need for nurses to do regular turns of patients. On some wards this represents such a significant part of the workload that actual staff savings can be realised by purchasing this type of bed.

Stand-up-Beds

The bed mattress and frame are pivoted on a mechanism that brings the foot board flat on the floor and the bed to a vertical position. The patient can then shuffle on to a foot board and then from there onto the floor. He can then operate the controls so that the bed returns to its horizontal position. A bar will hold the bedding (usually a quilt) and pillows can be attached with tapes or Velcro to stop them falling.

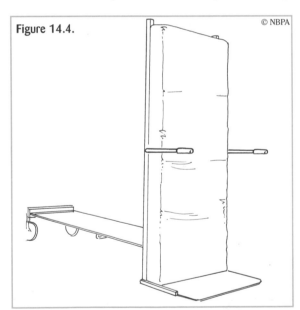

Figure 14.4.   © NBPA

This bed is appropriate for a range of patients:-

    Patients who have fixed hip joints,

    Patients who have undergone back surgery

    All patients whose post-operative management requires no flexion or movement of the spine.

    Patients who must be stood up as part of treatment

The bed is particularly appropriate for patients who have had hip replacements. There are a number of consultants who insist that when such patients are stood up for the first few times they must not be bent at the hip. If the consultant makes such a demand, then the only safe way of standing the patient is with a stand-up bed. A ward specialising in hip operations should have a number of stand up beds to allow the patients to be nursed on these beds for the first week post operatively.

Supine to Prone Turning Beds

These beds are designed to turn a patient over from supine to prone or vice versa. This is a completely different action from a normal turning bed which effectively rocks the patient from side to side. In this type of bed a second mattress is positioned on the frame over the top of the patient; both mattresses are turned completely over with the patient sandwiched in between; the first mattress is then removed. By this means it is possible to turn the patient from a supine to a prone position and vice versa, with a minimum disturbance to the patient and minimum effort for the nurse.

Supine to prone turning beds were originally designed for use with certain orthopaedic patients. They are now sometimes used in other fields.

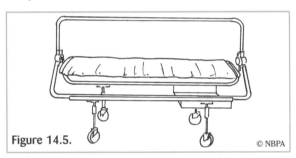

Figure 14.5.   © NBPA

Standard divan beds

The normal domestic divan bed is not suitable for people who need to be cared for by others. However, in the community it is sometimes necessary to extend the use of such a bed. There is a range of equipment that has been designed for this purpose; the bed can be raised to a safe working height; the patient's position in bed can be adjusted or even turned; the patient can be assisted to get into bed with a leg lifter.

Mattress Inclinators

These mattress inclinators are devices that are used in conjunction with a standard divan bed. Inclinators are used to sit a patient up in bed. They are electrically powered. They assist the nurse and keep the patient independent.

There are two different types of mattress variators.

Type 1. is placed under the mattress at the bedhead. These work best with foam or fibre filled mattresses. Hinged mattresses are useful as they allow a greater profiling action to be achieved. .

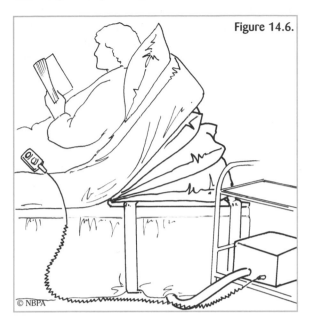

Figure 14.6.

Type 2. Is placed on top of the mattress with a foam pad on top.

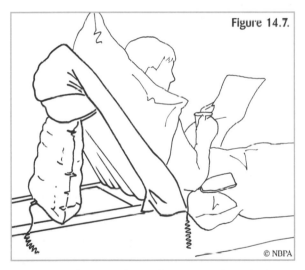

Figure 14.7.

Mattress inclinators do not form an angle at the knee. Therefore, the patient can be pushed down the bed.

Turning Frames

These are also devices that can be used with standard beds. Turning frames will turn the patient from side to side to avoid pressure sores, build up of fluid in the lungs, etc.

A frame is attached under the mattress. Attached to this frame are 2 air bags. Each airbag is the length of the frame and half of the width. One air bag is inflated and the patient is turned onto their side. Once deflated the patient lies on their back. The other air bag is inflated and the patient is turned onto the opposite side.

This piece of equipment can be programmed automatically and the patient can be turned at

predetermined intervals. This turning frame can be obtained with a mattress variator section.

The only limitation on the use of this frame is the girth and the weight of the patient.

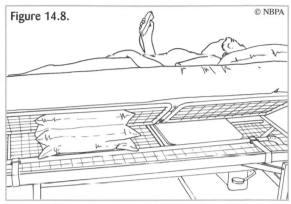

Figure 14.8.

View of airbag as the patient is turning onto their side

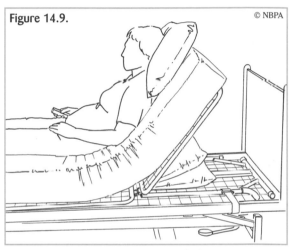

Figure 14.9.

Patient using mattress variator to sit up in bed.
Note: It is possible for the patient to slide down the bed

Bed Raisers for Divan beds

There are two types of device that can be used to change the height of a divan bed. The first type are simple bed blocks. These are extension legs that fit round the existing legs of the bed and raise the bed to a fixed height. This can be useful but has the usual disadvantage of a fixed height bed.

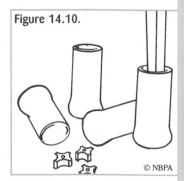

Figure 14.10.

The second type of bed raiser is a mechanical device that provides a variable height lift under the bed. These mimic some of the functions of a high low hospital bed. They do have the disadvantage that they sometimes reduce the stability of the bed and make it more likely to tip to one end. The price of these devices tends to be too high to justify their cost when compared with a hospital bed.

Heavy duty beds

All beds have maximum safe weights for patients. The limit varies from bed to bed. Most standard beds are designed to support patients up to 140 to 176kg (22 to 28 stone). There are some patients who weigh more than these safe limits.

There are beds that are designed to take these very heavy patients. These beds have some of the features of a profiling bed. However, they will usually also operate to move into the shape of an easy chair. This enables the patient to be effectively sat out of bed without being moved.

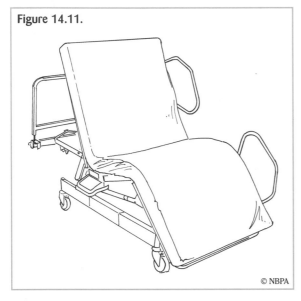

Figure 14.11.

© NBPA

MATTRESSES

The choice of mattress is as important as the choice of bed frame. The standard NHS mattress with a hard plastic surface was impervious to fluids and easy to clean. However, it is also an extremely hard surface to lie on. It is thought that this surface is so hard that it is responsible for a number of pressure sores (Ref 3).

Care must be taken that mattresses are not kept beyond their life span. Most foam mattresses have a life span of less than a year (4). After this point the foam will start to deteriorate and turn to crumbs.

Two recent reports by the Medical Devices Agency examined Static Mattress Overlays October 94 (Ref 4) and Alternating Pressure Overlays April 95 (5). These reports must be read for the detailed advice that they offer in this area. A number of common overlays were shown to be of little or no value in preventing pressure sores.

The choice of mattress can affect the choice of patient handling system. Many sliding systems do not work as effectively with soft mattresses as they do with firm mattresses.

Pressure Relieving Mattresses

There is now a wide range of pressure relieving mattresses ranging from simple foam overlays to sophisticated devices which inflate different sections in patterns to support and stimulate the patient's skin.

It is claimed that the early use of special mattresses can pay dividends. If patients are placed on a pressure relieving mattresses before anything goes wrong, the incidence of pressure sores will be significantly reduced. The misery and costs associated with pressure sores mean that even a small reduction in their incidence will pay for the investment in equipment.

Pressure relieving mattresses include:-

Static mattresses

Fibre filled overlay mattresses

Low air loss mattresses

Alternating pressure mattresses

Bead mattress. eg. a para glide

The amount of relief offered by these products range from simple comfort aids to those that provide a significant reduction in the pressure on the pressure points. The choice of such devices is a specialist subject and is outside the scope of this book.

The use of these mattresses should be approached with care and forethought by the nurse when handling the patient. Although they have great advantages for the patient, they often obstruct the use of handling devices. They also sometimes prevent the nurse from putting her knee on the bed to get close to the patient when sitting him up.

SERVICING AND MAINTENANCE OF BEDS AND MATTRESSES

It is essential for the safety of the patient and the nurses that the mechanisms of the bed are working at all times. Nurses have been injured where the brakes on a bed have failed and the bed has moved at the wrong moment. They have been injured because the bed could not be brought to the right height. Accidents have occurred getting patients off complex beds that have stuck in an awkward position.

The health services have traditionally had a very poor record over the maintenance of equipment. A piece of equipment is used until it falls apart and it is then thrown away. All that might have been needed to keep it serviceable was a few minutes attention with a screw driver and a spanner. Instead it is held together with expensive dressing tape until the nurses can't be bothered and it is too awful to have around. Then it is thrown away.

This culture has to change.

In part, the problem of the maintenance of equipment in hospitals is that to get anything done a 'requisition' has to be produced and passed through several hands. This is the wrong approach to the maintenance of equipment. Servicing and maintenance must be carried out before the piece of equipment is so broken that it becomes unserviceable. Servicing and maintenance or Planned Preventative Maintenance (PPM) is a positive process of checking and servicing the condition of a piece of equipment before anything has gone wrong. We are used to having our cars serviced. Beds need to be serviced as well.

Maintenance (PPM) is a budget item that is easy to cut. However, this is a matter of being penny wise and pound foolish. Anyone who misses out services on his car soon learns this lesson.

There must be an efficient system for repairing the bed. No faulty bed must be left in use.

The following must be properly maintained:-

- Back rests
- Brakes
- Wheels
- Height-adjustment mechanisms
- Profiling mechanisms
- Electric motors
- Hydraulics
- Batteries

Foam mattresses deteriorate quite quickly. They must be checked to ensure that they have not broken down. If they have, they must be discarded. All mattresses must be properly cleaned to maintain hygiene. Low air loss mattresses and similar mattresses where there are mechanical parts must be subjected to a positive servicing and maintenance schedule (PPM).

In addition to the logical case for implementing PPM, employers are required to implement proper maintenance under the Provision and Use of Work Equipment Regulations (1992) (Ref 5).

ANCILLARY EQUIPMENT REQUIRED FOR HANDLING PATIENTS IN BED

Having chosen the right bed for the patient, additional equipment will be required for specific handling.

The main piece of equipment needed to handle a patient in bed is a hoist. Managers must always ensure that there is a hoist available that will work with the bed. (N.B. Particular care should be taken with air fluidised beds where a specific hoist may be required.) A full range of hoists and slings must be available in all ward and nursing home situations. In the patient's own home a hoist must be provided wherever the patient will need lifting in bed.

In addition to hoists, there is a range of equipment that is available to move a patient in bed. These devices will often allow a patient to be handled without the need for a hoist. They fall into three groups:-

1. Devices to help the patient move himself (monkey pole, patient handling blocks, rope ladder etc.)

2. Sliding devices to help the nurse move the patient.

3. Special devices (e.g. leg lifters, female urinal, etc.)

Devices to help the patient move himself

The following aids can be used by patients who have good upper arm mobility, strength and grip.

A monkey pole

This is useful for bridging for the insertion of a bedpan or a fabric slide. It will not help the patient move up the bed.

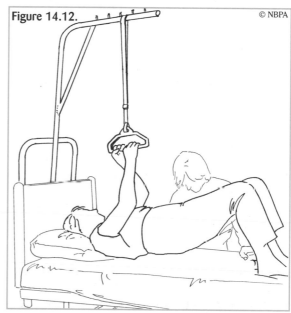
Figure 14.12.   © NBPA

Patient bridging for inserion of a bedpan or fabric slide

Patient Hand blocks

Providing that the patient can support his upper body and lean forward a little then he can use hand blocks to move himself up the bed. The patient must be able to push with his arms. If he cannot lift himself he may be able to slide himself up the bed on a fabric slide.

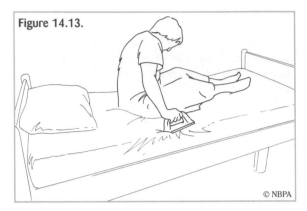

Figure 14.13.

© NBPA

Rope ladders

These are attached to the bottom of the bed. They allow a patient with upper arm strength to pull himself into a sitting position. Even if the patient does not have the strength to lift himself into a seated position he may be able to use a rope ladder to hold himself there whilst the nurse carries out some other action. This is a particularly cheap device. Most hospital will buy this for less than £5.

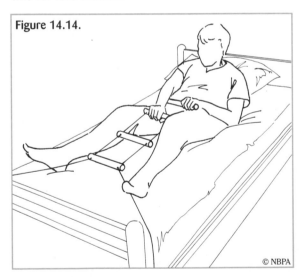

Figure 14.14.

© NBPA

Other devices

There is a wide range of bedside bars, grab rails and handles that should be considered. Some of these are particularly suitable for the long term patient in the community.

Sliding devices to help the nurse move the patient.

These consist of two groups (some devices can be in both groups):-

Sliding Devices for Moving the Recumbent Patient

Sliding Devices for Moving the patient in a sitting position

Both groups include three types:-

Hard sliding boards

Single skin fabric sheets

Cushioned sliding sheets

These devices have many applications in the handling of patients. This section deals only with their use in moving patients in bed.

Sliding Devices for Moving the Recumbent Patient

Lateral transfer systems

These systems move the patient from bed to trolley and bed to bed.

There are various lateral transfer systems and new ones continue to come onto the market. Some are made of material, others are made of board and others are made of rollers.

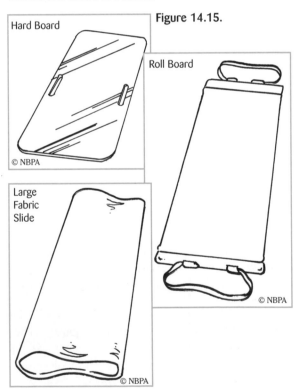

Figure 14.15.

Hard Board

Roll Board

Large Fabric Slide

© NBPA

Systems for moving patients up the bed

There are a variety of sliding sheets and cushioned sliding sheets that are designed to allow the patient to be slid up the bed.

N.B. if the patient is likely to slide back down the bed there are two solutions available. Firstly, it is possible to leave the patient on a one way slide. These stop the patient sliding in one direction but slide easily in the opposite direction. Secondly, the tilting mechanism of the bed can be used to tilt the bed a few degrees towards the head end.

Systems for turning patients in bed

These are cushioned sliding sheets that are designed to work from side to side. They allow the patient to be turned without the need for a turning bed. Providing padded cot sides are available one nurse can easily turn a patient on her own.

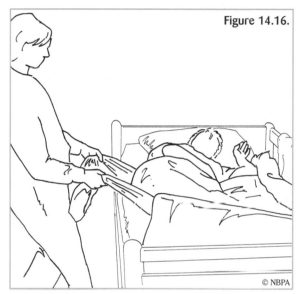

Figure 14.16.

© NBPA

Turning the patient in bed using a cushioned sliding sheet. Note that the cot side is up and padded to protect the patient during the turn.

Sliding Devices for Moving the patient in a sitting position

All devices in this group have uses in transfers other than those involving a patient in bed. They are therefore described in more detail elsewhere.

Sliding boards

These are smaller than the sliding boards used for lateral transfers. They can be used for bridging the gap between the bed and a wheelchair or commode.

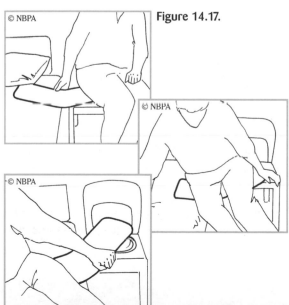

Figure 14.17.

© NBPA
© NBPA
© NBPA

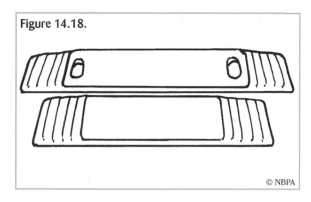

Figure 14.18.

© NBPA

Sliding sheets

Simple fabric sliding sheets consisting of a loop of fabric can be used in a number of ways. They can be used to move a patient up or down the bed. They can also be used in conjunction with sliding boards for transfers from bed to chair.

These slides can also be used to turn a seated patient so that he faces the side of the bed. This is useful for turning a patient who has been sat up from a recumbent position. The patient can be easily turned so that his feet are over the edge of the bed.

Cushioned sliding sheets

These can be used in all of the same circumstances as sliding sheets. In addition they can be used to bridge across a small gap to a wheelchair without the need for a sliding board.

Turntables

Until recently, all turntables were made of hard materials. These are not suitable for use in bed. There are now a number of fabric turntables that can be used in bed to turn a patient so that his legs are over the side of the bed ready for standing. Some of these are also designed to be used in car seats to facilitate turning the patient into the seat. Fabric turntables can also be used on the floor if at least one side has a non-slip surface.

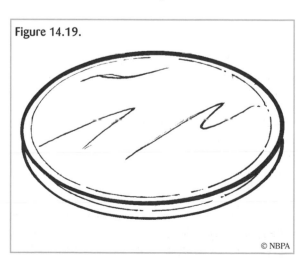

Figure 14.19.

© NBPA

HANDLING ON THE BED

Background

Most patient handling techniques do not follow the normal patterns of movement in the human body. This is necessary because the nurses would find it impossible to give assistance to the patient following the normal pattern of movement. An example is sitting up in bed. The methods described in this section show the patient being lifted from supine hinging at the waist. This is not a normal pattern. This move requires a great deal of strength even for a fit person. The normal pattern of sitting up in bed is for the person to roll to one side and push himself up with his arm.

The nurse should always consider this aspect when deciding to handle a patient. She should ask herself *"Will he be able to get himself up if I encourage him to move in the natural manner?"* If he can do this he will not need to be handled and will achieve at least some mobility.

Introduction

Nurses handle patients on the bed for 11 main reasons. These are to:-

- move the patient onto and off the bed in a supine position

- move the patient up the bed

- sit the patient up in bed

- turn the patient

- insert and remove bed pans

- change the bedding

- change dressings

- dress and undress the patient

- transfer the patient to a wheelchair or commode

- prepare a patient to stand up

- put the patient back to bed

There are two techniques that are used in many different situations. These are the log roll and sitting up in bed. They are described separately.

Log Rolling

This technique can be used to turn a patient to one side. In this position, equipment such as a sliding sheet can be inserted. The patient can then be rolled back and the manoeuvre completed. This technique is used for a variety of purposes including changing bedding and inserting hoist slings. It may also be part of the procedure for turning a patient in bed.

The bed is first brought to the nurse's waist level. The log roll is then done in four stages:-

Stage 1 The patient's head is turned to face the direction of intended movement.

Stage 2 The near side arm is bent at the elbow and placed out of the way. The upper arm should be pointing away from the patient's body, i.e. approximately parallel to the line of patient's shoulders.

The farthest arm is placed across the patient's chest.

Stage 3 The farthest leg is bent at the knee or crossed over the near side leg.

Stage 4 The nurse then rolls the patient towards herself by using the shoulder and the knee as levers.

Watch Points

1. Always move the patients towards you, never away.

2. Where there is a risk of the patient falling from the bed during the log roll, bed rails should be provided. This is particularly useful if he is being turned single-handed. In a domestic situation, an item of furniture can be used to stop the patient rolling too far. N.B. 1. Cot sides should not be left up unless they are required for other reasons. See the warning about bed rails or cot sides.

3. If the patient is large or awkward there should be two nurses to perform the manoeuvre. With these patients a third nurse is often needed to help from the opposite side.

A patient may be large or awkward if he:-

a) is unable to assist

b) is confused and or uncooperative

c) has multiple injuries or pathology

d) has pain

e) is attached to medical equipment

d) weighs over 152kg (24 stones)

There will be some patients who are not suitable for the log roll. These are extremely heavy patients,

patients who will resist the movement and those with frail shoulders and or knees. In these cases use a different approach. If the patient is to be moved he will have to be lifted using a slat type stretcher with a hoist.

4. In cases where rolling presents a risk, for example following hip surgery, the triangular wedge or the Immoturn can be used. The patient is always rolled on to his non-affected side. The Immoturn provides a handle to assist in pulling the patient over. There is no similar handle with the triangular wedge. In principle, patients with the wedge fitted are log rolled. However, as the knee cannot be bent the patient cannot follow the natural patterns of movement used in the log roll. Therefore, the use of the triangular wedge must be approached with caution. The nurses must avoid taking too great a load when lifting the patient's leg. If the patient cannot be moved safely another method must be used.

5. Patients who have had a fractured femur can be turned onto their affected side only. If the patient is large or awkward there should be two nurses to perform the manoeuvre.

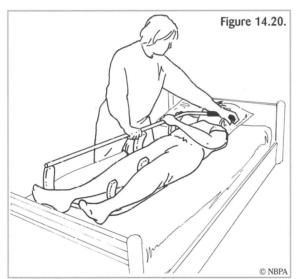

Figure 14.20.

Nurse using Immoturn device for turning patient onto right side.

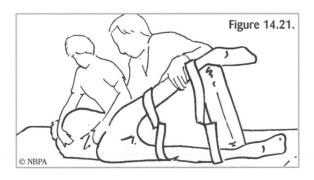

Figure 14.21.

Sitting the Patient Forward in Bed

It is normal practice in hospitals to sit a patient up by bending the patient's body up from a supine position. This is the easiest way of applying force to assist a person but it is not the natural way of sitting up. In normal life, a person rolls onto his side before sitting up. If a person sits up from supine without rolling, there are much greater demands on the stomach muscles. Even fit people do not always find this an easy manoeuvre. Nearly all people in hospital are going to require assistance if they are to sit up in this way. Before deciding to assist a patient to sit up, the nurse must always try to persuade the patient to use his natural body movements to sit up.

Sitting a patient up in bed is a task that must not be taken lightly. The torso, head and arms represent 60% of the weight of a person. Anyone sitting up a patient is at risk of being exposed to half of this weight. In a 70kg (154lbs) patient this represents a potential load of 21kg (46lbs). If there is muscle spasm or the patient is uncooperative the load can be higher.

If the patient is nursed in a profiling bed, the action of sitting the patient can be achieved by the bed. If the nurse wishes to attend to the patient's back the patient can be brought to a sitting position by raising the head end of the bed and held there whilst the bed is lowered to provide access to his back. A similar result can be obtained by the use of mattress variators or inclinators. Both profiling beds and mattress variators can push the patient down the bed. The foot end should be raised to stop this happening.

If possible, always allow the patient to move himself. A simple device such as the rope ladder, or alternatively a rope with knots in it can be fixed to the bottom of the bed to allow the patient to pull himself forward. (These devices may at least allow the patient to hold himself forward once he has been sat up.) Monkey poles are less useful in this situation as they are wrong for the biomechanics of sitting.

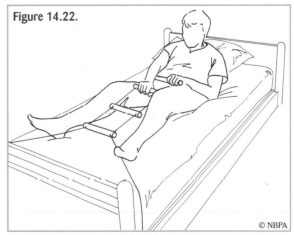

Figure 14.22.

Patient using rope ladder to sit up in bed.

The following manual procedures should only be used if the patient is able to use his stomach muscles to assist in the act of sitting up. If the nurse is providing more than 10kg (22lbs) of force the procedure should be changed to use mechanical assistance.

> Sitting the patient forward in bed for attention to pillows, back washing etc., is a seemingly simple procedure that can cause injury. A nurse who is behind the patient adjusting pillows is in a poor position to take the load if a weak patient flops against her.

With One Nurse

For the patient who can help himself. (He must be alert, able to follow instructions and not the type of patient who will fight the nurse.)

The nurse faces the patient. The bed must be in a low position. She places her nearest knee and foot on the bed at the level of the patient's hip and sits on her ankle. The nurse must be careful to get into this exact position otherwise the patient will not be brought up into the sitting position. She offers her near side arm and they use an elbow to elbow grip. The patient brings himself forwards by pulling against the nurse.

If the patient falls back or puts too much weight on the nurse she can simply extend her arm and let him go back onto the bed.

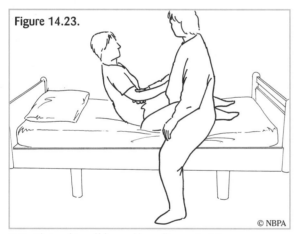

Figure 14.23.

Patient brings himself forward by pulling against the nurse.

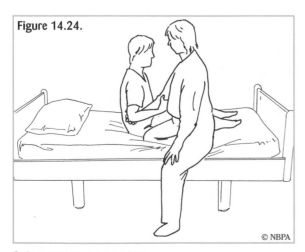

Figure 14.24.

Patient now into sitting position.

With Two Nurses

The nurses face the patient. The bed is adjusted to a low position. Each nurse places her nearest knee and foot on the bed and kneels on the bed. The nurse must place her knee at the level of the patient's hip. (see above) The other nurse is in a mirror position on the opposite side of the bed. They offer their near side arms and they use an elbow to elbow grip. (Fig 14.25). The other hand is kept to their side. The patient is brought forwards by the nurses sitting back on their heels.

Alternatively, a draw sheet or an additional folded bed sheet can be placed beneath the lying patient from the shoulders down to their hips. With the nurses kneeling on the bed as before, the top edges of the sheet can then be used as a sling for the nurse to grasp. They can pull the patient towards them into a sitting position in the same way as the elbow holds described above. A large towel can also be used for this manoeuvre. (Fig 14.26) In an emergency the sheet that the patient is lying on can be used. However, the nurse must be cautious as this sheet can tear. This risk is particularly relevant when the patient is being nursed in his own home.

The nurse must beware of reaching forward to bunch the sheet up close to the patient's shoulders as this would involve her in leaning too far forward. She should use the sheet to extend her reach and allow her to work in a safe posture.

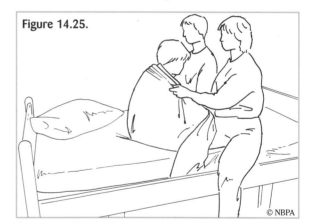

Figure 14.25.

Nurses using bottom sheet to assist patient into sitting

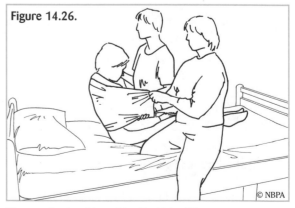

Figure 14.26.

Nurses using towel to assist patient into sitting

Supporting the patient in a sitting position

If the patient needs to be supported in the sitting position there are two methods that can be used.

Where there are two nurses the patient can then be 'hugged' while a second nurse sees to the pillows, etc.

Where there is only one nurse she moves her near arm across his back to keep him forward, placing her hand on the far side of the bed as a strut. This leaves her other hand free to adjust the pillows. This method should only be used with co-operative patients.

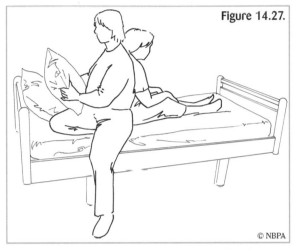

Figure 14.27.

Nurses holding patient in position whilst moving the pillows into position.

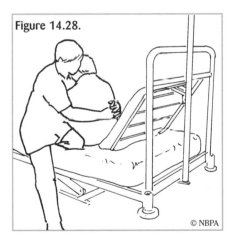

Figure 14.28.

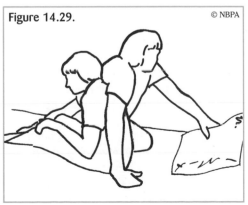

Figure 14.29.

© NBPA

Moving the Patient onto and off the Bed in a Supine Position

The lift from ambulance trolley to operating table is much loved by the producers of hospital drama. This manoeuvre is unsafe. There is no way in which a person can be manually lifted safely between a trolley and a bed.

Lifters at the head cannot hold the patient safely as he will bend in the middle.

Poles and canvas are also unsafe and must not be used.

The correct approach is to use a transfer system. There is a range of hard and soft sliding devices designed to allow such transfers. They are all used in substantially the same way. The patient is half rolled away from the direction of travel (see log rolling technique) and the slide is inserted. The patient is then rolled back onto the slide. He is then pushed and pulled across. The slide can then usually be removed without needing to roll the patient again. However, if necessary, he may be rolled slightly further in the direction of travel to release the slide.

Nurses should beware of leaning too far when pushing or pulling. It is best to have one nurse start the movement by pushing the patient away from herself. One or two nurses on the receiving side take over the effort by pulling the patient towards them when he comes within easy reach. Heavy patients may need four or more nurses to assist in this transfer.

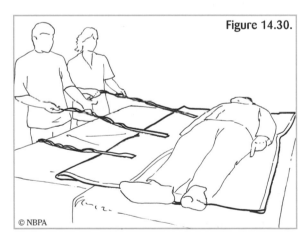

Figure 14.30.

The amount of reaching to pull the patient can be reduced if a strap can be extended for the nurses to grasp. In some cases there is a specially designed loose sheet with hand loops that goes between the patient and the sliding system. In other cases, the straps attach directly onto the sliding system. (An ordinary sheet can be used between the patient and the sliding device to provide the necessary extension. However, there is the risk that a sheet may tear and an accident could occur. This danger is particularly relevant in the community where the patient might be being nursed on his own sheets.)

N.B. 1. Do not lean over the patient or the bed to insert a slide. Move the trolley and bed apart to insert the slide.

2. Ensure that the brakes are on both the trolley and the bed.

3. Adjust the height of the trolley and bed so that the nurses do not have to stoop.

4. Bare flesh will stick on sliding boards therefore a sheet of some type should be placed between the patient and the sliding board.

5. When using sliding boards it must be noted that in most designs the board is not intended to move. Do not even consider lifting a board with a patient on it. Most boards have hand holes: these are not for lifting with the patient laying on the board. Where the manufacturer of the board says that it is intended to move with the patient on the board exercise great care in the use of handles, use extension straps and guard against pulling too hard.

6. If the patient sticks for any reason and does not complete the transit DO NOT LIFT HIM TO FINISH THE MOVE! Stop and re-assess the move and decide on a fresh strategy. It is often best to take the patient back to the starting position and work from there.

An alternative to the use of a sliding system is to use a trolley that carries out the transfer automatically. The AT2000 referred to in Chapter 18 should be considered as a way of carrying out all transfers.

Moving the Patient Up or Down in the Bed

If the patient is being nursed in a profiling bed there should be no need to manually move a patient up or down the bed. If the patient has slipped down in bed his position can be adjusted by operating the profiling mechanism to adjust the bed into a chair shape. The patient will automatically come into the correct position.

Moving the Supine Patient up or Down the Bed

If the patient is on some other bed or if the patient cannot be allowed to bend then he must be slid up the bed. There are two methods that can be used :-

Slide the patient up the bed using fabric slides

Lift the patient in a hoist with a stretcher attachment

Sliding the supine patient up the bed using fabric slides

There are a number of different slides available for this purpose. Some slides are long enough for one

slide to be used to move a supine patient up the bed. Others are smaller and two or three slides need to be used together to slide a supine patient. The advantage of the smaller slides is that they can also be used individually in other handling situations.

The procedure for the use of both types is the same. The following procedure requires two nurses:-

1. The patient is rolled to one side using the log rolling technique. He is held there by a nurse standing on the side of the bed that the patient is facing.

2. The second nurse places a sliding sheet on the bed behind the patient. The sheet is placed so that it forms a loop along the length of the bed and the open ends of the sheet are towards the sides of the bed

3. She then rolls up half of the sheet and places the roll behind the patient.

4. The patient is then lowered onto his back on top of the rolled up slide.

5. The first nurse slides her hands under the patient to pull out and unroll the sliding sheet. (N.B. This must be done from the opposite side. The second nurse must not lean over the patient to reach the slide.)

6. If the patient's heels are off the end of the sliding sheet, and therefore on the bed, there is a possibility of the heels dragging and causing sores. It is best to obtain a sliding sheet that is long enough or to use an additional sheet under the patient's heels. If this is not possible the risk of dragging the heels can be avoided by placing a small pillow under the patient's calves. The pillow will act as a roller and lift the heels away from the bed. (This pillow should be removed once the move has been completed.)

7. The bed is adjusted to a height where the nurses can face the foot of the bed and place one knee on the bed keeping the other leg firmly on the floor. They kneel and grasp the upper sheet.

8. Both nurses now sit back onto their heels holding on to the slide, moving the patient with them.

(N.B. Some sliding systems now have straps that can be attached and which will allow the nurses to pull the patient up the bed in a better posture.)

9. If he has not gone far enough the nurses reposition themselves and move again.

10. When the patient is in the right position the slide can be pulled out from under the patient

This move can be done by one nurse. However, she must beware of twisting the patient on the bed. If one nurse is working alone it can some times be better to push the patient's feet. If this method is chosen the nurse must beware of twisting, reaching or stooping to push the patient's feet.

If the patient cannot hold up his head then a small fabric slide must be placed under his head.

Lift the patient in a hoist with a stretcher attachment

If the patient is very heavy or cannot be rolled or bent for some other reason then the only safe way of moving the patient is with a hoist with a stretcher attachment. The stretcher must be either a scoop stretcher or the type with slats that can be individually slipped under the patient. The type of stretcher hoist that has a sling attached to a frame is not suitable for this type of patient as he would have to be rolled to allow the sling to be positioned.

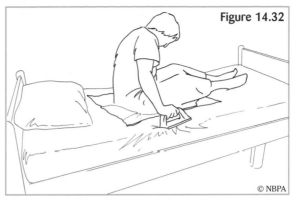

Figure 14.32

© NBPA

Patient moving herself up the bed using bed-blocks

If the patient simply needs a little help one nurse can assist as follows. Once he is sat up on the slide the patient is asked to steady himself with his arms. He places his hands on the bed on either side of his body. The patient's legs are bent. The nurse sits on the bed and holds the patient's feet. The command is given and the patient straightens his legs and thus moves himself up the bed.

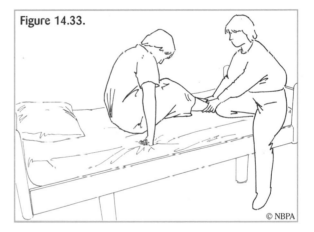

Figure 14.33.

© NBPA

If the patient is unable to move himself, two nurses are needed, one on each side. The nurses and the patient all face the same direction. The nurses place their near side knee on the bed and kneel. The other foot is placed firmly on the floor. Their offside hand holds the patient's hand with a palm to palm thumb grip or palm to palm grip and the near side hand grasps the handle of the fabric slide or the fabric slide itself. On the count of "ready Steady

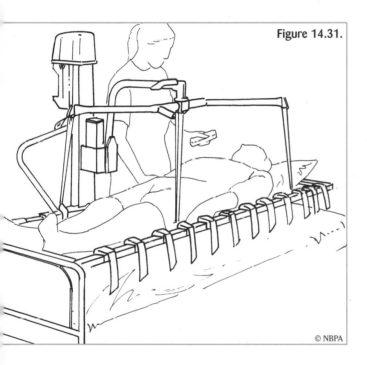

Figure 14.31.

© NBPA

Moving a Seated Patient up the Bed

The patient is rocked from side to side onto a fabric slide. In this case it is best to use a small slide under the patient's bottom. A slide must also be placed under the patient's heels or a pillow can be placed under the patient's calves as described above.

If at all possible the patient should be encouraged to move himself by pushing with his legs or by the use of hand blocks.

In some cases the patient can be encouraged to sit on the side of the bed; stand up and move sideways towards the head of the bed. He can then sit down in the right position.

SIT" they sit down. This moves the patient a little up the bed. The procedure is repeated to get the patient up the bed to the required position.

The position of the fabric slide is important. When the patient has moved he should be in a position where he has reached the end of the sliding sheet and very little is left under his bottom. The easiest way of doing this is to position the slide on the edge of the bed in the place where it is intended that the patient should be at the end of the move. The slide is then slipped down the bed to the starting position of the patient. This shows how it should be arranged when the slide is placed under the patient.

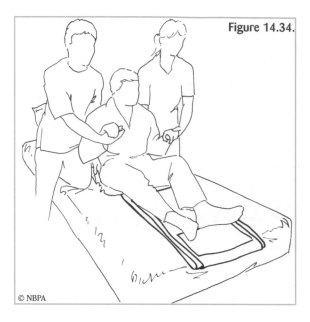

Figure 14.34.

© NBPA

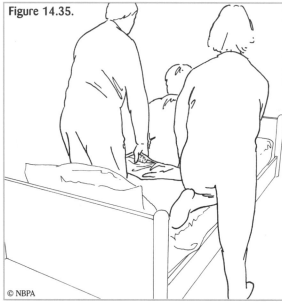

Figure 14.35.

© NBPA

Nurses holding fabric slide ready to sit down and pull patient up the bed.

It has been suggested that the through arm position can be used to assist a patient on a slide. This is not recommended for the following reasons:-

1. The patient's frail skin can be damaged

2. The pressure used by the nurses can hurt the patient

3. The nurses tend to use their shoulders to provide the force in this position. This can cause injuries to the nurses.

If the patient is unable to maintain a sitting posture by himself without direct support he must be moved in a supine position or a hoist must be used to move him up the bed.

N.B. the bed should be adjusted to waist level to insert the slide and then lowered to enable the nurses to place their knees on the bed for the actual move. If the nurse is stooping or bending to grasp the slide an extension strap should be used.

Sitting a patient up in bed

The methods to be used to sit a patient up in bed are described above. If the patient is to be left sat up, it will be necessary to support him from behind. If he is not in a profiling bed there are two ways in which this can be achieved:-

He can be slid back to the bed head or back support using one of the methods described above.

He may be propped up where he is :-

with extra pillows

with a portable back rest

with a small chair turned upside down to serve as a back rest

A small chair turned upside down to prop up the patient is particularly useful if the nurse is on her own or does not have appropriate equipment to hand.

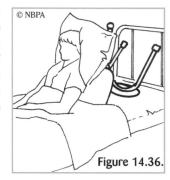

© NBPA

Figure 14.36.

WARNING

The use of footrests and similar devices to stop the patient slipping down the bed must be avoided as these can cause pressure sores and foot drop.

Turning the Patient

Whilst the patient should be encouraged to turn himself in bed it is often necessary to turn the patient to change his position regularly to reduce the risk of pressure sores.

Patients may also need to be turned for a variety of other reasons. e.g. Frequent turning is preferable and indeed secretions at the base of the lungs will be drained more effectively as long as the patient's breathing is not embarrassed in this position (Ref 6).

Patients who need regular turning should be nursed on a turning bed (or on a bed with a turning frame attached). This type of bed removes the risk inherent in any patient handling. A turning bed allows the patient to be turned more often than the conventional 'every two hours.' There is also the benefit of a reduced demand on the nurses' time.

In the absence of a mechanical turning bed, the following method should be used. The procedure starts from the position where he is lying on one side in the middle of the bed. The objective is to turn him so that he is in the middle of the bed lying on his other side.

There are two ways of turning patients in bed. One method uses fabric sliding sheets that are placed under the patient just for the duration of the turn. The other method uses a turning slide that is left permanently beneath the patient.

The 30 Degree Tilt

Traditionally it has been the practice to turn a patient completely onto his side. i.e. the patient is turned to 90 degrees or greater from the prone position. It is now thought that in some cases this posture creates new pressure areas on the side of the patient. t is thought that it is better to only turn the patient to 30 degrees as he is now supported down the whole of his side.

If this is to be done the patient is turned but the turn is stopped short of a full turn and pillows are inserted behind the patient to stop him rolling back.

The turn can be carried out using one of the methods for a full turn described in this chapter. The patient can be turned to a thirty degree position using the log roll or a fabric turning sheet. There is an alternative handling method that has been suggested for use when the patient is only being turned to 30 degrees:-

1. The patient's head is positioned in the direction of travel

2. The patient's far knee from the direction of tilt is lifted

3. The bottom sheet is then pulled out on the side that the patient will be turning away from. This sheet is passed over the patient and gasped by two nurses.

4. The sheet is pulled to roll the patient onto his side.

5. Another nurse inserts pillows to stop the patient falling back

There are a number of cautions which need to be observed when using this technique

1. Do not reach over the patient to grasp the sheet

2. Ensure that the pulling force is kept low. It is just as possible to suffer an injury from a pull as it is from a lift.

3. It is easy to achieve a turn that is significantly less than 30 degrees. The patient can also fall back if the pillows become compacted. Check that the full 30 degrees has been achieved and that the posture is maintained until he is turned again. If this is not done, the weight will remain on his pressure areas.

4. The nurse inserting the pillows must ensure that they are in a wedge shape and that there are no creases that will cause problems with the patient's skin

5. When the nurses start to turn him back the other way, they must first use the sheet to pull the patient up before removing the pillows. If this is not done, there is a risk of friction if the pillows are pulled out whilst the patient's weight is on them.

The thirty degree tilt or the full log roll are not substitutes for a proper turning bed or a full pressure relief mattress.

Turning a patient with a sliding sheet

The use of sliding sheets allows patients to be turned without any need to lift. The technique has the benefit of reducing the risks of skin to skin contact on delicate skin. There is also no risk of damage caused by the point loadings that occur from the nurses' arms when patients are lifted to turn them.

The following procedure is for two nurses, one on each side of the bed. Where the patient is light, the technique can be used by one nurse working alone. In this case there must be cot sides to stop the patient falling out of bed (or feeling that he is going to fall out of bed). (N.B. Cot sides must not be left up unless their use has been specified for some other reason.) Some patients may be able to turn themselves once the slide has been positioned.

1. The first nurse places a sliding sheet on the bed behind the patient. The sheet is placed so that it forms a loop across the bed and the open ends of the sheet are towards the ends of the bed

2. She then rolls up half of the sheet and places the roll behind the patient.

3. The patient is then lowered onto his back. This move is done towards the first nurse. The second nurse should be in front of the patient to reassure him as he is lowered.

Patients who are confused or simply asleep may resist being rolled onto their backs. Ensure the patient knows that the move is about to happen. Nurses have been injured where the patient resists a sudden pull onto his back.

If the patient is in a foetal position on his side he will need to be gently unravelled before he is laid on his back. Place his upper arm in line with his body and straighten his upper leg.

4. The second nurse slides her hands under the patient to pull out and unroll the sliding sheet. (N.B. This must be done from the side to which the patient was facing. The first nurse must not lean over the patient to reach the slide.)

5. The patient is now pulled and/or pushed across the bed. The patient is moved until he is on the edge of the bed.

6. The patient can now be log rolled onto his side in the middle of the bed.

7. The sliding sheet must now be removed by pulling it from under the patient.

N.B. The description above uses a single sliding sheet. It can also be carried out using three small sheets. One is placed under the head and shoulders. The second is placed under the buttocks and the third is placed under the patient's heels.

Turning a patient with a Turning Slide

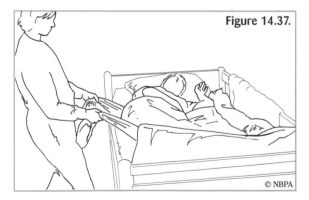

Figure 14.37.

© NBPA

Turning slides are full length slides that are specifically designed for turning patients. They are left permanently under the patient's sheet. Cot sides must always be used in conjunction with these slides to prevent the patient from falling out of bed. The procedure is similar to that for sliding sheets:-

1. If the patient is not on his side log roll him to one side.

2. Position the turning slide in behind him with the open ends towards the ends of the bed. Tuck the slide in behind the patient.

3. The nurse then lowers the patient onto his back on top of the turning slide.

4. He is pulled across the bed on his back so that he is near to the edge of the bed.

5. The patient is now positioned ready for being log rolled. The first three steps of the log roll are carried out.

6. The nurse now stands at the side of the bed to which the patient has just been moved. She grasps the upper surface of the turning sheet and pulls towards herself. This pull of the upper surface will turn the patient away from her into the middle of the bed.

The slide is then left in place. On subsequent turns the nurse follows steps 3 to 6.

Turning slides can easily be used by relatives nursing a patient at home.

Turning a patient using a hoist

When a patient is being returned to bed in a hoist there is a useful technique for placing him on his side at the same time. The patient is lowered onto his back on the bed. The connection of the sling to the hoist is rearranged. The side of the sling furthest from the hoist is disconnected and tucked close to the patient. The side nearest to the hoist is connected so that the spreader bar is turned to be parallel to the length of the patient. The hoops are hooked so that the pull will be even at both ends of the sling, i.e. there will be no tendency to bring the patient's head end up first as is normal. The hoist mechanism is now operated. The side of the patient nearest to the hoist will be lifted and the patient will roll on to his side. When the manoeuvre is completed the sling can be slipped out from under the patient.

N.B.
1. This will only work with simple material slings. It will not work with padded slings nor will it work with toiletting slings.

2. Practice this manoeuvre first before using it on a patient.

3. As with all manoeuvres explain carefully to the patient and reassure the patient thought out the manoeuvre.

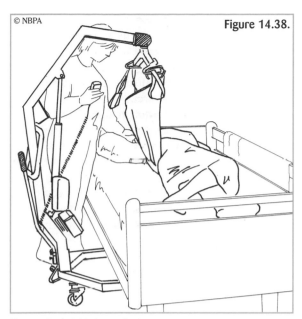

Figure 14.38.

© NBPA

Nurse using hoist to turn patient.

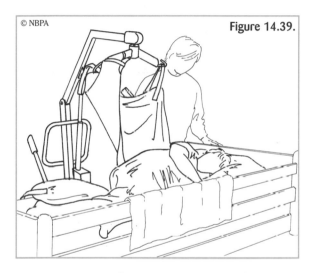

Figure 14.39.

© NBPA

Inserting and Removing Bed Pans

If the patient can bridge (see Figure 14.40) or raise his buttocks by holding onto the monkey pole (Fig 14.12) a bed pan can be slipped under him without any handling.

Where the patient only needs to pass urine male or female urinals should be used for those patients who are difficult to manoeuvre. Urinals are available for use in the lying position

If he cannot lift himself the bed pan should be inserted by rolling the patient towards the nurse, positioning the bed pan and rolling him back onto it.

If for some reason it is not feasible to roll the patient or if the patient is too heavy, then a hoist must be used.

The nurse should remember that the patient feels extremely precarious when left sitting on a bed pan and she should ensure that he has either a cot-side or hand-blocks to hold onto.

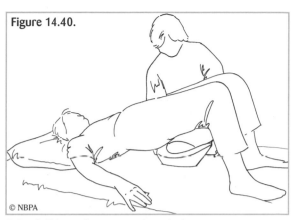

Figure 14.40.

© NBPA

Patient bridging so that nurse can insert bed pan.

Some special mattresses provide for sections to be removed or deflated to accommodate a bed pan. This can significantly simplify the handling needed to toilet the patient.

Changing the Bedding

Where the patient cannot be got out of bed whilst the bedding is changed the simplest solution is to use the log rolling technique described above.

The patient is rolled to one side. The soiled bed clothes are rolled up behind him. The clean sheet is then fitted on that side of the bed and the remainder is rolled up behind the patient. The patient is then log rolled backwards over both sets of linen. The soiled bed clothes can now be removed and the clean sheet can be rolled out

Some patients cannot be log rolled. When changing the bedding, these patients must be lifted using a stretcher hoist. The stretcher must be either a scoop stretcher or the type where individual slats can be slipped under the patient.

WARNING

On no account should the patient be lifted manually to change bedding. There have been many injuries where nurses have changed the bedding by lifting patients with handling slings. The loads involved are too great and the operation involves a twisted posture to change the sheets.

Changing Wound Dressings

Attending to patients' dressings on a bed is a potential source of postural stress and lifting injuries. If the site of the dressing is under the patient, use the Log Roll to get the patient into the right position to do the dressing. The use of height adjustable beds can reduce the dangers of stooping over the patient but they do not eliminate the risks. There are two main risks:-

Bent posture

Bending over the patient is a poor posture. Nurses must always try to work in a position where they have their back vertical. Where they must bend forward, they must not remain in this position for more than a few seconds.

Lifting part of the patient

It is often necessary to lift part of the patient to apply a dressing. For example, if the leg is being dressed it may be necessary to elevate the patient's leg for an extended period. This type of activity can lead to postural stress and permanent injury to the nurse.

If the patient's leg has to be supported for some time some external means of support must be used. This can be achieved by placing the leg on pillows, sand bags, or a device designed to suspend the leg, attached to the side of the bed.

Dressing and Undressing the Patient

Dressing an immobile patient can usually be achieved by use of log rolling back and forth as the clothes are pulled on. All the usual rules apply: avoid leaning over the bed and avoiding lifting the patient to get clothing into place. (Ref 8)

Consideration should be given to the objective of dressing the patient. Nurses must not be put at risk to obtain a social benefit.

Case History

Clothes may need to be adapted to suit the handling needs of the patient. A patient with Multiple Sclerosis liked to be dressed in trousers but these were not easy to remove for toileting. Eventually it was agreed that she should wear trousers with Velcro fittings so that they could be opened whilst the patient was in a toileting sling. Thus, a compromise was achieved that gave the patient the dignity that she needed and at the same time gave the nurses a safe system of work.

WARNING If a patient needs any support to keep him standing, do not attempt to dress him in a standing position. Patients who are holding on to a wall bar can suddenly collapse on the nurse and injure her even if she is not trying to support the patient.

Transferring the Patient from bed to a Wheelchair or Commode

Sliding sheets or fabric turntables can be used to turn the patient so that his legs are over the edge of the bed.

If the patient is lying on his back the first step is to insert the sliding device to be used in the turn. This can be done by rolling the patient or by asking him to bridge using a monkey pole. He must then be sat up. The procedure for sitting up is described above. If the patient is already sat up he can be rolled in the sitting position to allow the sliding device to be inserted or he may again be able to lift himself using a monkey pole. Once the patient is sat up and sat on the slide he can be turned by the nurse taking his legs and walking round to the front. This is only safe if the patient is very light. With all other patients place a sliding sheet under the patient's feet. The patient's feet can then be pulled round.

Always try to get the patient to make the move himself. Once on the sliding sheet, the patient requires very little effort to move round and he is of course rewarded by being able to do something for himself.

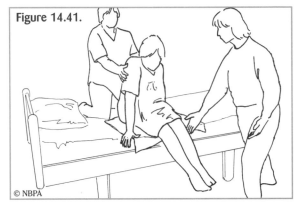

Figure 14.41.

Nurse kneeling on bed supporting patient whilst the other nurse moves legs to the edge of the bed.

Having got to the seated position on the edge of the bed the patient can now be transferred using one of the techniques shown.

(It is possible to use a turntable under the fabric slide. This can make the turn easier. However, beware that the patient can slide straight off the bed.)

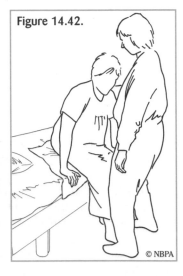

Figure 14.42.

N.B. 1. Beware that the legs can weight 30% (9) or more of the body weight of the patient. In heavy patients this may in itself be an unsafe load. Remember, this load is not being taken in the ideal position. There is a danger of stooping. If the patient is very heavy or is unable to co-operate, use a hoist for the transfer.

2. Sliding sheets can stick during the turn. A large sheet should be used. If the patient does stick turn him back and reposition the sheet.

Preparing a Patient to Stand Up from the Side of the Bed

This is essentially the same as Transferring the Patient to a Wheelchair or Commode above. However, there are two additional considerations:-

1. There are difficulties when handling patients who have had replacements of their hip joints and similar operations. Some consultants prefer patients such as these to be stood up without bending either at all or at best not beyond 90°. It is not possible to assist a person to stand without placing their nose over their toes. This means that the person must be stood by some other means. The solution to this problem is to use a standing bed (see above).

2. There are various techniques for standing a patient from a seated position. (See Chapter 15) However, if the patient is being nursed in an electrically operated profiling bed it is possible to assist the patient to stand in a completely different way. The patient is sat up and turned to the edge of the bed. He is then shuffled or rocked forward on his hips so that his feet are on the floor. The patient is brought forwards so that he is in the "nose over toes" position. His hands are on the bed to steady himself and one foot is slightly in front of the other.

The nurses stand on either side of the patient. They block the patient's feet with their feet to stop him from sliding.

With the bed in a fully profiled position the height mechanism is operated to raise the bed. The patient slips off the bed and is brought into a standing position without any support or assistance from the nurse. If the patient is using a walking frame this can be placed in front of him once he has been stood up. It should not be placed in front of him during the standing process as he may try to grab it and may fall. N.B. Do not try to stabilise the walking frame at the same time as supporting the patient.

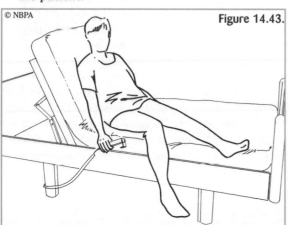

Figure 14.43.

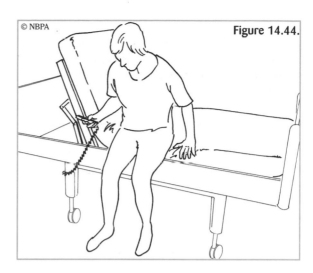

Figure 14.44.

Putting the Patient Back to Bed

This handling situation arises in two forms. 1.) When the patient is walking and 2.) When the patient is seated next to the bed.

In both cases the principle is similar. The patient needs to be sat on the bed on top of two slides. The top slide is a fabric slide positioned to move the patient across from the edge to the middle of the bed. Under this there will be a fabric turntable. This enables the patient to be turned through 90° to face down the bed. The same effect can be achieved by using two large (approx. 60 cms square) slides placed one on top of each the other.

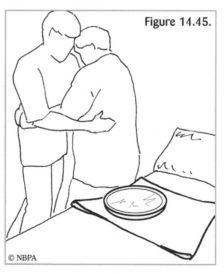

Figure 14.45.

The slides will need to be positioned before the patient is brought to the bed.

If the patient is ambulant he can just sit directly onto these two slides. If the patient is being transferred from some other seated position he will need to be slid onto the two slides. The methods of moving a patient from one seated position to another are described elsewhere.

If the patient is sitting down from a standing position the bed must be at a convenient sitting height for the patient. This will vary from patient to patient. Make sure that the patient is as far up the bed as possible to limit the amount of handling. If he sits in the right place it will not be necessary to move him up the bed.

Once the patient is on the two slides he is ready to be got into bed.

If he has any upper arm strength he may well be able to get himself into bed. (Hand blocks may help.)

Remember that legs can form a significant part of the weight of a patient. If the patient cannot lift his legs onto the bed, another slide can be placed for his legs and the legs can be slid onto the bed. In the community, the patient may need a leg lifter to place his own legs onto the bed.

If the nurse is going to assist the patient in getting his legs onto the bed, she must squat or kneel down and keep her back vertical. A towel can be used as a sling to lessen the stoop needed.

Having got the patient into the middle of the bed he should be in the correct position to be laid down or left sat up as appropriate. If he must now be moved up in bed use the methods above.

Air Fluidised Beds

The Air Fluidised type of bed requires specific handling techniques

Getting the patient into or out of the bed.

This bed would normally be occupied by patients requiring continuous bed rest. A hoist would usually be used to get them into and out of it.

Moving the Patient.

Because of the flotation effect of the bed, it is unnecessary to move the patient up or down the bed. If the patient has moved too near to the bottom of the bed a sliding sheet enables the nurses to pull the patient back without lifting. (See above)

Inserting a bed pan.

This is done by pushing part of the surface away to make a space for the bed pan. The mattress can then be solidified around the bed pan.

Wound dressing.

If it is necessary to get to the patient's back he can be log rolled onto one side. The surface can then be solidified to hold the patient in position while the dressings are changed.

Sitting the patient up.

A mechanical device is needed to achieve this safely. The latest beds have an electrical rising backrest. If the bed does not have such a device one should be obtained from the manufacturers.

Low Loss Air Mattresses

The details of these mattresses vary from model to model. However, most now seem to come with a cover for the air sacks. This cover is usually made of a slippery material. Some manufacturers supply an additional sliding sheet to work with their mattress. In general, the handling techniques described in above apply to low air loss beds.

When handling a patient on one of these beds use the controls to make the whole of the mattress fully inflate. This provides a hard even surface on which to move the patient.

Care should be taken to ensure that the bed is at a safe working height. The low air loss mattress may mean that the surface cannot be brought low enough for some techniques to be used. In this case the nurse must select alternative techniques. Checks must also be made to ensure that the hoists can lift patients off the bed with the mattress in place.

IF THE PATIENT ARRESTS, DEFLATE THE WHOLE BED SO THAT THE PATIENT IS LYING ON THE BASE. THIS PROVIDES A FIRM SURFACE FOR RESUSCITATION.

Profiling Beds.

The use of profiling beds can dramatically reduce the amount of handling required. In general the patient can be sat up or laid down with minimal effort. However, these beds are not simply Kings Fund beds that move. There are some different handling situations for the nurse to consider.

When sitting the patient up in bed it is usually only necessary to operate the controls to turn the bed into the profiled shape. Sometimes when the patient has been lying on the bed with the mechanism in a flat position he slips out of the central area. If he has slipped a little too far down the bed operate the mechanism to lift the foot end of the bed first. This will push the patient up the bed. Equally, if the patient is too far up the bed operate the mechanism to tilt the head end first. If the patient is a long way out of position it may be necessary to flatten the bed and use a slide to get him into the centre of the bed. An alternative method is to use the tilting mechanism of the bed. The bed is tipped down slightly in the direction of the intended movement to allow gravity to assist. The patient's condition must be assessed before using this method. Patients with low blood pressure may not be suitable for this manoeuvre.

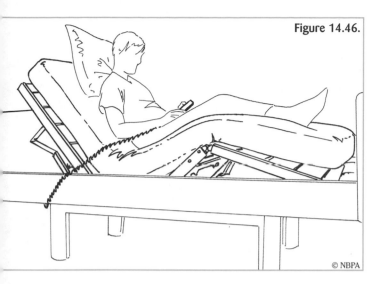

Figure 14.46.

© NBPA

Some times a patient, who is in the bed with the mechanism in a profiled position, collapses to one side. If he cannot be persuaded to straighten himself out when the bed is lowered, it may be necessary to use a slide to allow him to be pushed back into the middle of the bed.

WARNING

Bed rails should not be used to prevent patients getting out of bed. If they are used as a precaution during a handling procedure take them down again when the procedure is completed. Do not leave cotsides up unless it is written in the care plan for this patient. Patients and nurses have been injured when the patient has tried to climb over the cot sides.

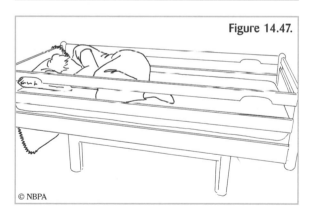

Figure 14.47.

© NBPA

Removing a sliding sheet.

A sliding sheet can be removed without any risk of the patient moving. The technique for doing this should be practiced. The nurse puts her hand through one end of the sliding sheet. She reaches through the sheet and grasps the opposite corner. The sheet is then pulled inside out in a diagonal direction. If this is done correctly it requires no force and the patient does not move.

Obtaining Special beds

Where special beds such as Low Air Loss, Turning Beds or Heavy Duty Beds, are required, they can be obtained at short notice.

Companies who specialise in the hiring of special beds can generally supply a bed within 4 to 6 hours. The companies operate 24 hour services. Employers should establish efficient systems that allow staff to take advantage of these services when they are needed. Nurses and patients must not be put at risk by bureaucratic inefficiencies limiting their access to appropriate equipment.

REFERENCES

1. NHS Estates, Health Building Note 40, Vol 2, Treatment areas, HMSO.

2. International Electronic Commission, International Standard 601-2-38, Medical Electrical Equipment Part 2, Particular Requirements for the Safety of Electrically Operated Hospital Beds, 1st Edition 1996-10.

3, Medical Devices Agency (MDA), Evaluation - Foam Mattresses PS2 August 93, MDA.

5. MDA, Evaluation - Static Mattress Overlays PS2 October 94, MDA,

5. MDA, Evaluation - Alternating Pressure Mattress Overlays PS3 April 95, MDA

6. HSE, Provision and Use of Work Equipment Regulations 1992 Guidance on Regulations, HMSO.

7. Hough A 1984, The effect of posture on lung function - Physiotherapy 70 101-104

8. Disabled Living Foundation, 1994, All Dressed Up, DLF

9. Pheasant Stephen, 1996, Bodyspace Anthropometry, Ergonomics and Design - Second Edition, Taylor Francis.

SITTING AND STANDING

by Christine Tarling

SUMMARY

The patient should be assessed for his ability to move himself, needing supervision and not assistance.

A variety of chairs should be made available where there are several potential users, and should suit individual needs.

A patient should not be lifted manually from a chair seat.

Mechanical hoists or transfer devices must be used when moving a patient who cannot move or support his own weight.

INTRODUCTION

To assess a patient's ability to stand from a seated position, a detailed assessment must be completed. This assessment must identify the potential risk to the patient and the carer. It must define whether the patient can get to his feet on his own. If he cannot rise with minimal supervision and assistance, then he must not be moved manually. The assessment must include details on the weight and disability of the patient; the location and design of the chair; the equipment that needs to be used; the environment in which the patient is sitting; and the capabilities of the carers.

To ensure that staff learn to avoid lifting a patient from a chair, they must be taught:

- the theory of the principles of handling

- practice the use of a range of equipment with colleagues and patients under the

- supervision of a competent trainer

- define and analyse the objectives of standing and sitting the patient.

TYPES OF CHAIR

A chair must be suited to a patient's individual needs, contributing to his comfort and independence. The incorrect choice of chair for use by a physically disabled patient often means he expects to have someone – a carer – to help him to stand.

If the patient is in a low chair, the helper cannot avoid adopting awkward and poor postures, with the risk of causing musculoskeletal strain. If the patient refuses to change his chair for one more suitable to his needs, carers must not use manual techniques to assist him.

CHOOSING A CHAIR TO REDUCE THE RISK : SPECIFICATIONS

THE SEAT

Height: Normally this should correspond with the leg length of the seated person, between 350 and 460mm (between 14 and 18 inches).

Some elderly people, or people who have weakness in their legs, sometimes need a seat 460mm (18 inches) high.

The height should allow the seated person to place his feet comfortably on the floor with the thighs level.

However, if the patient needs a higher seat so that he can stand without help, then pressure under the thighs may lead to swollen ankles. A footstool placed under the patient's feet avoids this problem. If a footstool could cause a hazard by being in the way when the patient moves, a chair with a riser seat will be a safer alternative.

The seat should be firm to help the seated person push up. Cushions under the seated person can cause instability, and should not be used.

Depth: A seat that is too deep encourages the patient to slump, and their hips to slide forwards. The appropriate depth is usually between 432 and 558mm (17 and 22 inches) and should correspond to the length from the back of the hips to the front of the knee. The addition of a lumbar support cushion will alter this measurement.

Angle: When the seated patient's hips are lower than the knees, extra muscle power is needed to move his body weight forwards and uphill against gravity as he prepares to stand.

CHAIR BACKS

The height depends on whether the user wishes to lean their head back – most elderly people need a head pillow or rest to support their head comfortably.

Wings at the side interfere with conversation, and they encourage people to lean sideways for support. It is said that wings keep out the draughts.

A lumbar cushion supports the lower spine. This may be part of the chair's construction. Some people prefer a separate cushion that they can place where they want. A cushion at the back brings a person forward towards the front of a deep seat. A choice of lumbar cushions is available: inflatable, sheepskin lined, shaped, or made of firm materials.

A head rest tilted at a slight backward angle gives extra comfort. The more upright the chair back, the more likely is the head to droop forwards. Further assessment will be required to determine whether a backward sloping head rest, together with a neck cushion, will give the required comfort.

A recliner chair with an adjustable back allows a person to sleep, or rest, and so avoid transfers which can be painful for the patient and stressful for the carer.

ARM RESTS

In an easy chair, the arm rest should come well forward so that a patient may grasp or lean on it to move forwards ready to stand. The front edge of the arm should be level with the edge of the seat, or in front of it.

Padding on the top of the arm will allow the patient to support elbow joints which may be painful. It is also more comfortable for people who press down on the arm rest to shift their weight. Constant pressure from an unpadded arm rest can induce a nerve palsy in the person's arm.

The arm rest should give good support to the elbows without distorting the position of the shoulders. Arm rests that are too high elevate the shoulders and reduce the person's ability to push down when rising. If too low, the user slumps sideways, and this depresses the shoulder joint, which may need support, particularly following a stroke.

CHAIR LEGS

The front legs should be vertical, and the rear legs angled backwards, for stability.

There should always be at least 130mm - 5 inches - clearance beneath a chair. The patient can then place the feet comfortably when rising independently.

This amount of clearance will enable a mobile hoist to be used as the chassis can then pass beneath the chair frame. This is particularly important when a small mobile hoist is being used in a patient's home. Most mobile hoists have width adjustable chassis legs. Many of these do not open wide enough to go

round a wide and low easy armchair. It is then easier for the first carer to operate the hoist while a second carer goes to the back of the chair to pull the suspended patient towards her. Some slings have hand loops on the centre back that can be used to pull on while other carers prefer to use both arms to pull both sides of the sling towards them. If the chair is too deep or the back too high, this second carer will be in a stooped position while reaching out to guide the patient's weight. In this case, the carer should work from the side of the chair and push the patient away from her. It is always possible to locate the patient's hips at the back of the chair while he is suspended in the hoist sling.

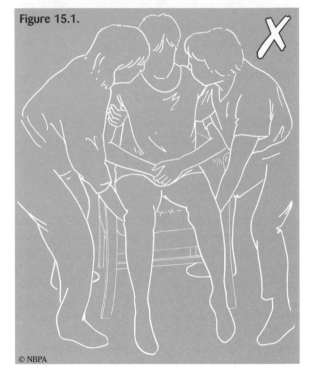

Figure 15.1.

© NBPA

WARNING

On no account should a carer, or both carers, do a manual lift to adjust the patient's position in the chair.

SIZE AND DESIGN

A variety of designs and sizes of chairs in a communal area will mean that people using the room will have more opportunity to find a seat to suit them.

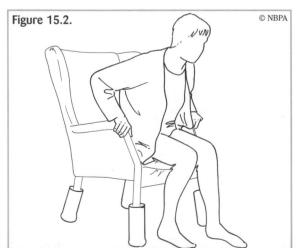

Figure 15.2.

© NBPA

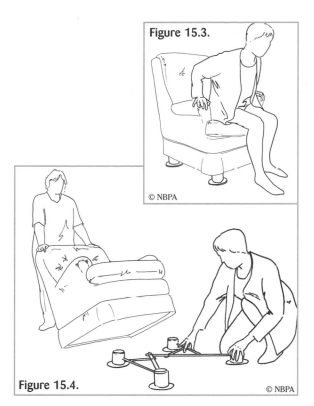

Figure 15.3.

© NBPA

Figure 15.4.   © NBPA

Some special chairs have a steeply backward sloping seat. They are mounted on a mobile base and have adjustable foot plates, arms, and trays. They are often too low, and are unsuitable for someone to rise from independently. Where a patient has his hips lower than his knees, his weak leg muscles will make it impossible for him to stand. It is unsafe for any carer to assist a patient to stand from one of these chairs. A hoist must be used.

WARNING

These chairs have been used for elderly mentally ill patients. They provide a form of restraint since it is impossible for frail, elderly people to stand up from them. It is assumed that the patients are kept in a comfortable and safe position where they cannot wander, fall or damage themselves. However, if left too long in one of these chairs, the patient develops contractures of the hips and knees so that he can no longer bear his own weight to stand.

FOR THE INDIVIDUAL

Altering the height-

people at home often reject the offer of a high seat chair from the equipment loan store since these usually have a metal frame and vinyl covered upholstery. Extra height can be added to their favourite chair, with sleeves for small chairs, or chair raisers for arm chairs and for small, two-seater sofas. Both types are available in a variety of heights.

Individual blocks should be avoided because they can be unstable.

RECLINING ARMCHAIRS

These are nearly always on unbraked castors. While this makes it easier to move themaround a room, they should never be moved when someone is sitting in them.

Chairs can be made to specific seat heights.

Some recliners have electric controls to alter the seat height and the inclination of the back and the leg rest.

A patient with swollen legs and ankles must have a recliner that allows his feet to be placed higher than his hips. A leg support that is too short, allowing the feet to hang over the edge, causes skin pressure.

SUPPORTIVE CHAIRS

A wide range of chairs offers a variety of special supportive seating positions, and chairs can be made to measure.

RISER AND ADJUSTABLE CHAIRS

These are essential where the person using them can still carry their own weight when standing, but who has weak muscles and painful joints - use of these chairs avoids the need for manual help to move a patient from sitting to standing.

Chairs with seats that rise and fall are widely used by people who have arthritic, painful or stiff joints. However, they are unsuitable for those who do not have control of their heads or trunks.

FOUR DESIGN CATEGORIES

- The seat that tilts upwards:

This may be operated by a spring system which is usually counterbalanced to the weight of the user and is specific to one person. It should not be used in a communal area. The spring system may or may not have brakes. The front edge usually stays at the same height while the back edge rises. This mechanism is available on a cushion which may be mounted in a separate chair base or as part of an armchair. People with weak or painful arms may find this type requires effort which causes discomfort.

- The seat that tilts forwards and rises upwards:

This type is often electrically powered. At the press of one or two buttons, the height is raised and the angle controlled as it tips forwards. These chairs can be used by people of different weights. The electrical systems make them easy to use for people who have no strength in their arms.

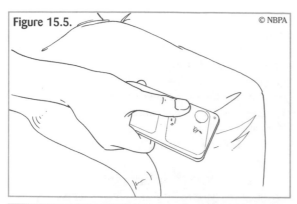

Figure 15.5.   © NBPA

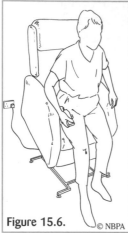

Figure 15.6.   © NBPA

- The seat that, together with the back rest, rises upwards and tilts forwards:

Some people need support at their backs while they are being placed on their feet. This design is useful for those who have stiff or painful knee joints and cannot put their feet back against the frame.

- The seat that moves from reclining to standing, and back again:

Some people cannot sit comfortably in a standard chair because they lack flexion in their arms, legs and spine. A range of chairs is available that can move them from standing to a resting and reclining position, and help them to stand again. The best of these are electrically operated.

When equipment is being put into a communal area, such as a hospital ward or the lounge of a sheltered housing complex, the provision of electric riser chairs must be considered since these should eliminate the stress of carers who help people rise, and should give seated people independence of movement.

UPHOLSTERY

Buyers prefer fabrics which are water and stain resistant, and easy to clean.

Some users find vinyl type materials assist them to move themselves into position of comfort. Others say that sitting on such fabrics becomes sticky and uncomfortable.

CHAIRS AT A DINING TABLE

A patient may need to be moved in the chair, possibly at a dining table, or to create space for a transfer to another chair. Chairs are available which have a turning mechanism so that the person can

face the table and, when ready, turn at a right angle to be in position to stand without help.

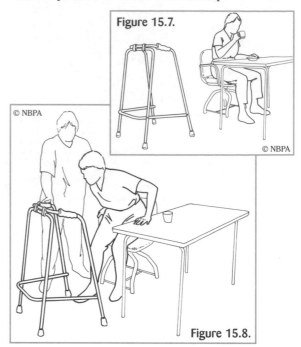

Figure 15.7.

© NBPA   © NBPA

Figure 15.8.

With glides or castors only on the back legs of a dining chair a person can be slid close to or away from the table without the need to lift them or the chair. However, an initial force is required by the carer and this must be assessed before using this method. A height adjustable mobile chair is available with transfer boards on both sides. This can be used when the patient is being transferred from bed to easy chair when both are at different heights.

The mobile seat height can be set high at the bed for the patient to move to it from the bed. Then the mobile chair seat is lowered to the same height as the easy chair for another, easier transfer. This mobile chair cannot be used by the patient independently but may be useful for a carer when the patient has only one or no legs but has strong arms. If the patient needs help to slide across to transfer between seats, a sliding sheet may make the task easier.

PROCEDURES FOR ASSISTING PATIENTS WITH CHAIRS

RISING FROM SITTING TO STANDING - INDEPENDENTLY

If a chair has been chosen to suit the patient, the move from sitting to standing will be easier, and often gives full independence to the patient. If the patient is not fully independent, the following process must be followed:

ASSESSMENT AND PREPARATION:

If the patient has been sitting a long time, or sleeping, he should not be rushed. The nurse should talk to the patient, gain his attention, talk about the reason for moving him, and look for clues as to his mobility - particularly important if the patient is unknown to her.

With a reassuring presence and verbal encouragement from the nurse, the independent patient will need little physical help.

Note that many patients will accept help even when they can move without it; some lose confidence because of a fall and this may contribute to them asking for help. The nurse must always assess the patient's ability and provide supervision to promote his independence. This avoids the possibility of his becoming dependent as a consequence of being given physical assistance which is no longer considered to be acceptable practice.

PREPARATION:

Is a walking stick or walking frame nearby? If not, ask whether the patient uses one.

See how the patient moves and prepares to stand. Ask him if he can manage on his own. If he moves forward in the chair and uses his feet and arms to balance himself, it may be that supervision and a spoken reminder are enough.

Is there enough space to move, or does anything need to be moved to give more space?

Is there room for the nurse to give help from the side?

Does the patient's footwear give support, and does it have non-slip soles?

THE MANOEUVRE:

The patient should shuffle his hips from the back of the seat towards the front, and lean forwards with his nose over his toes.

The feet should be positioned so that one foot is under him, with the knee at a right angle and the second foot should be just behind, with that knee at less than a right angle.

The patient should grasp the arms of the chair and push up to straighten his knees. As he stands up, his head should come up so that he looks ahead and stands erect.

When he is standing, the patient should pause to check his balance. He then makes sure he has a firm grip on his walking stick or frame before moving forwards.

RISING FROM SITTING TO STANDING - WITH HELP:

Before anything else, an assessment must be made to find out if the patient can bear his own weight through both legs, or whether his medical condition does not allow this. His ability may be affected by:

> contractures of the hips or knees so that the legs cannot be straightened, and so become load bearing

> muscular spasm that makes leg movement unreliable. Weight bearing may reduce spasm, but he may be unstable while getting the body upright and over the feet, and at risk from falling

> pain which makes him avoid movement

> joints which are fixed in a straight position at either the hips and knees, or both, in such a way that he cannot bring his feet back close to the chair to bring his weight up over them.

The nurse may be put at risk by patients who are unable to follow instructions or by those who have unpredictable movements or behaviour.

The most common reason for a patient to be unable to stand is paralysis or degeneration of muscles in one or both legs, so that the muscles are not strong enough to lift the body upright.

A patient must have thigh muscles strong enough to lift the body weight into a standing position.

Physiotherapists use these grades to denote muscle power:

> 0 = no movement seen

> 1 = a flicker of movement seen at the muscles of the thigh

> 2 = movement with gravity eliminated, as when lying on the bed and moving the legs from side to side

> 3 = movement against gravity, as being able to lift the leg while sitting

> 4 = movement against gravity and some resistance, as when lifting the leg while sitting and downward pressure is put on the knee.

> 5 = normal movement.

To be able to stand, the patient must have at least Grade 4 since his leg muscles are working against gravity and sustaining the weight of the body. If the patient's muscles are weaker than this, it will be more appropriate to use a sliding board – or some other system – that makes it unnecessary for the patient to stand.

During rehabilitation: a competent assessor must assess the patient's capabilities and determine how the individual members of the staff team are to handle him. The manual handling assessment includes the capabilities of the carers, and consequently at some stages of rehabilitation, different handlers may have to use different methods. Physiotherapists are the most skilled professionals at patient movement and they may use techniques that are not suitable for others to use because of the highly developed skills that are needed. The physiotherapist has a responsibility to keep a record of the patient's progress and to share it with the staff team so that everyone can handle him with safety.

This may result in some staff using equipment for transfers while others, such as the physiotherapist, are able to move him manually.

It is vitally important that a manual handling assessment sheet is completed for all patients, and made available to all staff who care for him. An important part of rehabilitation is the aim to have the patient as mobile as possible. The needs of the family, carers, or agency home care staff must be considered when deciding which transfer methods are to be used.

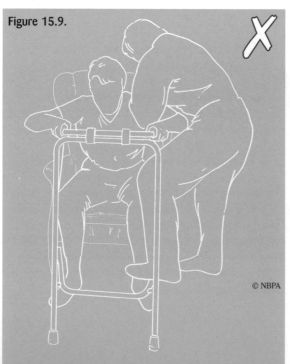

Figure 15.9.

© NBPA

ROCKING

For patients who can cooperate, bear weight through their legs, and control their head and arm positions, the stress of getting themselves from sitting to standing can be eased by gentle rocking before standing. Rocking gives the patient kinetic energy, and by controlling this, the nurse is relieved of most of the effort of moving the patient.

The patient sits towards the front of the chair. Then, with his feet slightly apart with one further forward than the other, one forward knee should be at 90 degrees flexion, the other at less than 90 degrees. He holds the forward arms of the chair to stabilise himself and then rocks gently forwards and backwards until his hips come up from the seat of the chair. As he comes up to stand, he pushes on the arms of the chair, and the nurse checks that he is stable on his feet before encouraging him to walk forwards. The nurse should avoid lifting or manually assisting the patient since he is bearing his weight and able to stand. If he cannot, then alternative and safer methods must be sought.

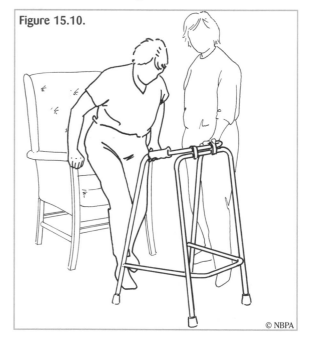

Figure 15.10.

© NBPA

HELPING THE PATIENT STAND FROM THE SIDE OF THE CHAIR

A handling belt around the seated patient's waist enables the nurse to support him without causing discomfort to his shoulders.

The nurse stands at the side of the chair facing the same direction as the patient. She should be on his weakest side to support him when he is standing.

When the patient is in position, his feet will be beneath the leading edge of the chair. His arm furthest away grasps the front of the chair arm; his near arm is supported by the nurse.

The nurse has her outer foot forward, level with the patient's feet, the other just behind the patient's hips and level with the centre of the chair seat.

One arm goes down to his waist at a position where she can hold the handling belt comfortably. Her knees are bent to avoid stooping, and her spine should be naturally erect, with her head held up.

The nurse's other hand supports the patient's nearest hand, with her palm facing up; the patient grasps her hand with his palm facing down, so that they are holding palm to palm.

Patient and nurse keep their heads up and face the direction of the move. Several gentle rocking movements should assist the patient to stand. As the patient gets to his feet, the nurse is in the supported standing position.

They take a moment's rest to check their balance and the direction of the next move forwards.

WARNING

This assisted move is only possible if the chair seat is of a height that allows the patient to give full assistance. Too low a chair seat makes a patient struggle to move his body against gravity, and makes the nurse lift part of his weight, if not most of it.

MOVING THE PATIENT BACK IN THE CHAIR

Once sitting, he should not be left until he is comfortable and secure in the back of the chair seat.

A patient who can lift his own body by his arms should be encouraged to do this, and position his hips well back in the chair. He may also be able to roll his body weight from side to side and move one buttock at a time backwards in the chair. The knees should be flexed and the feet flat on the floor close to the chair or on the footplates of a mobile chair.

Patients with conditions affecting the locomotor system frequently slide down in their chair, and this should be prevented. A one way sliding sheet on the chair seat can stop a forward sliding movement.

If the patient has additional problems such as leg muscle spasm, the angle of the hips should be decreased to 90 degrees or less. The patient may be comfortable in a chair with a seat that slopes backwards, or with a wedge under the seat cushion. This may give the patient relief from the leg muscle spasms but this gain has to be balanced against the loss of independence if he can no longer rise from the chair without help.

It is unsafe for a nurse to try to lift a patient's hips further back in a chair if he has slid forwards. This includes the unsafe technique of the nurse taking the patient's weight with a through-arm lift from the back of a chair.

It may be possible to encourage the patient who has slid to the front of the chair to lean forwards to the nose over toes position. The nurse can then encourage him to use the rocking method. But this is possible only where the patient can cooperate and take his weight through his legs to push himself back into the seat when his hips rock off the seat. If this is not possible then equipment must be used.

TWO NURSES HELPING A WEIGHT BEARING PATIENT

The technique is the same as for assisting a patient from the side of the chair (see earlier in this chapter, Helping the patient stand from the side of the chair). The chair needs to be in a position where both nurses have room to move.

If the patient is to stand to transfer to another seated position, the distance to be moved must be within his capability of standing or walking.

One nurse stands on each side of the chair and faces the same direction as the patient. In preparation for the move, the patient has moved forward so that his hips are close to the front edge of the seat. It may be helpful if he wears a handling belt.

The nurses support the patient using the hands nearest to him. If the chair seat is high enough, the nurses grasp the handling belt. They can put their other hands in front of the patient for him to hold, palm to palm.

Each nurse puts the outside foot forward of the chair, the other in line with the centre of the seat, so that the patient is between them when he stands up.

As the patient pushes up and stands, the nurses place their arms behind his back to support him. Pressure on his sacrum area at the bottom of the back will encourage him to stand and become established in an upright position, preventing him flexing his hips to flop back into the chair.

Once the patient is standing, he can have the support he needs - a walking frame, or the nurses helping him to turn slowly towards the next chair. When a patient has one side weaker than the other, the turning movements should be towards the weakest side.

The nurses should be slightly behind the patient while he is moving, each with one leg behind the patient's legs to stop him falling, (see Chapter 20).

When the patient arrives at his destination and is ready to sit, he should have his back to the chair so that he can feel the front edge of the seat. He should be encouraged to feel backwards for the arm rests with his hands, to grasp them, and then to lower himself as far back in the chair as possible.

Supporting this movement, the nurses should bend their knees while keeping upright. To get further back in the chair, the patient should rock his bottom from side to side while edging himself backwards.

However, the space needed by three people, and the instability of patient, are factors which, together, mean that it will be easier for him to stand and walk forwards a short distance while chairs are exchanged behind him by a third member of staff. This avoids a backwards or turning manoeuvre which could be unsafe.

OTHER TECHNIQUES

Bobath technique:

This requires extensive practical and theoretical training and an understanding of the principles of neurological rehabilitation processes. Staff should not undertake this type of move without that training. Accidents have occurred when a nurse who has watched a skilled therapist using the technique has tried to copy it without training. For these reasons, no description of the technique is attempted here.

Neuromuscular approach:

Some staff may have been taught other approaches to patient movement which need intensive skills training (see Chapter 6).

MECHANICAL ASSISTANCE FOR SEATED PATIENTS

The choice, to be made from a wide range of equipment, depends on how much assistance a patient needs.

It includes:

   an easy armchair with a removable arm

   sliding boards

   standing hoists.

The easy armchair:

the armchair with a removable arm aids a sideways transfer, with or without a transfer board, to a wheelchair or commode.

Sliding boards:

a range of different shaped sliding or transfer boards is available. The simplest is a wooden board which measures about 610mm by 305mm (24 by 12inches). This is used to bridge the gap between the patient's chair seat and the seat to which he is moving. The boards have chamfered edges and highly polished surfaces. Some are shaped to fit round the arms of chairs, and newer models have sliding inserts which reduce the friction caused by moving across the surface.

Standing hoists:

can lift a sitting person and transfer them to another seat - particularly useful for a movement from an easy chair to a wheelchair or a commode, or to a bed. It is also useful when a patient needs help with clothing or cleaning during toileting.

Most of these hoists have a chassis and mast similar to the total body lift hoists. At the base of the mast is usually a footplate where the patient puts his feet. His knees are braced against a padded cross plate, and a padded sling is put across his back and under his arms. The hoist's lifting boom is raised, lifting the patient into an almost standing position. Clothing can then be adjusted easily for the toilet, since there is no sling around the patient's hips. The patient must be able to bear his own weight but need not be able to lift his own weight,which is what the hoist does.

Patients with painful knees cannot tolerate this type of equipment.

TOILETING AND CLOTHING

by Christine Tarling

SUMMARY

A risk assessment of the toileting environment and a plan of action should reduce the stress associated with this difficult and personal task.

An assessment should be made of the space in which the toileting task is to be performed. If inadequate, privacy for the patient should be found by seeking alternative methods.

A patient should not be lifted manually from a chair to a WC or sanichair. When a patient is non weight bearing, a mechanical hoist and sling of appropriate design should be used.

INTRODUCTION

Toileting is a complex task requiring careful risk assessment, as a person must be able to pass waste body products in the right place at the right time, with dignity and privacy whenever possible.

Consequently, it is important to know how often the person is likely to use the toilet both for passing urine and for bowel motions. The same applies to a woman's menstrual flow and the changing of pads or appliances.

Nurses should be aware of a safe response to an urgent need and to know how to assist.

If someone suddenly becomes totally dependant, then a safe method of keeping him clean, dry and yet relieved must be considered. An example is when a new patient is referred to a community nursing service and is found to be excessively heavy, unable to move himself and unable to assist with any transfers. Until a full assessment is made and the results implemented - for instance the provision of a hoist or suitable sling - the response may be catheterisation, until the correct handling equipment is provided, to ensure safe transfers on and off the commode or W.C.

The prescription and supply of continence appliances should be checked, because outdated or outgrown appliances often cause difficulties and rejection by the user.

The Patient

Apart from knowing the pattern and timing of the patient's use of the WC, information about his ability to move himself, and postural control, is essential. The patient's wishes must be respected, since this is the task, above all others, that most people wish to do for themselves and for which they are reluctant to seek assistance. However, a safe system for handling the patient must take preference over his wishes.

The different options should be explained to the patient so that he can contribute to the discussion and to the resulting care plan.

The Environment

Toilet cubicles are danger areas in many hospitals, residential and day-care establishments, and are where many staff are injured. The cubicles have generally been designed and equipped without the benefit of either ergonomics or practical caring experience.

Assessing officers should be aware that the standard door width of 750mm (30 inches) is too narrow for self propelled wheelchairs and many pushed chairs. The result is that many staff have to struggle to move heavy and unsteady patients round through 180 degree turns in awkward and twisting postures.

A door width of 900mm (35 inches) is necessary. It should open outwards or have the type of hinges which allow it to do so, even if it is ordinarily an inward opening type.

A much larger cubicle is needed for an inward opening door, to enable it to be closed behind the user.

The door catch must be easily opened from the outside in case anyone inside should need assistance.

The methods that independent patients use are as varied as their disabilities. The five most common are listed here and may be used independently by the patient, or with the aid of a transfer board, or with a carer's supervision:

> from the side – a lateral transfer either left or right; both options should be provided in unisex toilets;

> forward facing – often used by double lower limb amputees, who choose to sit facing the

cistern, rather than turning all the way round;

through the back of the wheelchair, where the back rest has been adapted for this purpose

oblique, either left or right; opportunities for both methods should be provided

assisted frontal – where the person is turned round to sit facing the front.

Where an assessment of risk concludes that the toilet cubicle does not allow transfers to be made with safety, a mobile sanichair is a safer alternative. A transfer can then be achieved outside the cubicle where there is more space. This sometimes means using a lobby area outside several other cubicles, in which case a lock on the exterior door will ensure that the patient can be prepared in privacy.

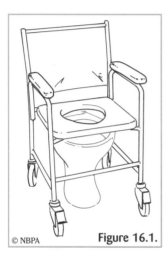

© NBPA   **Figure 16.1.**

There is a wide range of mobile sanichairs for use either in conjunction with a WC or replacing it. The type with a removable pan can be used beside the bed or in another private place, or the chair can be pushed through to the toilet cubicle, the pan removed and the chair then reversed over the WC pan.

WARNING

To use a mobile sanichair in a toilet cubicle, the height of the WC seat must not be altered from the standard in any way. Raising the bowl on a plinth or the installation of a much higher bowl is not recommended. If the primary reason for raising the seat is to make it easier for users to stand from sitting, then the addition of correctly sited grab rails or a fitted raised toilet seat is preferable, provided the mobile chair can still be wheeled over the standard height seat.

COMMODES

Mobile commodes

In the home of a dependent disabled person, a mobile commode is often provided as it is not always possible to enlarge the family bathroom. It is often possible, however, to knock down a partition wall between a separate WC and the bathroom to provide a larger space.

A mobile sanichair should be waterproof if it is likely to be used to move from the bedside to over the WC and then into a level access shower area.

There is a range of these chairs and the following design features should be considered:

wheels on a mobile commode should have brakes on all four castors. The braking mechanism should be easy to reach and able to be operated in soft slippers – particularly for carers in the home

a sanichair which is also used as a shower chair should be waterproof

removable arms for transfers which are either assisted, independent, or by hoist

the commode pan is removed for emptying from the top of the seat, the side or back, whichever is easiest for the nurse

footrests – are necessary and should be adjustable to the correct leg length for the user; if of a platform design, it should be possible to swing the footrest away so that the person can stand or transfer;

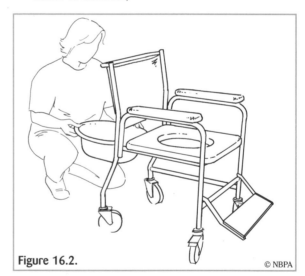

Figure 16.2.   © NBPA

the back rest should be straight. If it has handles to hold when the chair is being pushed, they must not protrude to come in contact with a low coupled WC cistern and so prevent the chair being positioned over the pan;

the seat can be flat with a shaped hole to fit the WC pan. Alternatives are a plastic toilet seat or a padded horse-shoe design. Padding gives comfort, and the horse-shoe shape is easier for the patient to clean himself after toilet use or during showering;

where the disabled person may be away from home on a visit or on holiday, a folding mobile sanichair, that fits into the back of a car, will enable him to use most WCs.

Static Commodes

Commodes should be sited in a private area and placed in such a way that there is space for easy and safe transfers. A frequent cause of falls by elderly people is when the commode is not beside the bed at night and they have to struggle to reach it when they are at their weakest and when they may also be under the effect of night medication, and confused.

A choice of design features makes it possible to suit the needs of most patients:

the legs should be adjustable so that the seat can be at a convenient height. The legs should be splayed out at the back for stability, but vertical in front for foot positioning

the arms should be removable for easier transfers on and off the bed, as fixed arms can get in the way. Some commodes fasten to the bed frame for stability for transfers during the night, when there may be minimal assistance available, or when the patient is able to move independently

emptying the commode should be done either from the back or side - space and usage may dictate which is preferable. In community settings, thought must be given to when and how the commode is to be emptied. If the pan is to be lifted out from the top, the user has to be transferred from the commode before it can be emptied. A carer may have to stoop to lift a used pan to remove it from the side or back. A chemical toilet, where the liquid is in the base, will eliminate smell and it can also be used several times before needing emptying; however, the more it is used, the heavier it becomes to empty.

whether the commode may be used in an establishment or by an individual person, it must be easy to clean

commodes are useful as a temporary measure, particularly for older people at night and when the toilet is some distance away from the bedroom, or where a person cannot gain access to the WC.

In the past commodes have been chosen because they can be removed from the bedside during the day and stacked in a small area, but the practice of lifting, carrying and stacking them away from the bedside can be stressful and must be discontinued.

When buying a commode, thought should be given to the increasing use of mobile sanichairs for use in a toilet cubicle. It is valuable to have a range of designs, so that the variety of patients' needs can be met.

Carers helping with toilet transfers must be trained in the various options and techniques, so that they are competent when the patient is most vulnerable. The equipment must be safe and accompanied by clear instructions, and carers must be knowledgeable in its use.

WARNING

Such practices as a carer manually supporting a patient up on his feet and at the same time trying to adjust clothing or clean him, are not acceptable and have been condemned for many years. Carers should not be asked to do more than one task at a time. If a standing patient has to be supported by one or two carers, another nurse should adjust clothing, remove pads, or clean him.

Figure 16.3.

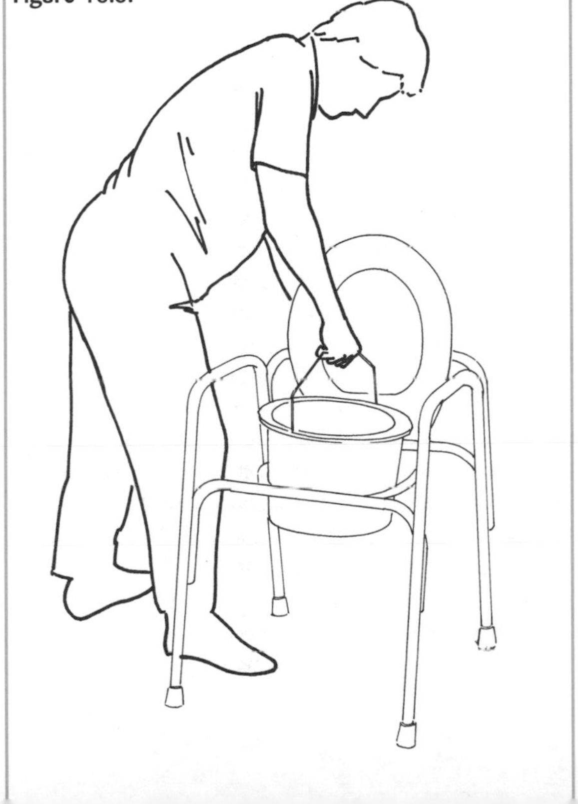

© NBPA

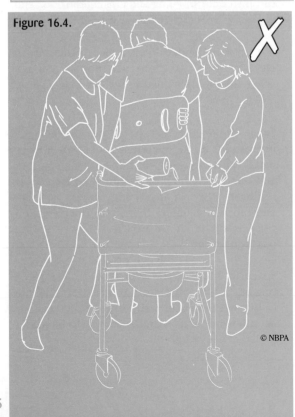

Figure 16.4.

© NBPA

If a patient cannot stand unsupported, mechanical assistance must be used.

Many nurses are still being injured while doing these personal tasks.

WC CUBICLE SIZES AND DESIGNS

Where the dependency level of the patient indicates that mechanical assistance is required for toilet transfers, space must be created to provide a private and suitable area. Joining two cubicles together can be a solution, or a wheeled sanichair could be used in the existing cubicle and pushed over the WC.

Where cubicles are to be used by several people who are dependent, the best use of limited space is made by having cubicles in which transfers can be made from one side only, some on one side, some on the other, rather than have all the cubicles wide enough for transfers on both sides. This gives patients and carers a choice.

When plans are being made to adapt or extend a bathroom, the method for transferring the patient on and off the WC, and its use by other members of the family and carers, must be taken into consideration. A bathroom may be enlarged by combining it with an adjacent WC, but this may cause privacy problems for those who want to use either facility when the disabled person is using the other one.

Key design features in planning adaptations or extensions to a bathroom to be taken into account are:

the size of the cubicle or toilet room for a wheelchair or mobile sanichair must allow for a turning circle, opening and closing the door, and space for the carer to move around the patient

if a hoist is needed it must be a ceiling track electric hoist, as there will not be enough space for a mobile hoist as well as a wheelchair and a carer

space beside the WC should be 1150mm - 45 inches - for an independent user to be able to make sideways or oblique transfers. An additional minimum of 900mm - 35 inches - is required for an assisting carer and an allowance of 400mm - 16 inches - if a side hand rinse basin is to be reached from a seated position on the WC

space in front of the WC should allow for a turning circle of a mobile chair of 1500mm (59 inches) diameter, without obstructions, for an independent user and 1600mm (63 inches) if assistance is required

the siting of a hand rinse basin is important: an independent user may want to wash his hands before handling the wheelchair or clothing; those having intermittent catheterisation need to approach the WC from the front and have immediate access to the basin; if the patient is always assisted, the basin need not be within reach of the seated person

where the WC is set to one side of the cubicle, a distance of 400mm (16 inches) is needed from the centre of the WC pan to the nearest side obstruction, including pipes, skirting boards and grab rails. This is so that a mobile sanichair can be easily pushed over the WC and centred over the pan

the door must be positioned so that direct access is gained to the WC and must be 900mm (35 inches) wide for an independent wheelchair. It should have a horizontal bar at handle height so it can be pulled shut. An outward opening door is preferred, with a lock which can be opened from both sides

the height of the WC pan must enable an elderly or disabled person to rest his feet on the ground. A standard fixed pan, 430mm (17 inches) high, is preferred, as the height of the seat can be adjusted with a raised seat of two inches, four inches, or six inches as required. A raised seat can be taken off or the normal seat can be replaced with a raised one that fixes on the back of the pan.

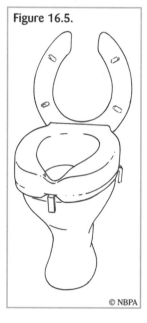

Figure 16.5.

© NBPA

A WC with a horse-shoe shaped seat, or with a dip in the front, makes it easier for users to clean themselves.

It is often preferable to have a seat without a lid, particularly when the WC is shared. Many people lean backwards for support and the lids are not designed either to take their weight or offer comfort, and often become soiled.

Support rails with a padded backrest can be supplied, especially where there is a high level cistern and a downpipe, which is uncomfortable to lean against.

Many independent users need a grab rail beside the seat to help them stand up. A rail should be mounted on the wall from a point level with the centre of the bowl, elbow height, and pointing forwards and upwards to a distance of some 250mm (10 inches) in front of the edge of the seat.

Rails can be hinged to fold down for side support beside the WC and lifted up to allow space for sideways transfers or for assistance. These rails are wall mounted at the rear of the WC and can also incorporate a paper holder.

Other rails can be provided in a variety of ways by means of floor mounted fixed frames which may get in the way of some people using the WC – or free-standing raised seats on a height adjustable frame.

The more adjustable and flexible the rail system the better. Some men may prefer to stand facing the WC and consequently need an upright rail close to one side.

Fixed rails are only suitable where the toilet cubicle can be reserved for ambulant patients, as they preclude transfers from wheelchairs and obstruct the handlers.

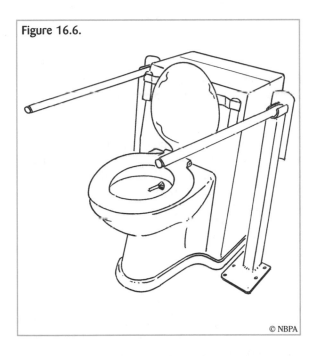

Figure 16.6.

© NBPA

A cantilever, wall hung, WC allows easier access for wheelchair footplates, and this aids transfers and makes it easier to clean the cubicle floor. A high level cistern often gives a few more inches of floor space than a low close coupled suite, which protrudes more from the wall.

CLEANSING

After using the toilet, cleansing is the most personal task – the majority of patients like to do it themselves to maintain dignity, privacy and

independence. When staff are assisting the patient, it must be regarded as a medium risk task, as they have to stoop.

There are several ways to assist the patient to remain independent.

Toilet paper must be within easy reach. Folded interlocking sheets are best for one-handed patients – and for assistants. The container must be sited to the front of the person and not on the back wall behind him.

Some WC support rails have a holder for a roll of paper, while others have devices to allow only one or two sheets to be pulled off at a time.

For people who cannot reach to clean themselves with the toilet paper, various holders are commercially available. These usually have a long, plastic angled handle, which has a clip or opening at the end to receive the paper. While some people find them useful, they must be used from the front towards the back of the perineal area to reduce the risk of infection.

A portable bidet, a plastic moulded dish, is designed to be placed on top of the WC bowl. It can be filled with warm water from a nearby wash basin. The patient can sit on it to wash himself without having to struggle to keep on his feet. The water is tipped down the pan afterwards. The patient can dry himself by transferring to a wheelchair or bathroom stool which has a towel spread on it, before the final transfer back to his own chair.

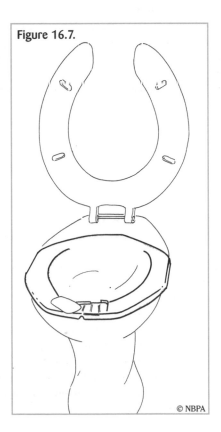

Figure 16.7.

© NBPA

Automatic WCs incorporating a washing and drying facility must be considered for use to maintain the patient's independence and to help carers with this difficult task. A WC pan is replaced by a whole unit, or there are modified units which can be fitted to existing pans.

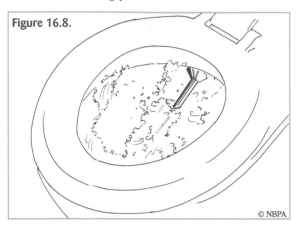

Figure 16.8.

© NBPA

After using the automatic WC, a douche spray can be operated. It has thermostatically heated water, with a temperature control, and can be angled to suit the individual. The task is completed by a warm air dryer. The spray and the warm air are controlled by a switch, which can be operated by a person's foot, fixed to the wall or hand held, and is designed and mounted to suit whatever is required.

This type of cleaning system is most welcome to many patients, wherever they live, as it maintains their independence, dignity, and privacy – and reduces, too, handling stress on carers. It should, however, be tested by the patient before installation, since it is not successful with all users. Those who suffer from muscular spasm in their lower limbs may find it increases the spasms and so makes them less stable while using the unit.

Assisting the dependent patient

The task of cleaning a patient after using the WC must be approached with caution. It involves stooping and twisting movements for the nurse and invariably three staff are needed if a patient can stand - two to support and the third to clean.

Apart from the loss of the patient's privacy in this circumstance, it may be difficult to find three staff available at the same time to help with the task, and it implies also that the staff may be handling a dependent patient in an inappropriate way which is no longer recommended.

As the methods of assisting patients are varied the following suggestions may be considered.

The patient, seated on the WC is moved forwards on the seat so that he can lean backwards towards the cistern or backrest. This action opens up the angle at the hip, and therefore, gives more space for the patient wishing to clean his own frontal area.

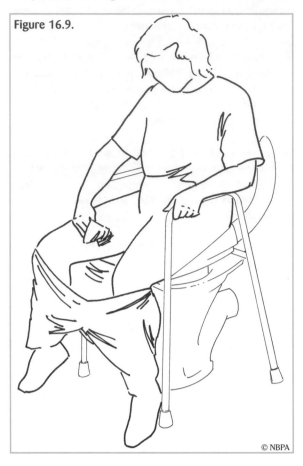

Figure 16.9.

© NBPA

For the same reason, it is also easier if the WC seat has a dipped access area at the front of the seat to allow a hand to get into the right area.

From the forward seated position, the patient can be assisted to lean forwards, giving a larger space behind, to help the carer clean the patient's anal area, which is difficult to reach if the patient is sitting back.

This method can be used on a WC, commode or sanichair, as the patient remains seated and so is stable. The task can usually be done by one carer and it helps the patient to retain some privacy and dignity.

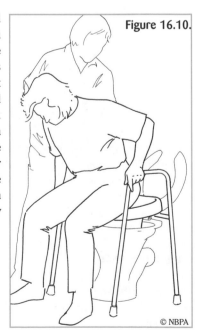

Figure 16.10.

© NBPA

For a patient who cannot move on the seat and cannot give any help, either a standing hoist is required or the patient is hoisted to a bed or changing couch so that the areas to be cleaned can be reached. Reaching beneath and behind a patient who is sitting on a commode or sanichair involves some risk of back or shoulder strain to the carer, apart from the difficulty of completing a task that cannot be seen.

If a standing mobile hoist is to be used there must be space for it inside the WC cubicle, otherwise transfers must be made outside the cubicle, but still with privacy.

Some WC seats are on frames which have an assisted rising action, either mechanical, or electrically powered. This riser toilet seat may help a patient rise to his feet and support himself on the frame while a member of staff helps to clean him.

Note: Increased use of the automatic washing and drying WC referred to earlier must be considered to alleviate this difficult task.

WHEELCHAIR DESIGN AND TOILET TRANSFERS

When people are transferring from wheelchair to WC certain design features must be considered when prescribing a wheelchair.

Back Rest

For the few people who like to transfer backwards on to the WC, a split back canvas can be supplied. Some amputee patients prefer this, if they are to sit facing the front.

Arm Rests

Arms should be easily removable, so that clothing can be adjusted, hoist slings positioned, or sideways transfers made.

Foot Rests

Foot rests should lift up and swing away from the front of the wheelchair and should also be detachable. There must be clear space around the feet to allow the patient to stand and move when being helped to transfer.

Cushions

A wheelchair cushion, with a cut-out at the front, allows a patient to use a hand-held urinal while seated. Adapted clothing is required for successful use, but it does allow a patient to micturate while sitting and without transferring, particularly one who spends long periods alone.

CLOTHING

The options for clothing management are:

Conventional

The person who wears strong cotton pants of a conventional style can often be supported and rolled from side to side while the skirt is eased up and the pants are eased down over the person's hips.

The nurse stands in front of the patient with her legs braced against and outside the patient's knees. The patient is supported by the nurse placing one arm around the shoulders and gently pulling the patient slightly forward and to the side being supported. With the free hand, the nurse pulls the skirt up so that it will be clear from underneath the seated person. The roll is then reversed so that the other side is then eased up. After the skirt is clear, then the side to side roll is continued but this time the waist band of the pants is pulled down until they are clear of the hips. Several rolls on each side may be required to get both sets of clothing clear of the hips.

Drop front

These can be made by a very simple clothing adaptation. All women's pants have a reinforced gusset. The front edge of this gusset is cut across and the two edges rejoined with a strip of appropriately coloured velcro. The hook part of the velcro faces away from the patient and the soft loop side can then be pressed into place against the patient. This type of design can be used by those people who are wheelchair bound and who wish to avoid transfer. They can wheel themselves (or be wheeled) into the WC cubicle. Lift the skirt, pull down the adapted gusset and place a hand-held urinal in place or use a funnel and tube over into the WC bowl.

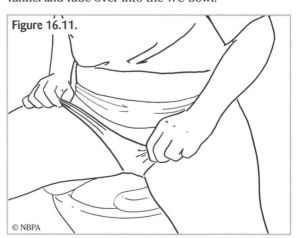
Figure 16.11.
© NBPA

Teddy

A commercially available design of an all-in- one, camisole and pants called a teddy can also serve in the same way as the previously described adaptation. The fastenings on the teddy may need strengthening or enlarging to make access easier.

Legged pants

Figure 16.12.

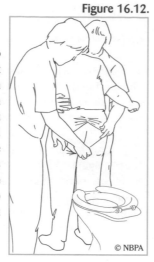

For older women who like a legged-pant design, an adaptation can be made which splits the back but allows full cover and dignity in front. To use this type, the person is again rocked but the pants are is pulled to one side with the waist band left in place.

© NBPA

TOILET TRANSFER - USING A HOIST

When a patient is to be transferred to a commode or WC and is non weight bearing, then a hoist must be used.

Where there is space, a mobile hoist can move a patient on to a mobile sanichair, or directly on to the WC.

If there is not enough floor space within a WC cubicle for a mobile hoist, it is usually possible to instal an overhead electric ceiling track hoist. This method may be preferred where there are many dependent people, such as in a residential home or nursing home. The track should pass over the centre of a wheelchair space and over the centre of the pan. Such a hoist will allow one carer to assist a patient with toilet transfers safely and privately.

Most manufacturers have developed slings designed to assist with toileting and the adjustment of clothing. They have a chest section with a velcro fastened band that fits around the user's chest wall. It does not have to be pulled tight nor does it restrict breathing. The sling has two side leg pieces that are pulled down each side of the user until each one can be passed under the nearest leg. These leg sections are usually padded to prevent any discomfort when the weight of the hoisted person is taken through the sling.

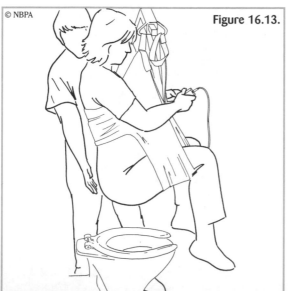

© NBPA

Figure 16.13.

When the sling is attached and the patient is lifted in the hoist, the sling leaves the hips free so that clothing can be adjusted downwards and clear of the area that needs to sit on the WC. Likewise, after using the WC the person can be lifted to make it easier to clean him and then readjust the clothing before returning him to the wheelchair.

Every person who is going to need a hoist should be assessed to determine the correct sling design. Generally, it has been found that the less muscle tone the person has, the less suitable is this particular type of sling, as its success depends on muscle tone holding the body in a sitting posture.

The slings are termed variously as Access, Dress, Independence, or Toileting slings by manufacturers.

The toileting sling has proved to be the most beneficial in a person's own home, where the task of assisting a dependent relative on and off the WC has previously been a stressful task. Many carers use this sling all the time since it is easy to use and requires much less effort to put on and off the patient.

The overhead scissor grip type of frame is also useful when a carer needs to adjust clothing. A metal frame, with body shaped supports, grips the patient around the side of the chest wall. Leg supports slide under the thighs from the inside of the leg, leaving the hip area free for the toileting tasks.

CHANGING INCONTINENCE PADS

If the patient is wearing protective pads, perhaps with special pants, it is easier to adjust clothing while lying him on a bed or changing couch.

A hoist should be used to transfer a non weight bearing patient from the wheelchair to the bed. The sling may then be removed to roll the patient from side to side to remove clothing, so as to reach the pants and pad. This also helps the carer to wash and dry the patient, while changing to a clean pad and pants.

The bed or couch must be height adjustable so that the carer does not have to stoop and stretch.

Easy access to a wash basin and a soiled pad disposal bin avoids carrying bowls of water and soiled pads and clothing through a public area.

STANDING TRANSFERS

A range of products has been developed specifically to assist with transferring a patient from one seated position to another, as in the toileting task. Most of them need co-operation from the patient, who should be able to take some of his own weight while being supported in a semi-standing position.

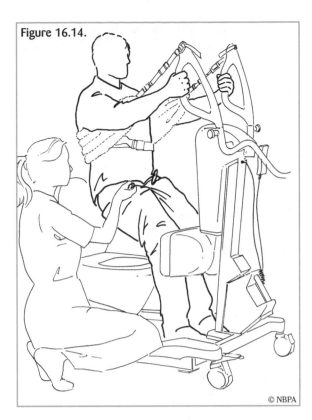

Figure 16.14.

© NBPA

The hoists have a padded band, often of sheepskin, which is placed across the lower part of the patient's back and forward under their axillae - the patient's feet having already been placed on the footrest of the hoist with the knees positioned close to the knee pad on the hoist mast. The padded band is attached to the front arms of the spreader bar and pulled tight. The bar is then lifted by operating the hoist, which may be done by a winding handle or an electrically powered hand control.

The patient is raised into a semi-upright position, where clothing can be adjusted, before being seated on the WC or the toilet seat attachment to the hoist or mobile sanichair.

Once the toileting is completed, the patient can be raised for cleansing and the clothing readjusted, before being returned to his own chair.

An advantage of this system is that the patient has the sensation of standing, even though being unable to bear his weight independently.

This type of product is most frequently used in residential or nursing homes or hospitals where several patients can benefit from it.

In a house where space in the bathroom or WC often dictates what equipment is selected, an overhead ceiling track electric hoist has many advantages. The track can be positioned to pass over the bath and the WC so that, with the use of an Access sling, transfers can be completed with minimal effort by the carer.

Some users have installed a folding changing platform over the bath, so that the changing of pads can be done in private, with suitable facilities on hand for washing, drying and the disposal of soiled pads.

MANUAL TRANSFERS

Unless the patient can rise from sitting, and then stand and bear his weight through his legs, transfers to the WC must be mechanically assisted. Any help given by a carer should follow the guidance given in Chapter 15.

Some patients can stand with the help of a horizontal wall bar on which to pull themselves upright. The carer can then exchange the wheelchair for a commode or a wheeled sanichair placed behind the patient.

For guidance on toileting a patient in bed, see Chapter 14.

WASHING AND BATHING

by Christine Tarling

SUMMARY

Washing and bathing are two of the most strenuous tasks for nurses, and care must be taken to reduce stress whenever possible.

IT IS NOT ACCEPTABLE THAT ANY CARER SHOULD LIFT A PATIENT OUT OF THE BATH.

For safety, a frail, disabled or elderly person should always enter and leave a bath while sitting, NOT by climbing over the side of the bath and balancing on one leg.

If none of the alternatives described here can be supplied or are unsuitable, either for the nurse or the patient, then a strip-wash or a bed-bath must be used. The difficulties of supporting and washing a patient are back threatening and must be avoided.

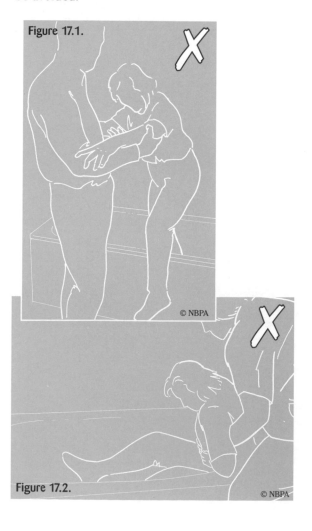

Figure 17.1.

© NBPA

Figure 17.2.

© NBPA

MAINTAINING PERSONAL HYGIENE

There are choices for the patient and the carer to make when deciding how to maintain the patient's personal hygiene.

The main choices are:

- a strip wash – in bed or sitting in a chair

- access to a bath using one of several types of bathing equipment. The patient must be able to lift, or have his legs moved, over the side of the bath

- a step-in shower with a wall fixed seat

- a level access shower base with an adjustable or mobile shower chair or stool

- a shower trolley, used either alone, or in conjunction with a height adjustable bath.

With this variety of bathing and washing alternatives, it should be possible to select a method that offers comfort and privacy to the patient.

More importantly, the chosen system must allow the carer to have a comfortable working posture.

Costs may be reduced by selecting the correct option since many patients may find that they can manage to bathe themselves independently, with the right equipment.

Whether the patient is in hospital, living in a residential home or at home in the community, a number of factors must be considered when making an assessment of the risks involved in bathing.

A person can be kept clean in many ways. In the community, this is not regarded as a high priority by a social services department when prioritising the needs of elderly or disabled clients. The person's needs that should be addressed quickly are: maintaining body warmth, having food to eat, getting to the WC, dressing and undressing, and the ability to move about in his own environment.

Services that enable people living in their own homes to continue bathing are often slow in arriving. Where a medical condition indicates that personal hygiene is important to promote health, an assessment of need is classed as a higher priority. Consequently, people with such conditions as incontinence or a skin condition which is being treated with prescribable emollients should be seen and assessed before people who have lost the physical skill of getting in and out of the bath.

A bathing assessment must be approached with sensitivity since many elderly people may reply in a way that they think is socially acceptable to questions on personal hygiene. The question "How do you manage with the bath?" implies that the bath is used, and elderly people may not wish to tell a stranger that they have not had a bath for years but have had strip washes at the kitchen sink. They see the task as keeping personally clean. Likewise, a question "How do you manage your washing?" might lead to a description of how difficult it is to operate a washing machine.

BATHROOM DESIGNS

In hospitals or residential homes, there are two types of bathroom layout. The first has the bath with its long side against a wall, and the second has the bath with the tap end at the wall but with room to move on both sides of the bath.

In the community, the bath is most often against the wall and any adaptations must take into account the needs of other users of the bathroom.

There must be space to undress, dry and dress again in the bathroom.

If water is required, often dressings or soiled pads are changed in the bathroom for privacy.

If a person is incontinent or has soiled himself, it is useful to have a WC in the bathroom, rather than in a separate room. However, if this is the only WC in the house, long occupancy of the bathroom by a disabled person may lead to friction in the family.

The bathroom is usually upstairs in a family house and then a decision needs to be made, by those participating in the assessment, about access to bedroom and bathing facilities.

If the disabled person cannot climb the stairs or use a stairlift to go upstairs, there may not be space in a family home for a vertical lift. In these circumstances, downstairs bathing and bedroom facilities may be the answer.

The provision of adaptations to houses in the community is complicated. If the house is owner-occupied or privately rented, it is usual to apply to the local authority for a disabled facilities grant. This is subject to a nationally agreed test of resources to calculate whether the disabled person and his family must contribute anything towards the cost of the work.

While most people who are living at benefit income level do not have to contribute anything, many people who have a private pension, and/or additional savings above the income support levels, may have to pay on a sliding scale of contributions.

A grant applicant who is employed and earning above family credit levels, usually must pay something.

For those people living in council housing, the local authority may pay for the adaptations from its own housing budget or use the disabled facilities grant to maximise local budgets. When the disabled person and his family feel that they cannot meet their financial contribution, they may apply to social services for a discretionary grant to assist them. In the current financial climate, many local authorities are unable to offer discretionary grants and this leaves the disabled person unable to make progress with the adaptations.

In all community cases, it is the responsibility of the social services department to assess need. For this type of adaptation, it is usually the community occupational therapy services that make the assessment and the recommendations. While most local authority social service departments employ occupational therapists, some still obtain these specialist skills from their local health care trust.

Where adaptations are required for a person to be discharged from hospital safely, carefully made plans for roles and responsibilities must be laid down.

The practice of minimising the patients' stays in hospital often results in them being discharged home months before adaptations can be provided. In these circumstances, patients are often living in a bed downstairs in the one living room with a bedside commode, and cannot use an upstairs bathroom and bedroom. This places a strain on carers and on the disabled person who loses privacy and dignity at a time when he is still recovering from the shock of the disability.

For the recently discharged patient attending rehabilitation as an outpatient, access to bathing facilities is an important part of treatment and care while adaptations are being assessed and provided. It can take six to twelve months for an adaptation funded through the disabled facilities grant to be completed. During this time, the needs of the patient for bathing should be discussed by those involved in providing his care and alternative services offered if facilities are not accessible at home.

Hospital or Multiple Use bathrooms:

In hospital or at home, the design of the bathroom must give the carers space to bathe the patient. It is best to plan for the needs of the most dependent patient so that there is adequate space for others. It should be easy to reach both sides of the patient in the bath without too much stretching and stooping. It must be assumed that frail, elderly or disabled people who live in hospital or residential or nursing homes, have difficulty in bathing. Since it is a physically complex task, most will require help, usually from a nurse, and often with equipment to get them into the water and out again.

Whether a bath or shower is used, each has advantages and disadvantages:

Bath advantages:

bathing is a familiar task to most older people who may not have had a shower before and who may be wary of a new experience

a long hot warm soak is said to be therapeutic and when used with bath water additives, such as those used by aromatherapists, can be beneficial to people who have aching and stiff joints. It also warms the body through, making it easier to relax and sleep afterwards. For people who cannot move themselves most of the day, a warm soak in a bath before bed is the best way there is to a beneficial sleep

in the community, retaining the bath is a cheaper and less disruptive way of providing bathing facilities

a variety of bathing equipment will help most people to reach and get into and out of the bath

carers often prefer assisting at a bath rather than a shower since they find it difficult to help the person to wash while keeping dry themselves.

Bath Disadvantages:

stooped postures have to be adopted by the carer if a height adjustable bath cannot be provided, for example, in the domestic home

it is slower than having a shower

some bath hoists and equipment are better not used with bath additives since they make it difficult to clean the equipment and make it slippery.

Shower Advantages:

a shower is easily accessible for most people

it is quicker than having a bath

it takes up less room if space is limited

a carer can reach most parts of the patient to assist, though there is some stretching and stooping to reach feet.

Shower Disadvantages:

it is generally a cooler experience than a bath since the patient has to sit while wet and undressed, and unless the bathroom is warm, may feel cold

in the domestic house, the provision of a shower may mean applying for housing adaptation work, and there are costs involved

where a shower is being considered in a domestic house, other users in the house must be considered, particularly where there are young children. It is not easy to wash an active young child in a shower, and his normal bath time and playtime activities are restricted

some older people who are nervous or frightened of new experiences will resist a shower if they have not had one previously.

Bathroom Flooring:

One of the greatest hazards in the bathroom is the wet floor. Floor covering materials must be non-slip and nurses should take extra care selecting suitable supportive non-slip footwear.

If a bathroom has been used for one patient and water spilled on the floor, it should be wiped and dried before the next patient is taken to be bathed.

The design of the bath:

The height of the bath, as well as its type of construction, can make the bath easier to use by any patient. The bath rim should be of a height which allows patients to sit and rise easily if bathing equipment is being used in the bath. The heights will be the same as those required for standing from sitting, that is about 18 inches (460mm) high.

The bath may be of enamel, metal, or acrylic. Some bathing equipment is not suitable for light weight acrylic baths although users report that these baths are warmer than the metal type.

Any grab rails on the sides of the bath should not protrude above the height of the rim so that any equipment which has to be fitted across the rim of the bath will sit flat. Any grab rails that stick up will also make it difficult when the patient is trying to move his legs across and into the bath.

The bath shape should be as simple as possible. Some of the newer and more curvaceous bath designs do not allow the use of bathing equipment. Because of the internal shape of the bath, there is not enough space on the floor of the bath.

A full size bath is preferred, 67ins to 75ins (1700mm to 1900mm) long by 32ins (800mm) wide. A bath that is shorter will restrict the use of certain types of bath hoists.

Some height adjustable baths allow the bath to be lowered to make it easier for the patient to get in, usually with a bath hoist, and be raised so that the nurse can assist without stooping. These are becoming much more widely used as the whole bathing activity becomes a much safer task for patient and nurse. Some models have a jacuzzi or bubble stream which tones and cleans the skin while it also stimulates the circulation.

Some other models can be mobile, with a fold down side panel which enables them to be used as a changing bench for people who are incontinent.

Other moulded baths have a removable side panel so that the patient can slide across to an internal seat. The panel is replaced and the bath can be angled backwards so that the greater proportion of the patient's body is immersed in warm water.

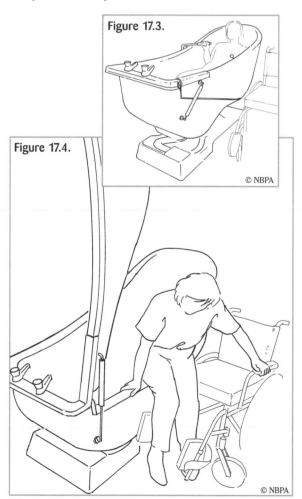

Figure 17.3.

Figure 17.4.

When choosing a specialist type of bath, it is important to check how the patient can enter and leave it safely. If it cannot be used with a hoist for the more dependent patients, then alternatives should be sought.

Sit-baths were once popular but are not frequently used now that alternatives allow patients to get into a more normal bath.

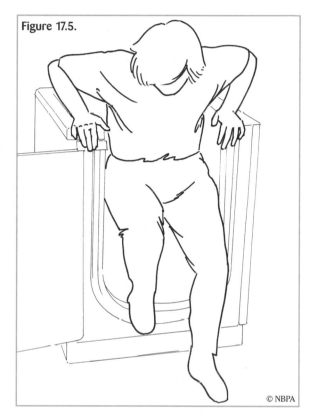

Figure 17.5.

© NBPA

Some mobile hoists transport the patient, who, while still seated, can be enclosed in a bath cabinet. Others require the patient to stand and step into the cabinet before the door can be closed and the water added.

While these designs may be useful for the confused patient or those who lack confidence to enter a full bath, they create postural problems for the nurse who has to assist the patient.

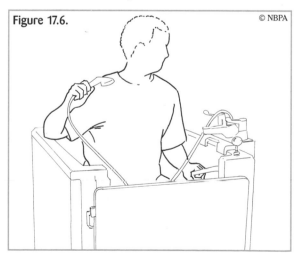

Figure 17.6.

© NBPA

The sides of the cabinet and the door are above waist height and the assisting nurse has to lean over them to reach the patient. Washing the patient's feet and legs is best left until the water has been released and the door can be opened. The nurse can then squat, or kneel down to reach into the footwell of the bath.

BATH EQUIPMENT

The options for resolving difficulties for patients getting into the bath are generally followed in a certain order that starts with basic equipment, such as the bath board and seat, which helps a patient with minimal mobility difficulties. It will then move through various other choices before considering the removal of a bath and the installation of a level access shower, as is needed by the most dependent patient.

In the community, social services departments will often have a policy that equipment must be tested with existing facilities before alternatives, such as a shower, are contemplated.

Bath Board and Seat:

This system is suitable for those people who can take their own body weight through their arms. If the patient has painful arms, in particular painful wrist and elbow joints, then this is not likely to be successful since the strain placed through the arm joints will cause more discomfort.

A simple test can be made by asking the patient to sit on a dining chair and then asking him to use his arms to lift himself up from the seat. If this check is not made before trying the equipment, there is a risk that the person will get into the bath and not be able to lift himself out again.

In addition to being able to take his own body weight through the arms, the person must be able to lift or move his legs over the side of the bath. This is made more difficult if he has poor balance so that sitting on the board while lifting the legs makes him unstable.

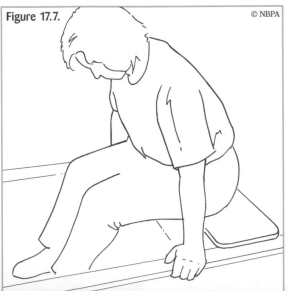

Figure 17.7.   © NBPA

Sometimes the bath board is used alone until another solution can be provided. Some people can have a sponge down while sitting on the board without attempting to go down on to a seat in the bath.

Points to watch

The height of the bath rim must be checked to give the patient seated access. He must be able to sit and stand from the board which is fitted across the top of the bath rim

Check whether the bath is metal or acrylic, since different types of bath seats may be required for an acrylic bath which cannot stand the strain of a seat adjustment bracket braced against the bath side.

Check the width of the bath since the bath board must not protrude beyond the width of the bath so that it does not tip if the patient sits on the outer edge. Also check if there are obstructions on the far side of the bath to prevent the board from being fitted firmly and flat; for example, a bath bar or extra row of edged tiling.

Check the depth of the bath since the bath seat will need to be about half way from the floor of the bath to the rim.

Bath boards are available slatted or solid, padded or firm; wood, plastic or cork coated. They all have adjustable brackets under the seat board which brace against the sides of the bath as near the head end as is possible.

Check the patient's weight since heavy duty boards may be required for those over 102kg (16st) in weight,

Bath seats are used together with a bath board if the person is to go down into the water. These also are slatted or solid and available in different heights. They usually have plastic suckers on the base, and these must adhere to the floor of the bath for safety.

BATH HOISTS

These require the patient to be able to get his legs over the rim of the bath. They take the effort out of the movement of getting down into the bath and up again. They may be operated either by the carer or by the patient, thus giving the opportunity for independence and privacy.

Bath hoists mounted on the floor:

Those that operate from a pillar mounted on the floor beside the bath are available with a range of seats including a commode seat that allows access to be made to wash beneath a seated person; some have detachable seats that can be mounted on a mobile frame to use as a mobile sani-chair over the WC or with a commode pan.

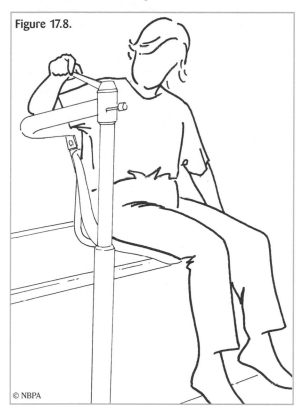

Figure 17.8.

© NBPA

Advantages:

since the seat can be swung clear of the bath, the other family members or users can use the bath without having to lift bathing equipment in and out

the seat provides good support for a person who has poor balance

it is easier for the carer to assist the person in and out of the bath. Hoists with gear winding mechanisms require more effort to use than the electrical models and the carer's needs must be taken into account

if the patient has difficulty in lifting his legs over the side of the bath, the hoist can be raised into a higher position. The seat height can also be altered to ease the task of standing or transferring on or off it.

Disadvantages:

there must be enough space in the bathroom for the seat part of the hoist to swing clear of the bath for the patient to get on and off. Many small domestic bathrooms, particularly those in the one bedroom bungalows provided for older people, lack space beside the bath

many patients find that they cannot operate the hoist themselves, particularly if it is a geared winding mechanism which is mounted on the top of the supporting pillar.

Bath hoists that fit inside the bath:

These are useful where there is limited space in the bathroom. A full length bath is needed since a short bath is not long enough for the base of the hoist to fit inside, nor for the patient's leg length.

> ## WARNING
>
> These are best used where only one person uses the bath and the bath hoist, since the lifting of the hoist in and out of the bath frequently is not recommended for the following reasons:

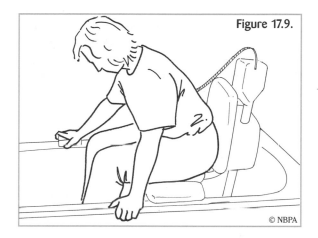

Figure 17.9.

© NBPA

very few hoists weigh less than 10kg (22lbs)

the hoist is fastened down in the bath by four suction cups which are difficult to release, resulting in the lifter struggling with a stuck load

the hoist is not a regular or box shaped load and its shape is irregular. This irregularity make it difficult to balance and hold when lifting from a low position

the position of the hoist in the bath means that the lifter has difficulty in positioning herself so that she can get the load close to or between her feet. The lifter is always forced into a stooped and often twisted posture

these hoists are not recommended where carers who are unfit and elderly have to move them in and out of the bath.

There is a wide range of internal bath hoists and each has its unique design features. There are advantages and disadvantages to each of them. When choosing a model, the following check list should be followed:

the length of the bath: a short bath makes it difficult for the patient to stretch his legs

the depth of the bath. Many bath hoists are mounted on a frame. This puts the patient a distance from the floor of the bath when fully lowered. If the bath is shallow, there is barely enough water to cover the person to the hips, let alone to the waist, which is what is perceived as 'having a bath.' The water tank may not provide enough hot water to fill the bath adequately

the backrest. Many designs do not allow the patient to lie down in the water if they have backrests which are not removable. The back rest may be necessary to give support to someone with poor balance, and not for someone who wants to lie back in the water

how the hoist is powered. Many have a hand control with an integral or adjacent battery pack that can be removed for recharging. Others have an air compressor that is plugged into a power socket outside the bathroom door. This results in a trailing air line that could be a hazard to some people and means a lack of privacy if the door cannot be shut

whether the person lives alone and the hoist can be left in the bath. Ask about who may clean it and who may move it

whether the person wishes to use bath additives such as a foam or creme bath mixture. Oils and creme mixtures in particular make the hoist seat slippery. Sitting on a small towel or flannel will sometimes give security. Some manufacturers do not recommend the use of such products with their equipment

the weight of the patient should be within the safe lifting load limits, which vary from 115 - 140kg (18 to 22stone), according to the type of hoist

whether the noise of the hoist disturbs the patient, as noise levels vary

the range of hand controls. If the patient is to be independent, his ability to operate the lever or press button controls is important.

The next stage in the choice of bathing options is the situation in which the patient cannot get his legs over the side of the bath while sitting on the hoist or bath board. There is an additional option to enable him to continue using the bath instead of a shower.

Ceiling Track electric hoist:

This hoist is suitable for the more severely disabled person. A sling or body support system holds the

person while a ceiling track hoist raises him high enough for his feet to clear the rim of the bath. Once down in the bath, a body support system may be needed since the person may not have enough postural control to sit comfortably and safely in the water. These support systems may be inflatables, vacuum bead cushions, made to measure or off the peg frames with a mesh hammock.

It is possible to leave the patient suspended in the hoist sling but this does not help the carer to reach all parts of the body to wash and is not relaxing for the patient.

Figure 17.10.

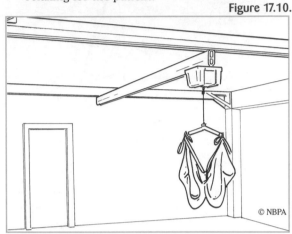

© NBPA

PROVIDING A SHOWER OVER A BATH

There may be domestic circumstances where the bath needs to be retained but the use of a bath hoist is not possible due to the problem of lifting it in and out of the bath.

Some people with severe back pain prefer to stand in the bath to shower rather than sit. If the patient prefers to sit while taking a shower over the bath then two options are possible:

a bath board across the bath, fitted as described earlier in this chapter. A slatted board or one with drainage holes avoids water running on to the bathroom floor

a swivel bather over the bath may raise the patient sufficiently high to allow his legs to clear the bath rim. This is a metal frame which is fitted astride the bath. A supportive seat moves and locks into four different positions. The seat faces the side of the bath and is locked. The patient transfers on to it. The lock is released and the seat is moved gently through 90 degrees and the patient's legs are lifted over the side of the bath. The seat can be locked into this position while a shower is used over the bath.

This equipment is useful where a carer is bathing a person who needs the confidence of a supportive seat. The seat, with arms, comforts and supports those who are confused or have short term memory loss. It also avoids the need for the carer to stoop since most of the patient's body is within easy reach.

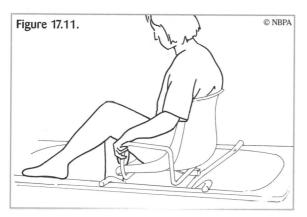

Figure 17.11.   © NBPA

PROVISION OF LEVEL ACCESS SHOWERS

In the community, showers are often regarded as a last resort since they require costly structural alterations to the house.

The design of level access bases has improved. It is usually possible to fit them to wooden or concrete bathroom floors. The shower base tray with a lip or step edge must be avoided.

A disabled person's ability to step in and out of a tray may deteriorate, and planning for wheeled access is always safer. The step in tray seldom gives enough space for the seated patient to bend forward and reach his feet.

There should be space for a carer to help a person wash. Cubicles and spaces of about 900mm (35inches) square are not large enough for a carer to reach all parts of the seated person. Where space is limited, it may be easier not to have a shower base but to cover the whole bathroom floor with a waterproof sealed flooring covering. One corner of this room should have an area where the floor slopes gently down towards the water outlet. A full length weighted curtain can be provided, together with moveable screens that protect the carer.

The following must be considered when planning these showers:

is there enough space for the patient and the carer?

is there a dry area where towels and clothing can be left?

the shower controls should be at a height that a seated person can reach, as well as the carer

the height and position of the shower head rail, because some dislike getting their head wet or washing their hair while showering

the type of water protection needed - from full length weighted curtains, or fixed or moveable screens - and at what height? If a cubicle is chosen because of a shortage of space, is there enough space for a carer to assist the seated person?

heating in the shower room, and an adequate extractor fan

a seat for the patient to sit on while showering. Fixed, wall mounted seats should be avoided. They require skill to locate them exactly in the area most comfortable for the patient. Most patients prefer a shower stool or mobile chair which they can move around in and position where they want it, with little effort. Some will be using a mobile sani-chair to which they will transfer from the bed, push through to locate over the WC and into the shower area.

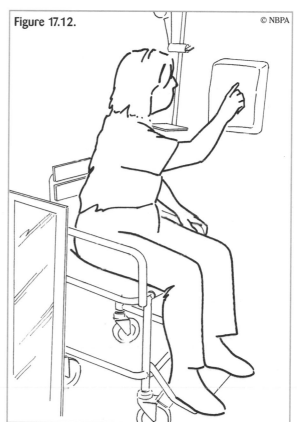

Figure 17.12.   © NBPA

Shower Trolleys

A mobile shower trolley, with a padded insert for the comfort of the dependent user, can be adjustable in height, and can be wheeled to the patient's bedside for transfers. The side of the trolley can be lowered to make the side transfer of the patient easier.

A full body sliding sheet may be used to move the adult patient from his bed to the trolley, so that he can be wheeled to the shower area.

The showering and drying of the patient is done at a height suitable to the carer, usually about waist height. This reduces the need for reaching and stooping, and reduces stress on the carer.

This equipment is in frequent use where there are high dependency patients. The padded inserts help prevent injury to patients with epilepsy or other uncontrollable body movements.

Changing benches and examination couches:

Areas where the patient may be required to be dressed and undressed include:

changing benches, which may be in bathrooms or adjacent areas where it is appropriate to change incontinence protective wear

changing benches in swimming or hydrotherapy pool areas

medical examination couches in hospitals, clinics, health centres, or general practitioner surgeries

treatment couches for other personal treatments such as physiotherapy, aromatherapy and chiropody.

For the person who has incontinence protective wear, the changing area needs to be private and with access to facilities for washing and the disposal of soiled pads and underwear, which is often done in the bathroom.

The changing of pads and pants is best done by using either a standing hoist or by lying the person on a changing couch. The standing hoist requires the person to be able to bear his own weight and to follow instructions, and co-operate in the task.

If the person cannot assist at all, then this is best done on a couch, and a hoist used for the transfers.

To save space, particularly in a bathroom, a ceiling track electric hoist would save space on the floor area (since it is sited on the ceiling) and time (since the hoist is always within reach and is easily operated).

Within the domestic home, carers sometimes use the client's bed to change pads. This may be acceptable if the bed is at a convenient height to avoid the need for stooping. However, some people may regard this as unacceptable since in normal practice the bathroom is the place where the toilet is used and washing takes place, and not the bedroom.

It may be possible to put a hinged changing table over the bath at a suitable height or in the shower area, so that a hoist can be used for transfers, and all other needs are to hand for the carer.

In a bathroom that is used by several people with incontinence, it may not be acceptable to use a showering bench also as a changing couch since keeping it clean and dry may present problems.

Since it is usually necessary to change a soiled pad soon after it is soiled, it may not be possible to wait until a shower bench is vacant and dry. A separate changing and drying area may be more useful than trying to combine the tasks into one small area.

Since many of these couches may be in restrictive spaces, transfers of patients on and off them must be planned. In hospitals or other health care places, the needs of the users will be the same.

If a patient cannot bear his own weight, and he normally use hoists where he lives, then visiting a swimming pool, a doctor's surgery or treatment area, will require a hoist if he is to transfer to a couch.

Since elderly and/or disabled people visit these facilities as part of everyday life, it is to be expected that adjustable height couches will be provided to enable the less active people to sit and lie down at the lower height, and for the doctor or treating therapist to raise the couch to the right height for the task they wish to perform.

SPECIAL HANDLING SITUATIONS

By Danielle Holmes

INTRODUCTION

This chapter considers at some of the special problems that arise in specific handling situations and with specific groups of patients. None of the sections in this chapter should be taken on their own. All of the advice in this chapter must be taken in conjunction with the advice in the rest of this book.

Most of the situations described in this section will apply at one time or another in any hospital, home or community trust. The managers of such organisations ought to consider each section to ensure that it is covered by their training and that they have the necessary equipment available.

THE UNCONSCIOUS PATIENT

The unconscious patient must be considered as a dead weight. Everything has to be done for him. There are three different types of unconscious patient to be considered:-

Long term unconscious for example, due to an accident

The patient who is unconscious recovering from anaesthesia

The collapsed person

The long term unconscious patient will need a high level of ongoing care. Proper equipment can reduce the amount of nursing effort required and also reduce the risk of pressure sores. This type of patient must be nursed in one of the automatic turning beds and/or on a pressure relieving system. When moving these patients, the nurse must use either horizontal transfer methods or hoists with scoop stretchers. N.B. When doing horizontal transfers, take extra care that the patient's head moves with the rest of the person's body. If his head is not moved properly the patient may suffer a neck injury.

When a patient is only unconscious for a short time, such as when recovering from anaesthetic, there is less need for direct intervention. However, if the patient has delicate skin, he may need to be moved to a pressure relieving mattress until he recovers. Again horizontal transfers must be done with sliding systems or scoop stretchers.

If a person has collapsed, the first priority is to establish why the collapse has occurred. In general, the rule is to leave the patient wherever he is until he has either been treated and/or he has regained consciousness.

DECEASED PATIENTS

People who have died must be treated with proper respect. However, there is never any reason to lift a body until the proper equipment is available. The lifting of bodies presents a hazard for the same reasons as the unconscious patient.

If the patient was in bed when he died, the body can be transferred using one of the lateral transfer systems or a scoop stretcher or a stretcher sling attachment. When transferring a body from the bed to the mortuary trolley, care should be taken to move obstructing furniture such as lockers. Ensure that the mortuary trolley can be brought to a safe height for the transfer. This means that mortuary trolley's must be height adjustable. Lateral transfer systems are not suitable for very heavy bodies.

WARNINGS

There are several types of concealment mortuary trolleys. There are two that present a handling risk.

1. The first type of trolley has a lid that sits on a trolley top. It opens to one side of the trolley.

When the trolley is placed up against the bed so that a body can be transferred on a sliding aid the nurse or porter cannot get to the side to pull the body as the lid is in the way. It is not possible to push the body all the way into the trolley as the reach from the far side of the bed is too far to be safe. This means that it is difficult to move a body safely into this type of trolley.

2. The second type of trolley is a box in the form of a square sided coffin. The body has to be lowered into the box. This is an unsafe lift. The only option would be to push and pull the body over the edge on a slide. This would be most undignified as the body would fall into the box with a thump. If the nurse or porter tried to stop the body from falling so hard and attempted to support its weight, they would be exposed to an unsafe load. It is then impossible to lift the body out safely on arrival at the mortuary.

N.B. It may be possible to place a body in both of these trolleys with a scoop stretcher or stretcher sling attachment. However, the stretcher could not be extracted safely. The scoop would have to be taken to the mortuary and returned when the body had been removed from the concealment trolley.

Concealment trolleys now exist that have drop sides. These allow full access for handling the body both on the ward and in the mortuary.

If a safe trolley is not available and the body is on a height adjustable bed, then the bed itself can be moved to the mortuary.

HANDLING OF DECEASED PATIENTS IN THE MORTUARY

The risks of handling and moving bodies is also an issue in the mortuary. The bodies have to be moved from whatever system they arrive on to the mortuary table and then to the storage refrigerator. When a body arrives in a mortuary it may be moved 5 or 6 times depending on whether a post-mortem is required

The only safe way of moving these bodies is with equipment. Ceiling tracking hoists are probably the best answer. There are different types, straight track or X Y systems (See Chapter 13). The type to be purchased must allow the bodies to be moved from the receiving trolley to the storage refrigerators and to the mortuary table. The solution selected must allow bodies to be moved into all levels of the storage without the operator having to twist and /or stretch to reach the top tray of the refrigerator.

Some mortuaries use special trolleys that lift the body to each level in the storage. However, these do not always solve the problem of moving the body on to the mortuary table.

Mobile hoists present problems in the mortuary. There is not enough space to manoeuvre them and they will often not be able to lift the body onto the top tray of the storage.

THE OPERATING THEATRE

There are especial problems in the operating theatre that need to be addressed to create a safe system of work. The nurse must be aware of these potential risks and make plans so that they can be carried out safely when the need arises.

Most surgeons have little knowledge of the issues of manual handling. Many surgeons expect the operating room technicians and nurses to lift. In addition to training nursing staff, managers of operating suites must undertake training programmes to ensure that surgeons and anaesthetists are trained in the safe handling of patients and other loads. This is necessary both to protect the surgeons and anaesthetists and to ensure that they do not make unsafe demands on other staff.

The manual handling tasks in theatres can be divided into 6 main groups:-

Getting the patient into theatre and onto the operating table

Moving equipment before during and after the operation

Moving the patient on the operating table

Taking the patient from the operating table to recovery

Caring for the patient in recovery

Sending the patient back to the ward.

Getting the patient into theatre and onto the operating table

Routines for transferring patients should be carefully examined. Moving the patient onto a surface for his operation, whether it be a minor or major operation, means the positioning of the patient on an operating table. Lateral transfer systems are often the simplest to use in this situation. There are concerns about infection control. This means that there is a preference for the hard sliding board type of system.

It should be noted that lateral transfer systems may not be appropriate for the very heaviest of patients. It is not unusual to find individual patients who weigh 222kg (35 stones) or more. The managers of an operating suite must expect to handle these patients from time to time. A strategy to move them must be established so that a solution is available before the problem arises. In some cases, the patient can be brought into the operating theatre on his bed. Simple operations may even be carried out with the patient on his bed. (N.B. The bed must be capable of being adjusted to a safe height for the surgeon to work. The surgeon must beware of getting into a stressful position by bending too far over the bed.)

Moving equipment before during and after the operation

The moving of sterile equipment such as theatre trays is a problem. The trays can weigh anything from a few kilos to over 25kg (56lbs). The heaviest trays must be stored at waist height. Steps must be taken to reduce the weight of trays that are too heavy to be handled. This is not easy as surgeons are used to the way in which trays are organised. It will be necessary to negotiate changes when the surgeons have been trained to understand the need for change.

In addition to the trays, operating theatres contain an increasing amount of equipment. Individual items can themselves weigh in excess of the guidance in appendix 1 of the Guidance to the Regulations. The Manual Handling Operations Regulations (1992) seems not to be a factor that is often considered in the design of these items! There are systems on the market that allow equipment to be suspended from the ceiling. The equipment can be hung from these systems and can then be easily

moved around by a light push. Alternatively, the equipment can be placed on appropriate trolleys. In either case, the initial positioning of the equipment presents a risk. There is a wide range of handling equipment available for use in factories handling materials and equipment. Managers of operating suites should equip themselves with an appropriate range of such handling devices to ensure that heavy equipment does not have to be lifted manually. (The site engineer will have a catalogue showing the wide range of devices available.)

Moving the patient on the operating table

The patient usually arrives in the operating theatre in a supine position. Some operations require the patient to be on one side or even prone.

The easiest way of turning a patient on a narrow surface such as an operating table is with a fabric turning slide. The slide is positioned before the patient is brought onto the table. He can then be turned using the normal methods for these devices (See Chapter 14).

There is some concern that fabric sheets can cause difficulties in infection control. The resistance of these devices to hot washing has improved. There is a tendency to prefer hard sliding boards because they can be cleaned more easily.

If the patient has to be on his side for the operation the correct position can be achieved as part of move from the trolley. Slide the patient part of the way across to the operating table. Then log roll him onto his side on the table. If the patient must be prone do not slide him quite as far. This requires careful planning! These moves must be practiced so that staff know how far to move the patient before starting the roll.

The operating theatre has other patient handling risks. The managers of theatres must continually review all patient handling to ensure that it is safe. A particular area to consider is the supporting of legs and arms both in preparation for and during surgery. Supporting legs or arms is posturally stressful therefore nurses must not be required to do so. There are a range of attachments available to be used in theatres. These must be available and must be used whenever a limb is to be supported. Some operating tables come with various supports that can be installed when needed. Alternatively, there are some devices that work like mini hoists attached to the side of any operating table.

Taking the patient from the operating table to recovery

This process is largely a reversal of the arrival procedure. There may, however, be additional drips and drains which can get in the way. The nurses need to include these in the process of planning the move.

Caring for the patient in recovery

Patients in recovery must be on height adjustable beds or trolleys so that they can be brought to the right height for care to be given. Most handling events in recovery are responding to some problem. The patient may need to be moved quickly to enable him to recover from such things as vomiting or a sudden shortness of breath or a coughing fit.

If the patient needs to be turned onto his side, there will need to be enough room to do a log roll. With most patients, the cot side can be put up and the patient log rolled towards the nurse. This manoeuvre has been timed in a real situation and was found to actually be quicker than going round to the other side of the patient and doing the (dangerous) flip turn. [The only disadvantage in this manoeuvre is that the nurse can get a shoe full of vomit!] Large patient's may be too big to turn on a theatre trolley, therefore, they must be moved to a bed whilst they recover.

Patients who need to be sat up present the same problems that are met in sitting patients up in bed. The techniques described in Chapter 14 should be used. Some patients may be too heavy for the nurses to sit them up safely. Such patients may need to be on a bed or trolley with a lifting section.

It is possible that the best solution will be to move patients from trolleys to proper beds as soon as they arrive in the recovery area. (See Chapter 14 for lateral transfer techniques)

Managers should consider these needs as part of their overall planning of patient handling. It may be desirable, for example, to bring the patient's own bed to recovery and move the patient onto that as soon as he comes out of the operating theatre.

(Some hospitals take the patient to theatre on his own bed and move him back onto the same bed for recovery. This approach saves two transfers for each patient.)

Sending the patient back to the ward.

The use of horizontal transfer aids is described in Chapter 14.

THE ITU

The problems in ITU are not really significantly different from problems that are met when caring for patients in other situations. The only difference is that all patients require the same high level of care. The high level of patient handling needed means that the managers of these units have no reason to make handling a secondary issue in their plans. All of their patients require handling and a safe system of work must be established to protect the nursing staff from injury and to protect the patients from bedsores and other injuries.

A handling assessment of an ITU unit should identify the following activities which need to be managed:-

turning the patient in bed

moving patients up in bed

tilting patients for drainage

moving patients to and from trolleys

positioning a patient for resuscitation

The unit manager must ensure that all bed spaces are equipped to allow these activities to be dealt with without manual lifting. Profiling beds allow the patient's position to be adjusted with minimal handling. Overhead "X/Y" tracking hoists will allow patients to be easily lifted to and from beds even when they are surrounded by equipment. Low air loss mattresses are necessary to reduce the need for turning patients. Ensure that Low air loss systems have fast deflation facilities for resuscitation.

THE X-RAY DEPARTMENT

In general, bed to bed transfers are applicable in transferring patients from trolleys to x-ray tables. There are specific problems when getting patients into the curved surface of the platform used to carry the patient into a scanner. The only system that is known to work is the System AT2000 formerly known as the Mobiliser. This device is able to lift a patient by insinuating a lifting surface under the patient. The mechanism can cope with the curved surfaces on scanner tables.

Radiographers must always beware of the weight of their lead aprons. These significantly increase the postural stress if the radiographer adopts a forward bend posture.

SPINAL INJURIES

In the acute stage of their treatment, patients with spinal injuries cannot be lifted manually. The patient's spine must be kept in alignment. The points of support from the nurses' arms cause the spine to bridge across and may cause further damage. Equally such patients cannot be lifted in conventional hoist slings. The normal slings used with hoists cause the patient to become bent and this can cause further damage to a patient with a spinal injury.

As a minimum, scoop stretchers and appropriate hoists must be available for moving this type of patient. There are also other pieces of equipment such as the System AT2000. This device formerly known as the Mobiliser is a sophisticated piece of equipment that insinuates a platform under the patient and then moves him sideways onto itself to move him to another place. The patient remains absolutely flat throughout the procedure. This device will handle patients weighing up to 228kg (36 stones).

Some types of automatic turning beds are also useful in the treatment of this type of patient.

Stand-up beds may be required at later stages.

ELDERLY

The elderly and in particular the elderly mentally ill represent a large proportion of the patients who need to be moved in hospitals and homes, etc. They present a number of specific problems when they are being handled.

They resist the use of equipment.

Some patients fight, kick and bite their nurses

Patients suddenly fail to stand when they have constantly stood in the past

They resist the use of equipment.

Elderly patients tend to take the view that some machine or other piece of equipment is frightening and strange and therefore less human than a nurse. The managers and staff caring for elderly people must not allow this sort of view to become established. It must be made clear to all patients that the hoists and other equipment are going to be used. It must be explained that this is as much in the interests of the patient as it is to protect the staff.

The attitude of the nurses is fundamental to "selling" the use of equipment. When a nurse approaches a patient with an injection that has to be administered, she does so with a determination that is firm but not aggressive. It is clear to the patient that the nurse will do her best to avoid pain but, in the end, the patient is going to be injected because that is best for the patient. (Most injections are after all painless today!) The nurse needs to think of handling aids in the same way. A determined, skilled and positive but none-the less reassuring approach will do as much to overcome

objections as an hour of reasoned argument.

If the patient continues to refuse to be handled using the handling aid it must be made clear that he will not be handled in any other way. The managers of any unit must be prepared to refuse to move a patient who will not accept safe handling.

One approach that has been particularly successful with the families of patients and with those elderly patients who are not confused is to provide a leaflet when they enter the home or ward. The leaflet says in friendly but firm terms that patients will not be lifted manually and that the patient has nothing to fear from the patient handling aids that will be used. If these leaflets are written with humour and sympathy they can do a lot to prepare the patient and their relatives and over come objections.

Some patients fight, kick and bite their nurses

Nurse must always beware of the tendency of elderly confused patients to attack in various ways the nurses who are caring for them. It is thought in some areas that these attacks are in fact motivated by the pain caused by bad handling such as the Orthodox lift and the Drag lift. The Care Plans for patients who are known to attack their nurses must be amended to provide handling solutions that accommodate the attacks without putting the nurses at risk.

Patients suddenly fail to stand when they are expected to be able to stand

Elderly patients are particularly subject to conditions that lead to deteriorating mobility. Nurses must always be aware that sooner or later all elderly patients are likely to reach the stage where they can no longer stand. The deterioration to this point can be very steady over a long period of time. This is one of the reasons for having formal reviews of care plans. This gives the nurses a chance to recognise the cumulative effects of small changes before they result in an accident. Having said that, nurses must always handle all patients in a way that allows them to cope with a sudden collapse. See Chapter 20.

The phrase "THE PATIENT CAN STAND" is one of the most dangerous in the whole of nursing. It can mean that the patient can stand himself from a seated position. It can equally mean that the patient is able to stand on his own two feet when he has been hauled up to his feet by nurses. Nurses writing care plans must be careful to ensure that they make the status of the patient absolutely clear. The nurse must use enough words to explain what the patient can actually do. See Chapters on risk assessment and sitting to standing.

When a patient who is expected to stand fails to do so, record the incident in the patient's records so that other nurses can be aware of the increased risk. The patient must be re-assessed to decide if the failure to stand was an isolated incident or a sign of the need to alter his care plan. Where there are repeated failures to stand the patient's handling must be changed.

NURSING ON THE FLOOR

Where a patient is thought to be likely to injure himself by throwing himself out of bed or by rubbing himself on the bed frame, it may be decided that the patient must be nursed on the floor in a separate room. Most such patients are capable of moving themselves. However, there are a minority who cannot or will not move themselves but never-the-less, it is thought that they cannot be left in a bed for their own safety.

This type of patient can present especial handling risks. Delivering care at floor level creates postural stress even if the patient is not handled. The simple log roll becomes much more dangerous in this position.

There are only two strategies when caring for these difficult patients:-

1. Decide to keep the patient in a bed all of the time and 'special' him to ensure that he does not damage himself. This may seem an expensive option but the costs pale into insignificance when compared with the costs of injuring nurses.

2. Lift the patient from the floor onto a bed using a scoop or slatted stretcher before giving any care. This lift can only be achieved with a ceiling hoist (or a ceiling hoist supported by an A-frame). Care must be taken that the nurses are not exposed to postural stress when positioning the stretcher. In particular it is not acceptable for the nurses to have to pull the mattress away from the wall before they can position the stretcher.

STROKES

Patients suffering from strokes are often not aware of one side of their body. This means that they must be helped to learn to control that half before they can move safely. Nurses handling such people need to consider this aspect at all times.

Physiotherapists have special therapy techniques that they use for assisting patients to regain control of their bodies. (One well-known group of techniques is known as the Bobath techniques from the name of the originator.) It is tempting for physiotherapists to teach a nurse or even a carer to use such a technique. This has the apparent benefit of extending the therapy throughout the day without using up physiotherapist's time. The problem is that these techniques are specialised and cannot be learned on their own. They are part of the whole skill profile of a physiotherapist. The physiotherapist knows how to assess the patient and how to vary the treatment to suit the changing condition of the patient. A nurse or carer is not equipped and often does not have the time to make these judgements. Therefore, there is an increased chance of something going wrong. Nurses must not be required to give such therapy unless they have had appropriate specialist training. Even when they are trained, nurses must not be required to actually lift stroke patients.

A particular problem has arisen in the case of these therapeutic treatments for stroke patients. The problem is that the techniques have been passed from one person to another and have changed in the process. A technique that may have been acceptable in the hands of a qualified physiotherapist is changed into a clearly unsafe lift in the hands of an untrained carer. An extreme example of this is that the drag lift has been described as a Bobath technique. The drag lift is, in fact, specifically criticised in Bobath literature. The only safe way of dealing with these techniques is to limit their use to those who are specifically trained and skilled in their use.

MATERNITY

It is often thought that as pregnant women are largely fit they do not present a handling risk to those who are caring for them. This is not the case. The following are some of the risk areas:-

The birthing process

Getting the mother on to the position where she wishes to give birth can require support. This may represent risks to those assisting. Once in position there is a risk of supporting legs during the process. [A midwife received severe injuries by holding a pregnant woman's leg for 20 minutes instead of putting the leg in a stirrup] Finally, it may be necessary to lift the mother out of wherever she has chosen to given birth. The midwife must assess the risks of any choice made by the mother to be. If things go wrong she may have to be lifted onto a trolley. The midwife must be sure that this can be achieved safely. If this is not the case the midwife must not give her consent.

Birthing pools present very significant handling risks. It must be possible for the mother to get easily into the pool without manual support. The midwife must be be able to work in a safe posture. It must be possible to get the mother and baby out of the pool without manual lifting. There must be facilities, when necessary, to get the mother out of the water in a hurry and move her to a birthing couch. These needs are foreseeable and therefore must be planned for in advance.

N.B. some older birthing couches do not provide enough control of the patient's posture. For example the stirrups are sometimes in the wrong position. The midwife has to remove them and take the force of the mothers leg on her side so that she can gain access to the baby as it is born. Another example is that mothers who have had epidurals are particularly susceptible to slipping down the couch. Modern couches allow the whole couch to be tilted to counteract this tendency. Out of date birthing couches must be replaced with proper equipment.

Baby's

It is quite easy to develop postural stress by bending and twisting over when handling and feeding babies. The weight of the nurse's upper body is enough to cause injury if she bends forward in an unsupported posture for a long time.

Equipment

This problem is particularly present in SCBU's but it also appears on normal maternity wards. The baby may only weight a few kilo''s but the special cot may weigh many kilograms. Monitors and other ancillary equipment can present a handling risk. Don't lift equipment onto high shelves.

Mothers with Disabilities

These people will need even more handling. Equipment must be provided that will move them safely into and out of ordinary beds and special couches. Procedures need to be in place for the ante-natal clinics to identify these mothers and discuss handling needs in good time.

General Postural Risks

The baby can take it's own time to be born. This leads to long periods of assisting the mother and waiting. Midwifes must review their activities and identify all points where they are at risk from their postures. They must change their working practices to ensure that they are always in a comfortable position.

KNOWN FALLERS

Very many patients are in hospital or in care elsewhere because they have begun to fall. Where a patient has a history of falling all of his handling must based be on the assumption that he will fall again. The failure to take this simple precaution has injured many nurses. KNOWN FALLERS ARE DANGEROUS!

The mobilisation of all patients must avoid using the nurse as a prop. Where the patient is a known faller, this rule has to be applied more rigorously. Patients must have a detailed mobilisation plan as part of their care plan. The mobilisation plan should go through a series of stages using appropriate supports for the patient.

The list should include such stages as rollator frames, walking frames, sticks, etc. This equipment must all be mastered before the nurse is used to give support in walking

Consider use of a walking hoist or a walking harness in conjunction with a mobile hoist or an over head hoist (N.B. Not all hoist manufacturers provide this option.)

It is better to walk a patient back from a toilet rather than walk him to the toilet. If a patient is beginning to mobilise but has some way to go it is best to avoid stress. When going to the toilet the patient is worried that he will not get there in time. The stress of this can lead to a fall. He should be taken to the toilet in a wheelchair and then allowed to walk back when he is not under pressure.

SEE WALKING A PATIENT AND THE FALLING PATIENT FOR MORE INFORMATION ON THIS SUBJECT.

PODIATRISTS

This group of people have been chosen to illustrate the range of handling situations that have to be considered in the health services. The following notes show that even jobs that would not be considered intrinsically dangerous have significant handling risks that must be addressed by managers. All jobs must be considered in the same depth. There are four risk areas to be considered in the case of podiatrists.

Moving patients into treatment seats

> The techniques for moving patients from one seated position to another are discussed in Chapter 16. One particular problem for Podiatrists is that they see very many patient's and do not have time to carry out individual assessments. They must be provided with care plan information that they can rely on. Podiatrists must not handle patients if they do not have a copy of the patient's Care Plan.

> It may be possible to change the working practises so that the patient can be treated in the wheelchair in which he arrived.

Lifting limbs

It has been noted elsewhere that limbs themselves can be quite heavy. A whole leg and foot represents 16.7 per cent of the body weight of an average person. If this weight is lifted at waist height it can be safe providing the patient is not very heavy or there is not some disease that causes the leg to be overweight.

However, the podiatrist is lifting near to the floor. In this position the lifter's capacity is much reduced. Even the legs of an average patient can represent unsafe loads. Therefore, lifting legs near floor level is a potentially hazardous lift and must be removed. Mechanisms for lifting legs should be provided. There are chairs that have sections that can lift the patient's legs. There are also devices that attach to standard chairs to provide the same function.

Whatever the weight of the leg, it is known to be dangerous to support any load for extended periods. If the podiatrist has to hold the leg, she is at further risk of injury. There must always be a means of support available.

Poor Posture

Bending down to work is posturally unsound and can in itself lead to back injury. Squatting can improve posture but is not always practicable for extended periods. A squatting posture can cause damage to knees and ankles. Kneeling on one knee can also be helpful but is not always acceptable if the floor is dirt

The danger from this and the lifting of limbs can be reduced by changing the working environment. Where podiatrists are working in a fixed location, the environment can be altered to enable the patients to be at a higher level than the podiatrist. This can be done by raising the patient's chairs on some form of lifting platform or by wheeling a wheelchair onto higher level staging.

Carrying her own Equipment

When the podiatrist is visiting patients in their homes she will be carrying her equipment with her. Care must be taken to ensure that the equipment bags are not too heavy. A heavy bag carried in one hand is an unbalanced load. See Chapter 6 for the effects on the spine of carrying such loads.

There are three solutions. The first is to reduce the load. It is very tempting to go on adding items to the bag on the basis that they might be useful and there is still some space. A detailed analysis should be made of what is actually used. Anything that is not used on a regular basis ought to be left out of the bag. The second solution is to put the

bag on wheels. These wheels must be big enough to cope with the terrain that will be encountered visiting clients. The miniature wheels on some suitcases and bags are only designed to cross the marbled halls at airports. They are not designed to go up the average garden path! The third solution is for the load to be split over two bags so as to balance the load on the spine.

PATIENTS IN SPASMS

Patients who go into spasm are always difficult to handle safely. It has been known for a nurse to be thrown across the room by a patient's violent spasm but as yet, nurses know little about how to control it. The following principles should be applied:

Handle the patient firmly and avoid sudden movements.

'Fold him up' before attempting to move him. Extended positions predispose to spasm, flexed positions inhibit spasm.

Encourage the patient to initiate movement; spasm commonly occurs as a reflex response to the nurse's movements.

Preparatory movements such as rocking forward to or thrusting the patient's foot hard down onto the floor will inhibit spasm. Weight-bearing through the arm or leg also reduces it.

If the spasm is not under control, do not try to move the patient. Wait until the spasms have subsided. If the spasms do not subside, change the working environment or chose a different method of movement so that handling is not needed.

Patients who have spasm are often strapped into their wheelchairs during the day. Care must be taken by the nurse when handling the patient. Always keep the patient in a folded position. If the patient goes into spasm and then extends it is safer to undo the strap and allow the patient to slide to the floor. When straps are used, the nurse must ensure that they are correctly positioned to stop the patient sliding out and/or jack knifing. It must be possible to release such straps quickly under load.

If the frequency of spasms increase medical advice should be sought to bring them under control. In severe cases specialist treatment may be required.

PATIENTS IN TRACTION

Patients in traction tend to slip down in the bed. This is caused by the pull exerted by the weights. Nurses find that these patients need to be continually moved back up the bed.

There are two approaches to solving this problem. The first is to find a way of moving the patient back up the bed without lifting him or risking sores from dragging him over the sheets. The second is to stop him moving down the bed. The section on moving the patient in bed provides a discussion on the techniques that can be used for moving the patient back up the bed. Stopping him sliding down the bed in the first place can be achieved in two ways:-

Use a one way sliding sheet

These special sliding sheets are slippery in one direction but lock in the other direction. If the patient is placed on such a glide, he will tend to stay in place. If he does slip down, the glide can be used to move him back up the bed.

Tilt the bed

Most hospital beds provide for some degree of tilting. A small tilt of 3∫ to 5∫ down at the head end will usually not disturb the patient. However, this will provide a counter pull of gravity to stop the patient sliding towards the foot of the bed.

VERY HEAVY PATIENTS

Most patient handling equipment and beds will handle up to 127 or 159kg (20 or 25 stones). However, some pieces of equipment have lower limits. Managers need to be aware of the weight limits of their equipment. They must not exceed the capacity of their equipment by using it to handle very heavy patients.

There are an increasing number of very heavy people. People who weight 222kg (35 stones) whilst still being relatively unusual are not the rarity they once were. Any large hospital or community trust must expect to have to treat several patients weighing more than 127kg (20 stones) in the course of a year.

In planning the equipment needs of a trust, the managers must obtain some equipment that is capable of lifting heavy patients. This equipment can be in normal use for all patients but must be made available when a very heavy patient arrives.

The managers must ensure that all staff known that equipment for heavy patients is available. In particular the appropriate staff must know how to obtain this equipment when it is required outside normal office hours.

See Chapters 13 and 14.

DISABLED PATIENTS

There are many different disabilities that a nurse may encounter. It would take a separate book to discuss the handling needs of all possible disabilities. In general, the nurse must be prepared to use the full range of techniques and equipment in supporting disabled patients.

If the limitations of their disability can be overcome some disabled patients are able to live full and active lives. These people need support in achieving their objectives. They rightly make strong demands for facilities to give them freedom. However, one person's need for freedom cannot be bought at the risk of injuring another. Nurses and others working with this group of people must be able to find solutions to handling problems that do not put carers at risk. They must be able to explain the need for this approach to the disabled person. A dictatorial attitude will only lead to conflict.

There are specific sources of information on equipment for the disabled. There are several Disabled Living Centres. They welcome practitioners who wish to become familiar with the wide ranges of equipment available. Various exhibitions are also valuable sources of information on equipment for disabled people.

Equipment that can assist in day to day living.

The handling techniques and rules that are described in this book apply to disabled patients as much as they apply to other patients. Much of the equipment described in this book is essential to providing a safe and caring environment. However these will not always be enough The range of equipment that is available to assist the disabled person live a fuller life expands almost daily.

An example of specialised equipment is the standing wheelchair. This chair will allow the patient to either sit as in a normal wheelchair or to it will bring him to a standing position. This gives him independence and confidence when out shopping. He can reach shelves etc. Most importantly it is possible to interact with other people at eye level.

The full range of such equipment is beyond this book.

The correct piece of equipment gives self esteem and improves confidence and independence. Failure to provide the correct piece of equipment and allowing the person to be 'man handled' degrades and brings more attention to him as well as putting the nurses at risk.

LEARNING DISABILITIES

People with learning disabilities may have either mental or physical disabilities or both. There has to be a way of giving these people as full a life as possible. We must not lock these people away. It is important to rehabilitate them into society. However, it is also important that those caring for these people are not themselves injured or incapacitated. It is equally important that the disabled person does not have an injury caused by bad handling added to his problems.

Normalization

Over the years the idea of normalization has led to some people believing that people with learning difficulties should do everything that it is possible to do in society. This is sometimes taken to extremes. It is possible for any person to try bungy jumping but most people will choose not to do it. Many people play rugby football, but there are many more who do not. Normalization does not have to mean making people do everything that is possible.

Those caring for disabled people need to establish a strategy that takes account of the 'art of the possible' and the real needs and wishes of the disabled person.

If it is decided that the person really has to undertake a particular activity then it must be done safely for both the nurses and the disabled person.

THE PATIENT WHO IS UNWILLING TO CO-OPERATE

Patients who are cared for in mental health units present a wide range of handling risks. The issues raised in discussing elderly patients, known fallers and others in this chapter apply to the care of these patients.

This section concentrates on some basic principles which nurses need to bear in mind when faced with a patient who, for a variety of reasons, may not be a willing partner in the transfer.

There are specific groups of patients to whom these principles particularly apply:

People with learning disabilities

People with acute mental health needs

People with organic dementia's and disorders characterised by disorientation

People who are violent, disorientated or disturbed due to substance abuse, alcohol or drugs.

People who are violent due to a personality problem.

Over many years, most if not all Mental Health Nurse courses omitted all mention of patient handling. This is very dangerous as many patients in the care of a Registered Mental Nurse present special handling problems. Managers of such nurses must ensure that these nurses are given basic patient handling training. Up dates are not sufficient for people who have not had the foundation training that they ought to have received. Those responsible for training new nurses in this demanding area must ensure that handling of patients is given a proper place in their syllabus. Where experienced staff are employed, managers must make positive checks on the quality of the person's knowledge of safe handling. Where the need is identified full training must be given immediately.

A nurse has a basic duty of care to her patient or client. She has to be responsive to the patient's needs and provide competent care at all times. In meeting this challenge the nurse must not be asked to put herself at risk of injury.

The ward manager/team leader should assess the competence of the nurse in:

Her ability to communicate effectively with the patient.

Her assertion skills in declaring her right as a practitioner to decide whether or not to become immediately involved in any situation.

Her risk assessment skills. This implies that the nurse can take a calculated course of action following an assessment of the situation consistent with the available resources and the urgency of the situation.

In meeting these criteria, nurses have a responsibility to exercise judgement. The nurse should wait rather than rush in as a matter of principle. The nurse should seek to calm a situation, adopt an encouraging and reassuring manner and call for or await the arrival of help.

It is the duty of the employer to ensure that adequate help is readily available when this is needed and called for.

The overriding rule is that nurses dealing with aggressive or unco-operative patients should not place themselves at risk any more than nurse in any other situation.

Handing Skills Required for the Confused or Frightened Patient

Confusion, fear and aggression are closely inter-linked and each state may present the nurse with a handling problem. This is usually found in the patient who has difficulty in co-operating and tends to struggle or react against the carer involuntarily.

The skill, one of the most challenging in nursing, is to enable this person to feel calm and safe, and in a mood to help. Sometimes this might mean leaving him alone for a while; at other times nothing more than a confident tone of voice, or even just a smile; or yet again, a particular way of holding him that makes him feel the nurse is with him, not against him. There are no rules for this situation, only principles and empathy.

A person who is not able to behave or think logically is extra sensitive to mood and non-verbal signals coming from other people. If the carer is tense or nervous, he also is likely to feel tense and his fears may come to the surface, possibly resulting in aggression. Even if he only stiffens up he will be more difficult to handle. The first principle then is to relax, and assume a confident attitude. When the patient starts to relax and co-operate, confidence will increase.

People who are deeply anxious sometimes feel they are being 'crowded.' This makes them want to hit out. Their need for space must be respected. Other people who are frightened need the reassurance of a kindly touch, which means more to them than words.

Confusion and fear may be caused simply by sensory loss and disorientation. The nurse can make a handling task easier for herself by ensuring that her patient knows where he is and what is expected of him; that he can see the chair that he is being moved to; that he understands, from instruction clearly and quietly repeated, in which direction he is to turn or where he is to put his hands.

Some flooring can create fearful usual impressions. To a disorientated mind, the space in a ward can seem so immense as to be impassable and big blocks of colour may appear as barriers that stop the patient in his tracks, while a very gentle slope may seem like a precipice.

A person who is in pain or frightened needs to be given as much control of his own movements as possible: encourage him to take the initiative; invite him to stand up, or turn over. An elderly lady with learning difficulties who was going blind and becoming unmanageable in her residential home appeared to be unable to move at all on admission to hospital and nurses found it very difficult to stand her up. Enquiries at the home obtained the information that she had been ambulant until that week, but seemed frightened because she could not see. The next morning the nurse asked this lady if she would like to walk with her out to the toilet. The patient stood up, took her hand and walked out with her – thus a patient-handling problem was averted. But, the nurse knows only too well that some patients respond best to a voice of authority. So, there are no rules, but it is essential that a sensitive assessment of the patient's capabilities and responses is made and useful information recorded in the Care Plan.

A 'confrontational' approach tends to set up resistance from a confused or frightened patient, while with the 'indirect' approach the patient feels the sympathetic touch of the nurse's hands on his skin and by reflex responses 'gathers' himself in the intended direction of movement before any actual lift is attempted. But, if there is any threat of hurt or sense of being outnumbered his reflex response will be in the opposite direction, away from the nurse. Nurses should avoid gripping the patient's arms for this reason. Guiding with the palm of the hand is recommended.

When helping these patients to move, the nurse should position herself very close to give a feeling of security.

The dependent patient for whom a mobile hoist is called for, may, initially need reassurance. Though the hoist offers a very comfortable and safe mode of transfer, it may not look like it to the patient: he may be scared of it. The first experience of the hoist must therefore be good. The time taken to overcome any fears will be well spent.

Handling Skills Required for the Maliciously Aggressive Patient

This guide does not address the issue of control and restraint of violent or aggressive patients who are detained in security institutions. People who are caring for this type of person should receive appropriate specialist training. This section, however, deals with the patient who may be confused, irrational or malicious.

Such patients may withhold their co-operation intentionally from the outset of a handling task or during it. The patient may attack the nurse by biting, scratching, deliberately falling or throwing their weight onto the nurse. Other problems known to arise are caused when the patient lifts his feet off the floor and swings on the nurse arms. This can only arise if the nurse is unwise enough to put herself in the position of supporting such a patient. It is particularly common where the nurse is using the drag lift/hold. This is one of the many reasons for condemning the use of the drag lift.

All handling tasks involving such patients require the nurse to proceed with considerable caution if the nurse is to avoid injury. If the handling technique is likely to be uncomfortable the patient may resent being handled. For these reasons wherever an aggressive, confused, irrational or malicious patient is to be handled the procedure should be carefully considered and planned beforehand.

Whenever the patient lies on the floor out of choice (as distinct from falling) it is invariably safer to leave him where he is. If it is imperative to get him up again, the techniques described in Chapter 20, should be adopted.

When escorting an aggressive patient two nurses should hold the patient's wrists, one on either side, with their other arms around the patient's waist. This will restrain the patient from striking out at the nurses. Should the patient fall, the nurses should then go down to the floor with him.

Whenever such patients need to be lifted from the floor a hoist must be used with the correct sling.

PATIENTS WITH HIP FRACTURES

Patients with fractured hips and those shortly after hip surgery cannot be log rolled in the normal way. These patients must be moved with their legs held straight and without any twisting of their hips. There are three ways of moving these patients.

1. The Immoturn is a frame that has been specifically designed for this purpose. It can be used to turn a patient without a risk of bending his legs. The frame can be slipped quickly into place on the unaffected side. The patient is rolled by pulling on the built in bar and the broken hip rises safely. Nurses must beware when pulling on the bar. They must ensure that they keep their back upright. They must also ensure that the patient is not too heavy to pull. The manufacturers recommend that the Immoturn should not be used for patients who weigh more than 114kg (18 stones). (The Immoturn comes in pairs consisting of left and right hand versions depending upon which leg has been operated upon.) See Chapter 14.

2. The Charnley wedge can be strapped to the patient's legs. In principle patients with the wedge fitted are log rolled. However as the knee cannot be bent the patient cannot follow the natural patterns of movement used in the log roll. Therefore the use of the Charnley wedge ought to be approached with caution. The nurses must avoid taking too great a load when lifting the patient's leg. If the patient cannot be moved safely another method must be used.

3. A hoist with a scoop stretcher or a stretcher made up of slats is useful for heavy patients and patients whose condition is not suitable for the Immoturn or Charnley wedge.

When patients with hip fractures are to be stood up they may need a standing bed. See bed chapter.

THE AMPUTEE

There are many reasons for patients to have had amputations. In the younger patient the frequent cause is acute trauma as the result of an accident. In the majority of these cases, the patient is well and fit very soon after surgery. His rehabilitation process will be thorough and independent patient movement is achieved quickly.

With the older patient, the cause of the amputation is more usually because of vascular difficulties or the failure of severely infected sores to heal. In these cases, the other remaining limbs of the patient are often not strong enough to compensate for the loss. There may be other medical problems, such as a 'stroke' that affects the ability of the remaining limbs to assist. Many elderly patients are not able to regain their strength to become competent artificial limb users but do manage to undertake independent sliding transfers. The use of various transfer boards, sometimes with an additional sliding sheet, can be successfully taught and used. The compatibility of chair, wheelchair, bed and WC seat heights are critical to success.

If the amputation is close to the knees, the patient may be transferred from bed to chair using a sliding sheet that has been introduced by rolling the patient from side to side; the chair should be turned in towards the bed, and the patient slid to the edge of the bed with his back to the chair. The nurses can then put one knee on the bed, and while facing each other, take hold of the sliding sheet on either side and then slide the patient backwards into the chair.

The effort needed by a carer to use a sliding sheet with such a patient must be assessed and a hoist used with all heavy or large patients. The sling must be appropriate to the body shape of the patient. If only one leg has been amputated just above the knee and a good length stump is present, then a divided leg sling is often used. It is helpful if the divided leg sling has quilted leg pieces so that they form a firmer and wider sitting base that does not crease while being hoisted.

If a patient has a double leg amputation and the resulting stumps are very short, then the whole balance of the patient's body is affected and their centre of gravity moves much higher into their chest. Most hoist slings will not be suitable for a double leg amputee since the mechanics of the sling rely on the patient's legs to both hold the sling in place and the body in an upright seated position. Several hoist manufacturers make 'amputee' slings and these should be assessed with the individual patient.

Where a 'one-piece' sling is used as a short term measure to transfer a patient in and out of a hospital bed, then this should be lined with sheepskin or other pressure relieving materials since the patient will remain sitting on it while in his chair. 'One-piece' slings cannot be removed from under a seated patient but only positioned by rolling the patient while in bed. Some elderly carers may prefer this option since they find it stressful to place slings on and off the patient.

In many elderly patients, an added complication following an amputation due to vascular insufficiency, is an additional pressure sore. It has proved to be very difficult to place an amputee or divided leg hoist sling around a patient without dislodging any treatment dressing on the patient's hips. A decision must be made about the healing of the pressure sore by remaining in bed on a specialist mattress, or the need to hoist the patient in and out of bed to progress their rehabilitation. In severe cases, it may be difficult to roll the patient to use a 'one-piece' sling so that bed rest is the only safe and comfortable option for both staff and the patient.

GETTING IN AND OUT OF TRANSPORT

This section will consider the options of transferring a disabled person and, where appropriate, his wheelchair onto transport.

Many disabled people use the Mobility part of their Disability Living Allowance to access the 'Motability' scheme which will provide a car under a leasing or hire purchase agreement. There is a wide range of cars available through this scheme. Some cars are adapted to carry wheel chairs whilst others are simply adapted to allow the person to sit in a normal seat.

There are a number of mobility assessment centres around the UK who provide expert advice and guidance on choosing a suitable car. They are able to undertake assessments for a disabled driver or for a disabled passenger. They can also give information on adapted vehicles where several disabled people may be sharing transport.

However, the problems of getting in and out of transport are not limited to people who purchase cars.

In and out of a car:

For standing and weight bearing patients

For a disabled person who can stand from sitting, then car transfers do not present many problems. The wheelchair must be positioned close to the seat where they are to sit. A two door car will provide much more space for the transfer to the front seats than a four door car will.

A person with mobility problems must not be transferred into the rear seats of a two door car

since, if they need assistance, it is impossible for the helper to position themselves without creating a handling risk.

People who have unpredictable behaviour but full mobility may be positioned on the rear seat, with an escort, in order to restrict their interference with the driver. If a risk assessment shows that this behaviour is frequent, then the close confines of a normal car may be unsuitable and alternatives must be considered.

One problem faced by many elderly or disabled people is that of positioning themselves on the seat once they have sat down in the car. The turning action, to face the front of the car is difficult if clothing hinders the rotating sliding action.

Two alternatives are worth trying to aid the turning action on the seat. Either a good quality carrier bag placed on the seat will act as a substitute sliding sheet or a soft turning disc can be purchased. The soft turning discs can be of floppy and slippery material or be a sheepskin covered cushion on a firmer rotating base. The carrier bag not be left under the patient for the journey as the patient may slide too easily in the event of an accident.

An adaptation to the car seat will allow it to rotate outwards so that extra space is created around it. This may not be suitable for people with long legs who have stiff knee joints since as the seat returns to its position inside the car, the legs still have to clear the car door opening.

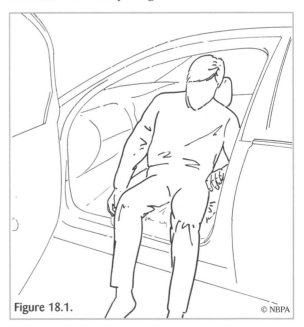

Figure 18.1.

© NBPA

For non-weight bearing patients :

The simplest transfer is done by the use of a sliding board. This method will enable the patient to use almost any car, either their -own, a relatives or a hire car on holiday.

- The car is parked so that the car and the wheelchair are on the same level ground. Parking beside a kerb with the wheelchair higher than the car seat will cause problems.

- The car door is opened. A two door car will give a better opening width. The passenger seat (or the seat to be used) is pushed back as far as possible to increase the leg room in front of the seat. If the seat has deep contours with side pads to the seat back1 then it may ease the sideways movement if the seat is reclined a little so that the side pads of the seat are not sticking so far forward.

- The wheelchair is positioned so that the foot plates are swung back and the patient's feet are placed so that they are resting on the door sill. The seated patient's hips should be level with the back of the car seat. The inside arm rest is removed from the wheelchair to allow a sideways transfer.

- The patient leans away from the car seat and the transfer board is slid underneath his hips so that it spans the gap between wheelchair and car seat. In order for the slide across to be successful, the board must reach at least halfway under the patient's hips.

- In order to ensure that the maximum amount of the patient's weight is taken on the board, he should lean forwards. If he has strong upper limbs, then he should be able to shuffle himself sideways across the board and into the car seat. His legs will follow and fall into place if they have been placed on the car sill to begin with. Alternatively a disc under the feet will assist them to move.

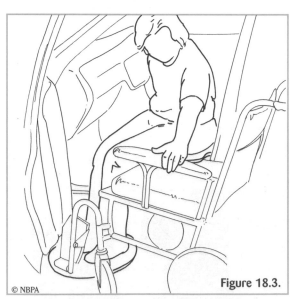

Figure 18.3.

© NBPA

- If the patient does not have strong enough arms and is of a light enough weight, the helper can position the board and the patient as above.

The helper then goes around the car and kneels on the driver's seat. The left hand is braced along the back of the passenger seat and the right hand grasps the patient's trousers at a point where maximum weight is taken on them, i.e. under the hips.

As the patient leans forwards, the helper pulls smoothly towards her and the patient will slide across and into the seat. This sliding action can be eased by use of a sliding sheet under the patient's hips. Or by use of a nylon mat which is positioned on the wheelchair cushion before the patient sits on it. The board can be slid beneath it and the handles at the ends of the mat provide a good hold for the helper. This is particularly useful when the helper cannot grasp the patient's clothing because it is too tight or may tear. A patient handling belt may also be useful in providing a means of pulling the patient.

To leave the car, the procedure is reversed.

- If there is a difference in levels between the car seat and the wheelchair seat, the addition of a 2" wheelchair cushion on the car seat will often raise it sufficiently to create a level transfer.

- If the helper is assisting to pull the patient across the board and out of the car, then an arm should be braced on the car roof while the other pulls. Once the patient is fully on the board and partly across the two seats, then the helper will find it easier to readjust her position and use two hands to pull the patient.

WARNING

A careful assessment must be made of the effort involved in using the method of pulling a patient across the sliding board. If there is any resistance, then the method must be re-evaluated to lighten the load.

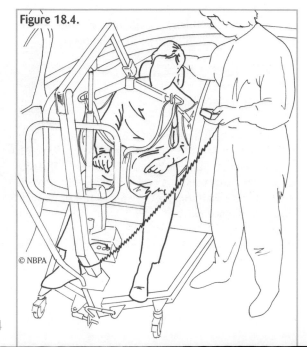

Figure 18.4.

© NBPA

An alternative method that could be used is the combination of a rotating seat with a mobile hoist. The action of the seat swinging outside of the car provides much more space in which to use a mobile hoist to transfer a patient on and off the seat.

Unless there is a mobile hoist at the destination, this may only be useful if the disabled passenger is to stay sitting in the car. A light hoist can be disassembled and put in the boot of a car so that it may be used for several transfers in different places.

Car hoists

These may be mounted inside the car to take either the disabled person from their outside wheelchair into the car seat. Alternatively, there can be a system whereby the car seat is totally removed and the disabled person sits in a special wheelchair. This adapted wheelchair can be hoisted up and into the space left for a seat.

Other car hoists may be mounted on the roof of the car. A retractable hoist boom can be extended over the seated patient in his wheelchair and he is then hoisted and the boom retracted so that the patient's hips can be positioned over the car seat.

Alternative Transport:

Some patients may be much safer and more comfortable if they travel in their own wheelchairs. This alternative option considers the provision of adapted vehicles. The most common of these is the converted van which allows a wheelchair to be pushed up a ramp (or on a tail lift) into the back of a van that has additional windows for all round vision. Some vans may be converted so that the wheelchair driver can access a tail lift at the rear of the van, drive forwards across the floor of the van and then position themselves to drive from their wheelchair. This method allows a family to go out together without the stress of wheelchair to car seat transfers.

In planning home visits from hospital, the method of transport must be assessed. If the patient is a wheelchair user, or still in a weakened state and not fully weight bearing, then most NHS Trusts will have a transport contract with an outside firm. These contractors should be able to provide a 'black cab' taxi that will allow the patient to travel in their wheelchair together with the escorting member of staff. The more general use of wheelchair accessible 'black cabs' has enabled many disabled people to use taxis in the same way as their able bodied friends. Many Local Authorities will now only grant hackney carriage licences to those taxi drivers with such accessible vehicles.

Wheelchairs into the car

Once the disabled person is seated inside the car, the helper has usually to get the wheelchair into the car, either in the boot or between the front and back seats inside. N.B. This problem can be avoided by the use of services such as Shopabilty whereby wheelchairs can be obtained at the destination.

Into the boot

The car should have a level entry into the boot which is not too high off the ground, i.e. no higher than the helper's knee. Where the boot has a high lip then a manual lift should not be attempted. There are mechanical winching systems that can assist with lifting a wheelchair into the boot.

To manually lift a wheelchair into a hatch back type of boot, the boot should be opened and cleared of obstructions.

The wheelchair should be stripped of its armrests and foot plates in order to reduce its weight. The wheelchair can then be folded and the backrest is also folded down (on all newer models). The wheelchair now resembles a square on wheels.

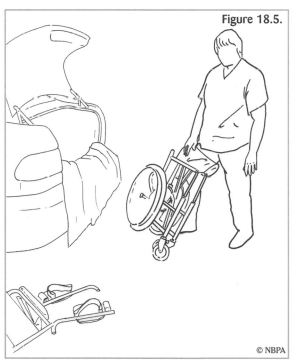

Figure 18.5.

© NBPA

A carpet or travel rug should be pulled forwards from the floor of the boot and draped over the rear body work and bumper of the car. This will protect the car from any scratches when the wheelchair is slid in.

The brakes are applied to the wheelchair wheels. The helper positions the folded wheelchair so that the heaviest sides (usually the self-propelling wheels) are on their strongest side, i.e. on the right side if the helper is right handed. The helper grasps the wheelchair with one hand holding the wheel rim furthest from her and the other hand holding the seat frame next to her.

The helper uses her knee to pivot the wheelchair base away from her and up so that the lower part of the wheelchair frame is resting on the edge of the boot space. The top part of the wheelchair is held close to the handler's body. The helper must avoid a vertical dead lift and an action that lifts the wheelchair away from her.

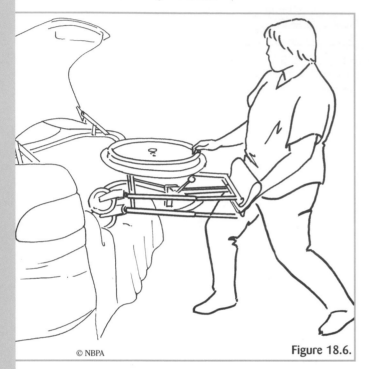

© NBPA   Figure 18.6.

Once the weight of the wheelchair is resting on the edge of the boot (and the protective rug) then it can be slid into the boot to position it for travelling. It is best if the wheelchair stays lying flat but the boot shape may require it to be stood up. In this case the travel rug will be useful to drape over the top half of the wheelchair to prevent it rattling on the back window as the boot lid is shut.

To get the wheelchair out of the boot, the boot is first opened and the rug repositioned for protection. The helper pulls the folded wheelchair towards her so that only the castors and lower part of the larger wheels are resting on the boot edge. The helper then positions her feet so that one is forward and the other is behind. As the weight of the wheelchair is pulled out, the front foot swings backwards so that the weight of the wheelchair lands between the helper's feet.

In all these procedures, it should be possible for the helper to work with an erect posture. There should be no need to stoop or twist while lifting the wheelchair in or out of the boot. However, this procedure does involve a manual lift and most wheelchairs are heavy. The helper must make an assessment of whether this is within their

capabilities. If an elderly carer is being shown how to travel with a wheelchair, then the second method inside the car and between the seats may be more suitable,

The wheelchair is stripped of its armrests and foot plates as before. This time the brakes are left off as the rolling action of the wheels assists in getting it inside the car. The back door of the car is opened, or the front seat is slid forwards in a two door car. It may be useful to put a travel rug for protection over the front edge of the back seat. The wheelchair is tipped back on to its larger wheels and the front castors are placed resting on the sill of the car. The helper then holds both back wheels of the wheelchair and rolls it forwards so that it rolls 'head over heels' into an upside down position between the front and back seats of the car. With practice, this method can eliminate any lifting of the wheelchair and can be managed by most elderly carers.

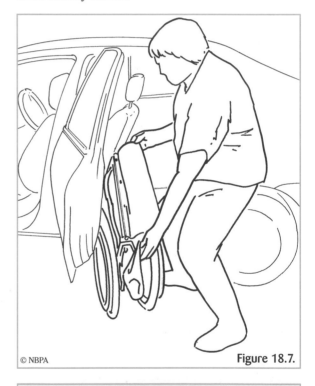

© NBPA   Figure 18.7.

WARNING

If these methods of getting a wheelchair in and out of the car prove to be awkward or heavy, then the carer is best advised to reconsider their choice of transport or to mechanise the lifting of the wheelchair.

Various mechanical systems are available to lift the wheelchair either into the boot or up and on to the roof of the car. Disabled Living Centres and other disability reference bases will give more detailed information about these options.

This has been only a brief introduction to the issue of transporting a patient beyond the hospital or home. A full discussion of this area would involve a book as large as this one. Some of the possible sources of information are mentioned below. Wherever the patient is transported it is essential that the principles of handling described in this book are followed. The operators of buses, trains, ships and planes must not be allowed to pretend that their circumstances allow them to ignore safe handling. Safe solutions are possible everywhere.

SOURCES OF FURTHER INFORMATION

Association of Transport Co-ordinating Officers (1996) Safe Journey Home to School Transport for children in Wheelchairs. A guide Community Transport Association

Disabled Living Foundation (1993) Wheelchair information DLF

Mells A (1996) Ins and Outs of Choosing a car. A guide for elderly and Disabled people RICA

NHS Estates Health Building Note 6 (1992) Radiology Department H.M.S.O.

NHS Estates Health Building Note 20 (1991) Mortuary and Post Mortem Room H.M.S.O.

NHS Estates Health Building Note 21 (1989) Maternity H.M.S.O.

NHS Estates Health Building Note 22 (1995) Accident and emergency Department H.M.S.O.

NHS Estates Health Building Note 27 (1992) Intensive Therapy Unit H.M.S.O.

NHS Estates Health Building Note 35 (1988) Accommodation for people with Acute Mental Illness H.M.S.O.

NHS Estates Health Building Note 39 (1981) Hospital Accommodation for Elderly People H.M.S.O.

NHS Estates Health Building Note 40 (1995) Common Activity Spaces Vol.1 Public Areas H.M.S.O.

The above publications are reviewed from time to time

O'Brien J Lyle C (1990) Five essential accomplishments for a human service as in frame work for accomplishments Responsive Systems Associates Lithania Georgia

RCN (1992) Focus on Restraint 2nd Edition

Wolfensberger W (1972) The Principles of Normalization in Human Services National Institute of Mental Retardation Toronto

HANDLING BABIES AND YOUNG CHILDREN

By Pat Alexander

SUMMARY

Staff and parents should not put their own health and safety at risk in the belief that the continuing welfare and development of the child is more important.

Children should be encouraged to help move themselves, but even normal babies require total care in their daily life.

The risks of musculo-skeletal problems to which all who work with children are exposed should be recognised, whether they come from continual lifting, stooping, or working at an awkward level.

The work place must be well planned, to reduce the need for hazardous actions.

Before buying new equipment, it should be examined to ensure its suitability for staff and children, in the place where the work is to be done.

It is a legal requirement that staff must have regular training in moving and handling where it is part of their job.

INTRODUCTION

Back pain is a common problem for those working with babies and small children.

This work is not often seen as a problem to carers and nurses, but as an extension of parenting, dealing only with small weights.

A survey in 1996 showed that only 3 per cent of nurses reported first taking sick leave for back pain or injury when working in paediatrics, as opposed to 18 per cent who were working with the elderly (Ref 16). However, many of the problems met while working with children may be due to an ergonomic mismatch rather than a lifting accident.

Most parents produce, lift and carry their own children without any apparent ill effects, although research shows that 20 per cent of women with low back pain attribute this to pregnancy and childbirth (Ref 4). Most parents see their children learn to crawl and eventually to walk, but those who work with small children grow older while the group of children they work with is always young.

This chapter deals with problems arising from working with normal babies in a mainstream setting, such as a nursery, as well as those with disabilities. It continues with sick children in hospital, those with multiple handicaps, and those discharged into the community with a long term disability who may need special equipment wherever they are, at home, in hospital, at school, for therapy, travel, and leisure activities.

INFANTS IN NURSERIES AND CRECHES

Nursery nurses, teachers and care staff in mainstream nurseries and creches stoop, lift or squat and work at awkward levels to reach the children. Staff with good knee joints and strong thigh muscles will not find squatting a problem while they are young and fit, but older staff may need to use a low seat to avoid stooping and putting their spine at risk. An ergonomic approach to these situations will be useful

Wise selection of nursery equipment – cots, high chairs, low chairs, and playpens – should reduce the risks of back injury for staff.

An example of when adult backs could be at risk is when clearing away toys at the end of each day, when backs are tired. A solution is to make this a game for small children, but if adult staff have to do it, they can sweep the toys into a pile with a broom before kneeling to gather them and put them away.

INFANTS IN CAR AND CARRY SEATS

Dual purpose infant carry seats, which can also be used as car seats, often cause strain on the backs and shoulders of carers who carry them. These should be tried out with the infant before purchasing, preferably ones which can be held safely with both arms close to the trunk, bearing in mind that the child will become heavier in a short time. An alternative could be to use a back carrier.

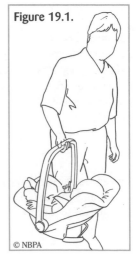

Figure 19.1.

© NBPA

Many infant car seats can be fitted to the front passenger seat facing backwards, and then the adult carer does not have to twist and stretch to put a child into the back seat. At six months, a child can be placed in a front facing seat in the front of a car.

CHILDREN IN HOSPITAL

Cots and beds

An acutely ill or disabled child in hospital may be a handling problem for staff and parents. The child may be put in a cot or bed. Height adjustable cots are not readily available, but a raising mechanism, which can adjust the height of a cot, can be obtained. Many nursing procedures and observations require a nurse to stoop over a cot for a long time. Until height adjustable cots are provided routinely, kneeling, or sitting on a low chair alongside is the way to help reduce any risk. All cots should have adjustable sides which can be lowered sufficiently to allow the infant to be reached without stooping.

Children should be encouraged to help move themselves around in a cot or a bed, and parents are often able to help them. A sliding sheet rolled under the child makes it easier to move one who needs more help.

To allay a child's anxiety and fear of being parted from his parents, many paediatric units have facilities for parents to stay with their child. These range from complete en suite facilities to a Z bed by the child's bed or cot. A bed for parents at the child's bedside can add to the handling difficulties. It has to be lifted and carried from the store; it is often heavy, and once in place, it restricts the access to each side of the child's bed or cot. Also, to avoid disturbing parents, the nurse may have to adopt an awkward posture to reach the child. Consequently, it is important that units provide overnight accommodation which is away from the bed or cot side or allows sufficient space for the nurse to handle the child safely.

Incubators

Height adjustable incubators are a necessity in a special care neonatal unit, where staff may stand for up to an hour at a time for some nursing procedures. The monitors are positioned above the incubators so that there is no need to stoop to read the display windows.

Neonates at risk can be carried in portable incubators from home to hospital in an emergency, or between hospitals. These incubators may weigh up to 10kgs (22lbs) and are carried on special trolleys; self loading trolleys should be used to load these incubators into ambulances and helicopters.

Bathing and showering

Bathing facilities in hospital are often unsuitable for small children who need more than supervision from the nurse. Plastic bath inserts, making the bath shallower, or children's bath or shower seats, can be used to support a dependent child. Other aids, such as inflatable or hydraulic adjustable seats, may also be used.

A shower cubicle should have level access, so that a wheeled shower seat can be moved into it, and should slope back to a drain. Height adjustable shower trolleys can be taken to the bedside for a sliding transfer to be made. Trolley and child are taken to the bathroom where the child can be washed with a hand held shower at a height convenient for the attendant.

Height adjustable changing tables should be provided to allow staff to work at comfortable levels.

THE DEVELOPING INFANT WITH MULTIPLE AND COMPLEX NEEDS

In hospital

Staff should consider all aspects of a child's development when formulating care plans. The child's emotional growth, development of movement, intellectual stimulation, recreation and the need for assistance with personal care should all be taken into account when the staff team is assessing handling needs, The plan needs to be revised and kept up to date as the child develops.

As with all children, it is important to establish bonding between parents and a child with special needs (Ref 12). Parents should be shown how to handle and cuddle their baby without interfering with naso gastric tubes, gastrostomy tubes or a ventilator, and how to feed, wash and dress them.

Older children with complex needs are sometimes in special care units in hospital because they are being ventilated, and this can lead to risks to staff when they encourage developmental play and learning. Equipment must be used – for example, to encourage standing – that will allow the child to develop skills while also allowing for safe positioning of tubes, without putting staff at risk of injury.

The problems for staff presented by very dependent children are increasing with the survival of damaged neonates due to technological advances in obstetric care (Ref 11). Anxiety to improve their quality of life should not allow staff to risk their own health and safety and staff should try to use suitable equipment, such as tilt tables and other motor assisted standing aids, to encourage a child's development.

In the community

Children with chronic disabling conditions such as cerebral palsy, spina bifida or muscular dystrophy now commonly live in the community. Their complex needs require assessment by a specialist team. Health visitors, nursery nurses, physiotherapists, occupational therapists, psychologists and teachers who all may work with the paediatrician should devise a plan of care that meets all the child's special needs without putting carers or staff at risk.

The therapist will advise the parents on how to handle a small baby or infant to counter any delay in the child's development and to minimise spasm and the risk of contractures. As with any professional advice and treatment, staff must be aware of their responsibility for the safety of family and other carers when teaching them how to handle and carry children with disabilities (Ref 7). They must be certain that the people they are teaching know exactly what to do, and use the techniques correctly, and staff should keep a written record of what they have taught.

THE CHILD WITH VARIABLE MUSCLE TONE

Many disabled children show abnormal patterns of movement that result from disorders of coordination and muscle tone (Ref 5). Small children with variable muscle tone need to be handled in a consistent way. The methods used should be known to all the carers.

Conditions such as cerebral palsy may produce an exaggerated startle reflex, which though normal in young infants may persist in some cases (Ref 14) and require special handling techniques to reduce its potentially harmful effects. Handling the resulting rigid star-shaped child could be risky for the inexperienced handler.

Certain key points on the body may need special control as their position may affect the child's

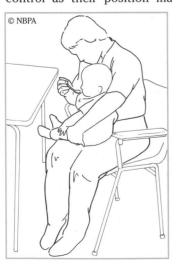

muscle tone in the rest of the body (Ref 9). If the seated nurse's arm is around the sitting child's back and shoulders keeping them in a rounded position, the gross extension pattern (Ref 6), common in some neurological disorders, may be prevented. This position may be useful for feeding

Figure 19.2.

some children with a persistent tongue-thrust, which is often related to the head dropping back and increasing the extensor tone in the back and neck (Ref 10).

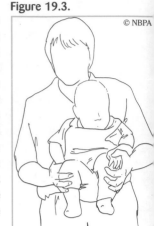

Figure 19.3.

Carrying small children like these may be easier if they are curled up in a flexed position to prevent their legs being held in an extended, adducted pattern. Some infants with spastic diplegia, in which the legs are stiffer than the arms show a reduction in muscle tone if the infant is carried astride across the nurse's hips. This method must be viewed with caution if it puts the handler's spine in a twisted position for too long. The infant can be carried on alternate sides to ease this.

If a very small child has windswept hips (where both hips are rotated to the same side) the uppermost hip may be dislocated and professional advice on handling should be sought from the therapist as cradling the child across the carer's body may increase this deformity.

Figure 19.4.

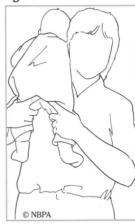

An alternative method of reducing spasm when carrying a very small cerebrally palsied child is to let the child's arms hang down the nurse's back, facing in to the nurse, with both legs gently parted and held across the nurse's chest. Many small children may require specific methods of being handled, and this should be known to all the team.

TOYS AND PLAY

Most infants, regardless of their physical ability, spend much of their waking time on the floor. Many older disabled children will spend a large part of their day lying on the floor on their front or side, and may require special position aids to encourage them to lift their heads. Wedges or side-liers can help these children achieve a stable position for play, and toys to encourage reaching and grasping should be provided for them.

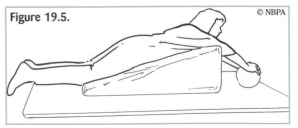

Figure 19.5.

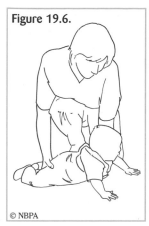

Figure 19.6.

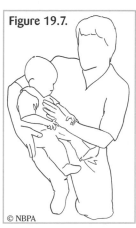

Figure 19.7.

© NBPA

A small prone child may be lifted from the floor by the nurse placing one hand up between the child's legs and supporting its abdomen, and the other arm down between its head and shoulder or from the side and on its chest. The nurse can then pull the child to sit on her knee, facing outwards, and then either stand upright or edge backwards to sit on a small stool or bench. From this position the child can either be put in a chair or passed to another nurse, and neither nurse needs to stoop. Like all handling techniques, these procedures should be written in the care plan, to avoid misunderstandings, such as suspicion of abuse.

Older children can be raised from the floor by rolling them on to an inflatable cushion seat. Once sitting on the deflated cushion, the child can activate the control to raise himself enough to allow a sideways transfer to be made. Alternatively a hoist could be used. If an older child needs help to stand up in long leg callipers, these can be applied when the child is lying on a height adjustable plinth which is raised until the child can slide over the side, with assistance, to stand on the floor.

DEMANDS OF A THERAPEUTIC ROUTINE

Risks to parents and staff

Specialists in neuro-developmental therapy prescribe spasm-inhibiting postures, repetitive exercises, and equipment to help children make movements (Ref 9). These techniques take many months for health professionals to learn and perfect.

Parents and care staff start from a different knowledge base and may be tempted to risk their own health and safety to give the child every opportunity to develop. The child's continued improvement depends on them providing care and consistent attention. If they injure themselves they may be unable to help their child make progress.

It is sometimes useful to make a distinction between handling done for therapeutic reasons

and handling giving routine care. Many people working with children believe that a child's improvement depends on everyone handling the child in the same way, but there may be times when the welfare of the carer is the more important consideration.

When the child is too tired to co-operate, there is no point in attempting to elicit or facilitate normal patterns of movement.

Risks for therapists

Therapists may believe it is their duty to take personal risks to continue the progress of rehabilitation, but these risks should be assessed in line with the Manual Handling Operations Regulations, 1992 (see Chapter 1). They are responsible not only for their own health and safety but are obliged to use safe systems of work. Their professional opinion as to the safety of their actions must be recorded, along with their aims and the risk (Ref 8). Careful thought must be given to safe practices, especially when instructing unqualified staff, such as school welfare assistants, to carry out complex treatment regimes or use equipment without supervision (Ref 7).

Aids to mobility

Many walking or standing aids are difficult to put the child into, and safe prcedures must be used for this. Once a disabled child is bigger than a toddler, picking him up and putting him down on the floor may be hazardous for carers and the use of a hoist should be considered, especially as many children will be wearing heavy appliances such as callipers. Children with progressive disorders must be assessed carefully to help them maintain function without putting carers at risk.

The HSE guidance accompanying Manual Handling Operations Regulations, 1992, says the lifting and lowering of objects to and from the floor close to the feet, weighing over 10kgs (22lbs) for men and approximately 7kgs (14lbs) for women, present some risk and a written assessment must be made before deciding whether it is safe to do this. The same guidance says that few fit, well trained people can lift more than double these weights in safety, even when all other conditions are ideal.

These weight guidelines are different at different heights and distances from the trunk, and the full assessment will take account of the amount of cooperation the child can give, the nature of the task, the environment, and the capabilities of carers (Ref 13).

Many therapists put children on mats on the floor for treatment. A ceiling mounted hoist is ideal for this, but a mobile hoist may be used if its legs are pushed under the edges of the mat and the edges are flicked up. The child is then lowered to the mat. In a treatment room, children can be put on wide, height adjustable plinths.

Figure 19.8.

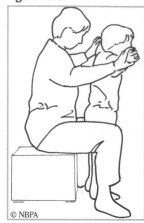

© NBPA

Assisted walking

Many staff find that helping a small child to walk by holding its hands from in front can cause strain. Instead, the therapist can sit on a small stool on castors and can paddle about with her feet while supporting the child. It is not recommended that children are supported by holding their arms above their heads; this can damage vunerable shoulder joints and can put an unexpected strain on the carer's back if the child stumbles. Carers should be taught safe ways to encourage walking.

Toileting safely

If pads and a changing table are not appropriate, a commode seat or a moulded plastic throne seat placed over a toilet can support the floppy child. This design could cause problems because the child must be lifted over the pommel at the front, which is a splash guard and stops the child's legs scissoring in an involuntary spasm. It has a wide base to make it stable, and the use of a hoist avoids the need for the handler having to lift the child at a distance from her own trunk.

Figure 19.9.

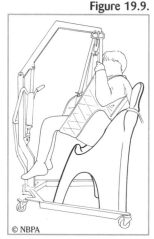

© NBPA

Slings must be selected with care for safety and comfort as well as allowing access to clothing. Toileting slings should be assessed carefully for suitability; a child with low muscle tone or who cannot keep both arms outside the sling may slip through some types. Children who need the support of moulded seating can have an extra mould made with perforations and a commode aperture, mounted on a wheeled frame, for toileting and showering.

IN SCHOOL

Disabled children in a mainstream school may be accompanied by their own welfare assistant. This person should be trained in the general principles of moving and handling as well as the techniques specific to the child in her care.

Some teachers feel that special equipment draws attention to the child's disability. It is preferable to provide equipment that meets their needs and enables them to learn and play with other children.

In special schools, equipment is more likely to be provided routinely. Ideally, there should be a tracking system of hoisting across and along each room used by children with disabilities to make it easier to move them. Where there is no tracking system, several mobile hoists may be necessary. Special care classrooms must have enough space for bulky equipment.

Time to use the equipment should be built into the timetable.

All the equipment should be chosen to meet the varying needs of children and staff.

Standing aids in the classroom

Standing and positioning aids are often part of a treatment regime for children who cannot stand without help. They should be accessible from all sides.

Standing is important (Ref 2). It is believed to:

reduce the risks of osteoporosis due to the child not bearing his own weight

enhance bladder and kidney function

reduce spasm and stimulate balance reactions

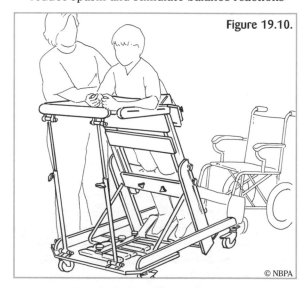

Figure 19.10.

© NBPA

reduce the likelihood of contractures

give the child a different perspective on the class room and provide a suitable position for observation and learning.

In many standing aids the child slopes slightly forward and is strapped in securely with the head level with that of the standing person. The child's feet may be a foot or more above the ground.

At present many staff hold the child upright and lift him on to the apparatus by stretching across its base. Even with two staff this is hazardous because of the possibility of musculoskeletal strain when handling all but the smallest child at arm's length.

In schools for children with learning disabilities the oldest may be nineteen years old, and as heavy as adults. Few hoists can lift a child prone on to this apparatus, so safer, alternative aids must be sought (Ref 1).

Alternatives could be:

    tilt tables,

    supine standers,

    flexible standers,

    standing wheelchairs.

With tilt-tables and supine standers the child is transferred or hoisted on in a supine position, secured, and then tilted to the desired angle. A table can then be attached. The resulting position is a few degrees back from vertical, instead of a few degrees forward, but this may be suitable for many children.

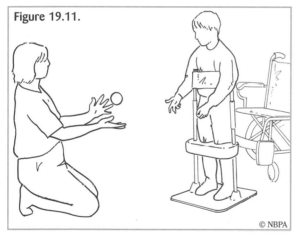

Figure 19.11.

The flexible stander can be reached from a wheelchair. The child's feet must be secured to the base, which is at floor level, then the child is helped to stand, either by carers, or a motorised lifter, before being secured to hold the correct position. Young adults can also use a standing wheelchair.

Although this equipment will meet most of the requirements of a standing regime, it may not help some who have poor head control. If a larger child needs to be encouraged to control his head, lying him prone over a wedge on the floor, or putting a wedge on a height adjustable plinth for part of the day, may help. A hoist could place the child on his back, and he is then rolled over to the prone position. A variety of positions should be used during the day (Ref 17).

Special seating

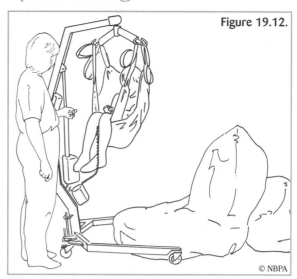

Figure 19.12.

Children sitting in matrix or moulded seating, or in bean bags which conform with an irregular shape, may be difficult to handle. Putting them back into their chairs often means that carers lean over the fixed head support and leg extension supports to lift at a considerable distance from their body.

A sling should be left in position behind these children after hoisting them into their chairs, so that they are ready for any other transfers. This sling could be applied after dressing, before getting them off the bed. It is difficult for the carer to remove and re-apply this sling, and this can cause discomfort to the child.

Mesh slings are often cooler and more suitable to mould around these children, and a sheepskin lining may prevent pressure problems occurring.

Slings must be close fitting and not wrinkled up when left in place, particularly when the child has a lack of sensation or cannot tell his carer he is uncomfortable. Manufacturers will tailor-make slings to suit an individual, and a seating engineer should allow space for the thickness of the sling when adjusting the matrix or making a new mould.

Many of these seats can be tipped back temporarily on the chassis (Ref 15), allowing the child's pelvis to be positioned correctly when the hoist is being used, as well as giving an opportunity for pressure relief.

School playgrounds

Playground equipment such as swings and roundabouts can have ramps for a wheelchair, and impact absorbing floor surfaces are useful when there are children who may fall from losing their balance or having convulsions. There are wendy houses with doors wide enough for wheelchairs.

Multi-sensory environments

Sensory rooms are often provided for children with sensory impairments. These can have padded floors and walls, and disco-type lights projected on to the ceiling, music and lights that vibrate, and mobiles and inflatable shapes that make noises when squeezed. Children with limited mobility can have some control by using a large button on the wall to change the light pattern or music.

When places like this are being planned, access with tracking hoists must be considered. For existing areas, hoist access under a raised padded floor, or removable mats at the entrance, should be arranged, to allow a mobile hoist to lower a child to the edge of the padded floor, and from there a carer can slide him into the room.

TRAVEL

School transport

Minibuses and ambulances used for school should have tail-lifts for children in wheelchairs. The tail lift should be large enough to accommodate chair and escort. Drivers and escorts should not be expected to lift children who cannot bear their own weight into a seat on the bus. There should be enough space in the vehicle for all the wheelchairs to be secured so that there is no need for risky transfers.

For children who can stand for a short time, swivel discs for the floor, or seat cushions that swivel, may be necessary so that they can be moved safely from wheelchair to seat.

Seat belts and wheelchair locking clamps must be provided, and buggy type push chairs must be of a type that can be safely strapped down, with the correct straps.

The most able children should be seated next to the windows so that escorts do not need to stretch to the window seats to assist those who have disabilities. The aisle seats should be for those who need help. Small children who need special seat inserts may have to sit in single rows.

Routes may need to be planned so that children are collected in a sequence that suits these seating arrangements.

No drivers or escorts should be expected to work in a stooped position in a bus that is not tall enough to stand up in.

School outings should be planned to ensure safe access for disabled children and their carers, and schedules should allow time for staff to have sufficient rest.

Wheelchairs should be selected and maintained so that they can be used safely on school outings and should not be overloaded with picnic bags. Staff should be familiar with their use.

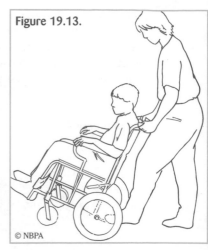

Figure 19.13.

© NBPA

Family travel

Some parents choose vehicles that allow children to be pushed up ramps in their chairs through a rear door, then secured in place. Some manufacturers will put the front passenger seat on a transfer beam, to swing out over the pavement, making seated transfers easier. A child's seat with head supports and pommel can be fitted to this seat, so that parents do not need to stretch to put the child into the back seat.

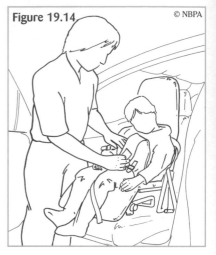

Figure 19.14.

© NBPA

A special seat for a child can be mounted on a frame over the car seat, and it can rotate through 90 degrees to face outwards and then to slide out a short distance on a rail, so that carers do not have to stoop or stretch.

Buses and trains

Public transport is still difficult for many families who have a disabled child.

Buses which have a low floor are easier to get on and off.

Many underground stations are inaccessible to wheelchairs, but some main line stations will provide help for a disabled person to travel if notified in advance, providing ramps and extra helpers as necessary, though each line may have different arrangements.

SPORT AND RECREATION

In all sports there is a risk of injury to the participants, so special care is needed in the preparation and planning of recreation for disabled children accompanied by carers.

Care should be taken to find out whether children who have difficulty understanding or expressing themselves, or have learning disabilities, are fully informed about activities that some other children find exciting, and that they understand what to expect. It cannot be assumed that all children enjoy them.

Access to recreational facilities for disabled people is slowly improving.

Swimming

Swimming can be beneficial to disabled children, physically and socially.

Many swimming pools have special clubs for disabled swimmers, and provide a hoist seat or stretcher for the disabled person to go in or out of the water safely. Where pools slope into the water, shower chairs can carry the person far enough in to float off.

Many pools have inflatable toys, rings and floats which can be used for fun and therapy.

Changing rooms which disabled people can use are not often provided. They may need height adjustable changing tables and hoists, at present usually provided only in special schools or special holiday centres.

Horse riding

Riding may be beneficial for disabled children. Many therapists believe the rhythmic movements of the horse, coupled with the wide stride sitting position, can relieve spasm and improve balance, as well as be fun (Ref 3).

Many centres for riding for the disabled offer lessons, and have volunteer staff who work under the direction of trained instructors.

Staff and volunteers should be trained in handling children with physical and other disabilities, and the centre should be prepared to refuse to accept children whose handling problems cannot be overcome.

Staff and volunteers are covered by the Management of Health and Safety at Work Regulations, 1992, which states that employers are responsible for anyone exposed to risks in the workplace, whether an employee or not.

Instead of the traditional mounting block, the horse may walk between two parallel ramps and down a slope, like a train between two platforms, and the child is wheeled up to the correct level for mounting. The child is helped to stand beside the horse, then laid face down across the saddle, and staff help him to sit astride.

Some riding centres with an indoor exercise area have overhead tracking hoists so that riders can be lifted from their wheelchair to the saddle.

The use of hoists is encouraged.

Cycling

Cycling helps disabled children move around faster, have fun and be like other children.

Helping larger children to mount a three or four wheeled cycle can be awkward. A height adjustable plinth can raise them to the correct saddle height and may make it possible to transfer them sideways, especially when the child has strong arms. Alternatively a tracking hoist can be used.

Ball pools

Ball pools, frequently used for exercise and recreation, may be difficult for some children to use. If the pool is sunken into the ground the child can be hoisted to the floor, then slid over the edge of the pool. If the pool stands above floor level, a tracking hoist may be needed to lower the child into it, or a small removable section provided at one side to allow the child to be slid in and out. A large sliding board or similar could be slid across the surface to enable the carer to slide the child to the edge before getting him out.

Boating

It is sometimes possible to get a disabled child into a canal boat in a wheelchair over a ramped gangplank and an elevating platform which lowers to deck level.

Washing and toilet facilities can be provided on the boat for disabled people.

Holiday centres

Some holiday centres cater exclusively for people with disabilities and their families, with hoists and other equipment supplied routinely. A holiday for a disabled child should not put carers at risk, struggling in unfamiliar surroundings and coping without the necessary equipment.

Asking questions in advance, and a preliminary visit, will discover what is available and whether the place is wheelchair friendly.

Exciting sports are possible, but safety must be paramount, and, as with any activity holiday, inquiries should be made about the centre's safety record and the level of skill and training of the staff.

CHALLENGING BEHAVIOUR

Children with challenging behaviour present social, ethical and physical problems for the handler. The children may throw themselves to the floor, run into the road or attempt to harm themselves and others. Any risks arising to staff from this behaviour should be assessed, under the Management of Health and Safety at Work Regulations, 1992, and staff should trained to deal with this.

Ethically it is permissible to move someone against their wishes if they are endangering their own or someone else's health and safety. Moving them in other circumstances could technically be considered an assault.

Procedures for managing children with challenging behaviour should be discussed by the team and written records should be kept so that staff are protected from misinterpretation of their motives. Careful observation to discover triggers for this behaviour may allow for behaviour modification programmes to be devised.

Children's behaviour may be modified by a variety of methods, but special techniques may be needed to prevent them injuring themselves or others, and specific psychological guidance should be sought.

USEFUL CONTACTS AND ADDRESSES

Chailey Heritage, North Chailey, Near Lewes, East Sussex BN8 4EF

Follifoot Riding for the Disabled, 23 Cavendish Ave., Harrogate, North Yorkshire HG2 8HY

Strategies for Crisis Intervention and Prevention, Loddon School, Wildmoor, Sherfield-on-Loddon, Hook, Hampshire, RG27 0JD

Muscular Dystrophy Association, Prescott House, Prescott Place, London SW4

Riding for the Disabled Association, Avenue R, National Agricultural Centre, Kenilworth, Warwickshire CV8 2LY

Scope (for people with cerebral palsy), 12 Park Crescent, London W4

The author wishes to acknowledge the contribution to this chapter by Rosemary Pearce and Maggie Williams of the RCN Advisory Panel for Back Pain in Nurses.

REFERENCES

1. Alexander P., (1996). Problems in Paediatric Situations. The Column, 8 2. London. National Back Exchange.

2. Bell E., and Lamont J.E., (1993). Profound and Multiple Disability. In: Eckersley P., (ed.) Elements of Paediatric Physiotherapy, Edinburgh. Churchill Livingstone.

3. Bertoti D.B., (1988). Effects of therapeutic horseback riding on patients with cerebral palsy. Physical Therapy, 68 (10) 1505-1510.

4. Biering-Sorensen, (1983a). A prospective study of low back pain in a general population: 1, occurrence, recurrence, and aetiology. Scandinavian Journal of Rehabilitation, 15,71079.

5. Bobath K., (1966). The Motor Deficit in Patients with Cerebral Palsy. Suffolk. The Lavenham Press.

6. Bobath B., (1971). Abnormal Postural Reflex Activity caused by Brain Lesions, 2nd edition. London. Heinemann Medical Books.

7. Chartered Society of Physiotherapy, (1996). The delegation of tasks to physiotherapy assistants and other support workers. Professional Affairs Information Paper PA6. London. Chartered Society of Physiotherapy.

8. Chartered Society of Physiotherapy, (1996). Treatments involving manual handling. Professional Affairs Information Paper no. 35. London. Chartered Society of Physiotherapy.

9. Eckersley P., and King L., (1993). Treatment Systems. In: Eckersley P., (ed.) Elements of Paediatric Physiotherapy, Edinburgh. Churchill Livingstone.

10. Finnie N., (1974). Handling the cerebral palsied child at home, 2nd edition. London. Butterworth-Heinemann.

11. Grimley A.M.D., (1993). A historical perspective. In: Eckersley P., (ed.) Elements of Paediatric Physiotherapy, Edinburgh. Churchill Livingstone.

12. Hall G., (1993). Living skills and the environment. In: Eckersley P., (ed.) Elements of Paediatric Physiotherapy, Edinburgh. Churchill Livingstone.

13. Manual Handling Operations Regulations (1992) and guidance on Regulations L23, HMSO (1992).

14. Illingwoth R.S., (1987). The Development of the Infant and Young Child, 9th edition. Edinburgh. Churchill Livingstone.

15. Pope P.M., (1996). Postural Management and special seating. In: Edwards S. (ed.) Neurological Physiotherapy - a Problem-solving Approach. London. Churchill Livingstone.

16. Seccombe I., and Smith G., (1996). Manual Handling and Lifting, a review for the Royal College of Nursing. London. Royal College of Nursing.

17. Shepherd R.B., (1995). Physiotherapy in Paediatrics, 3rd edition. Oxford. Butterworth Heinemann.

GLOSSARY

Adducted: held close to the midline of the body, or crossed over,common in neurological disorders.

Contractures: fixed deformities, usually caused by shortened muscles or ligaments.

Extended: part of the body held in a straightened position.

Extensor: producing straightening of the body or limb.

Neonate: newborn infant.

Neurodevelopmental therapy: treatment based on normalising patterns of movement by inhibiting abnormal reflex movements.

Prone: lying face down.

Scissoring: a position of the legs, in which they are stiff, straightened and crossed over each other.

Side-lier: a piece of equipment that enables a child to achieve a stable position lying on its side.

Supine: lying face up.

SUPPORT IN WALKING AND THE FALLING OR FALLEN PATIENT

By Danielle Holmes

SUMMARY

This chapter addresses the techniques to be used to assist a patient in walking. There is particular emphasis on the ways of achieving rehabilitation in patients who have lost their ability to walk. The danger to the nurse is that the patient may fall. At no time must the nurse support a collapsing patient. The chapter describes what to do when the patient fails to walk and collapses to the floor.

MOBILISING PATIENTS

Many patients who are in hospital or otherwise in care have lost some or all of their mobility. Some of these are capable of regaining mobility. It is, of course, desirable to achieve as much restoration of mobility as each individual can achieve. There is a danger that this is taken to mean that every patient must walk again. Rehabilitation must be planned and monitored to ensure that the patient achieves as much as he can without being forced to attempt levels of mobilisation that are beyond his abilities. Falls, resulting from trying to go too far or too fast, discourage the patient from trying to mobilise again. After several falls, the patient becomes convinced that he cannot regain his mobility and gives up. He expects and allows the nurses to lift him.

There has to be a safe plan for the restoration of mobility with realistic goals. A patient may be able to achieve considerable independent mobility with the help of sliding equipment. There is no need to force this person to try to walk if he cannot do so. The concentration on walking may even deprive the patient of what limited mobility he was capable of developing.

Every patient who is being rehabilitated must have a clear written plan that progresses from one goal to the next in a logical sequence. The plan should be created by all disciplines involved in the care of the patient. There are three safe handling rules to be followed in creating the plan:-

1. Do not put nurses and carers at risk by using them as props.

2. Patients must be supported by devices that will not let them down when they feel too weak to continue.

3. The transition to the next stage must only happen when the previous goal has been achieved.

The starting point for a rehabilitation programme and the steps within it must be chosen for each individual. The following list contains some of the steps that may prove useful. The list must not be treated as prescriptive. At each stage a positive decision must be made that it is worthwhile proceeding to the next stage.

On every occasion that a patient is mobilised the nurse must assess his current condition. Whilst assessing the patient she should consider the following points:-

The patient's mental and physical condition.

How good is the patient's sense of balance?

Whether the patient is particularly tired for example at the end of the day

Is it the first time/day that the patient has walked?

Is there anything else that may increase the stress on this occasion?

e.g. 1. A patient hurrying to get to the toilet is under greater stress than the same patient returning from the toilet. Take the patient to the toilet in a wheelchair and let him walk back.

2. A patient may be disorientated when he wakes at night. It may be safer to slide or hoist on these occasions even though he is capable of walking.

The first steps are to improve pre walking mobility.

STAGE	METHOD	COMMENTS
1.	Sliding Systems	Nurses may already be using sliding devices for some transfers. It is quite natural to go on to letting the patient use the sliding system without the nurse assisting him. This can progress to the patient learning to position the device himself. See Chapter 13 & 14 for more details on sliding devices
2.	Self propelled wheelchairs	There is a tendency for all wheelchairs on a ward to be of the small wheeled variety. Patients cannot move these themselves. If a few large wheeled chairs are available, patients can be encouraged to move themselves.

The most dangerous time during the rehabilitation of a patient is in the initial attempts to stand. This phase must be approached with the greatest care. The method of actually bringing the patient to his feet must be chosen to avoid risk of injury.

STAGE	METHOD	COMMENTS
3.	Standaids	There are a number of standaid hoists on the market. These can be used as part of a rehabilitation plan to transfer a patient in a tanding position from one seated position to another. N.B. Some standaids require the patient to lean back in the sling. This is not desirable in a rehabilitation programme as it does not encourage a normal pattern of movement.

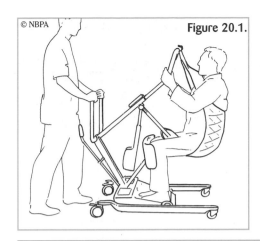

© NBPA

Figure 20.1.

STAGE	METHOD	COMMENTS
4.	Walking hoists	There are a variety of mechanical devices that can be used to stand a patient up from a seated position and support him whilst walking. These fall into two main groups. The first group is a frame that is placed around the patient. These do not have any over head element. The second group consists of patient holsts that have a walking harness. (N.B. not all hoists are capable of this adaptation.) The main characteristic of either group is that the patient can only slip a few inches before he is supported. He can be walking nearly fully supported or completely unsupported. However, as soon as he slips, he can be confident that the hoist will support him. See box D - Standaids as a walking aid

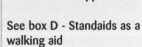
Figure 20.3.

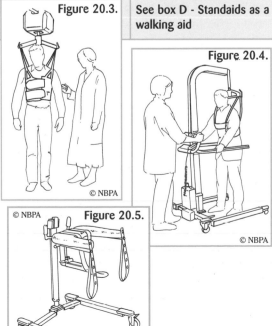
Figure 20.4.

© NBPA

© NBPA

Figure 20.5.

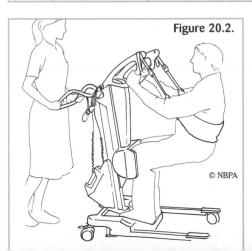
Figure 20.2.

© NBPA

5.	Rollators	These wheeled walking frames save the patient from the chore of lifting the walking frame and repositioning.
6.	Walking frames	These are universally known as Zimmer frames. They provide invaluable support to the patient. When a patient is first using a walking frame or a rollator a nurse should follow with a wheelchair. If the patient feels weak, he can quickly sit down without an accident.
7.	Tripods, walking sticks and crutches	Some or all of these may form useful stages in the plan for individual patients.

Box D - Standaids as a walking aid

Most "Standaids" transfer the patient whilst he is standing on a small platform. It is not possible to use these in walking a patient.

Some standaids now come with a standing platform that can be removed and a support that can be fastened all the way round the patient. It has been suggested that these particular devices can be used to support a patient in re-learning to walk. In some cases, it is suggested that the patient can be lifted from behind over a small chair which is removed when the patient has been lifted. The patient is supported by the stand aid with the whole of the mechanism behind him. He can use a rollator or zimmer frame to walk whilst supported by the stand aid.

These may provide an effective approach but, as there is little experience of using standaids in this way, they should be approached with caution.

No attempt should be made to use a stand aid as a walking aid unless the manufacturer has said that it can be used in this way. Make sure that the sling will support the patient even if he throws his arms straight up in the air. It is essential that nurses practice using this method before using it with patients. If the device is used over a small chair make sure that the chair is small and light enough to lift safely.

SUPPORT IN WALKING

Once the patient has exhausted the list of walkingaids he may need a final helping hand. He may need the nurse to support him during walking exercises.

The benefit of support in walking is that the nurse is able to give encouragement to a hesitant walker. The nurse is close by but not taking the patient's weight. She must recognise that she cannot give more than minimal support in this situation and if the patient does collapse the nurse must be ready to lower him to the ground.

Can the Patient Get to His Feet?

The nurse must assess the patient's ability to stand and walk. Before commencing to assist the patient it is a good idea to check if the patient can stand. A patient who has been in a home for a long time, or a patient who is hospitalised may have lost a lot of muscle power. The nurse must ensure that an assessment is made.

1. Ask the patient if he can walk. Remember that the patient may think he can walk and in reality not be able to do so.

2. Ask the patient to move his leg. The following scale will assist the nurse to assess the patient's ability to stand. This is described in greater detail in Chapter 15.

  0. no movement seen

  1. a flicker movement seen at the muscles of the thigh

  2. movement with the effects of gravity eliminated - as in lying on the bed and moving the legs from side to side

  3. Movement against gravity - is able to lift the leg while sitting

  4. Movement against gravity and some resistance in the sitting position - can lift the leg whilst pressure is put on the knee.

  5. normal movement

If the patient is in category 0,1, 2, or 3 he will not be able to stand.

If the nurse is confident that the patient can stand she should use one of the techniques described elsewhere in this book to bring him to his feet. (See Chairs and Bed Chapters)

Planning Support in Walking

If a nurse decides to walk with a patient and provide support, she must consider carefully the extent of that support and how she is going to react when the patient relies on her too much or actually collapses.

The ergonomics of support in walking are not favourable. The nurse is providing support at or about her waist height. This is the safest height for taking any load. However, when supporting a patient who is walking, the load must be taken to one side. This is a bad position as the load is unbalanced on the spine. If the patient actually collapses, the nurse has to move very quickly or she will be taking the load in a twisted posture. Even if she manages to move to the correct position the load will be too heavy for her to safely support the patient.

It is also important to consider the environment in which the patient will be walking with the nurse. Is there enough space for two (or three) people to pass throughout the intended route? If it is necessary to pass some furniture where there is not enough space, the furniture must be moved first. The nurses must not try to go through a single width door. If there is such a door on the proposed route then another route must be chosen. If there are doors on the route ensure that they can be wedged open or that someone else will open them whilst the nurses and the patient pass through. Nurses must not try to open doors at the same time as they are assisting the patient. If the patient is being taken to the toilet the nurse must ensure that there will be enough room for her and the patient in the toilet. (N.B. Nurses should always consider taking the patient to the toilet in a wheelchair and walking back. This puts a lot less stress on the patient.) If there is not enough space for the nurses to safely support the patient throughout the journey then they must not do it.

Nurses should be aware of their limitations when supporting patients if they are not matched for height and build. This is particularly the case when the patient or the nurse is unusually short or tall.

Giving Support in Walking

If possible, the patient should wear a belt. The nurse, or nurses, should stand close to the patient using the Palm-to-Palm Thumb Grip.

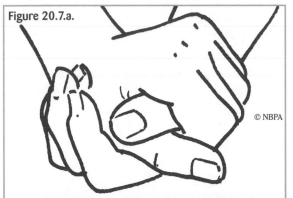

Figure 20.7.a.

© NBPA

If there is only one nurse, she should be on the weaker side. On the right side of the patient, the nurse holds the patient's right hand in her right hand and on the left vice versa. The patient's arms should be straight, pressing down with his palm onto the nurse's palm with their thumbs interlocked (with a clinging patient the nurse may prefer to avoid the thumb hold).

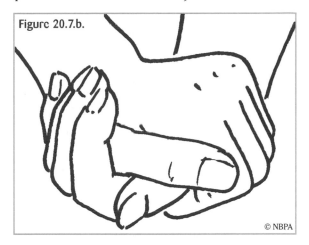

Figure 20.7.b.

© NBPA

The nurse's other hand can be used to keep the patient's elbow straight, but without gripping his arm painfully or putting pressure under his armpit. Alternatively, she can hold him round the waist. If a belt is being used to hold the patient, the nurse's hand should be inserted from underneath. The hand should not go all the way through the belt. This avoids the nurse's hand being trapped if the patient collapses. The nurse must be close to the patient to avoid unnecessary stress on her back, but also to support the patient. Both must face in the direction in which they are walking.

> ### WARNING
>
> The palm to palm thumb grip is not suitable for all patients. For those patients who are aggressive and likely to grab the nurses thumb use the techniques described in Chapter 18.

The backward leaner

This phrase is used to describe a patient who has a tendency to lean back in a hyper extended posture when standing or walking. Any attempt to pull the patient by the hand, arm or body from in front tends to result in the patient resisting by recoiling or pulling away from the nurse.

When mobilizing such a patient, it is safer to stand at their side facing in the same direction and to ensure that the patient initiates the moves to stand and walk.

As with all support in walking, there should be a body belt in position around the patient's waist. Two nurses are often required, one on each side.

When walking, the patient's arms should be down at his sides with the hand clasped in the hands of the nurses (see above). Their near side arms should be holding the body belt round the waist. The nurses should stand close for reassurance and support should the patient become unsteady. If the patient does start to fall, the nurses should proceed as described below.

Following with a Wheelchair

In the early stages of walking with a patient or if the patient has a known tendency to collapse a helper should walk behind pushing a wheel chair. This will enable the patient to sit down, should the need arise.

THE FALLING PATIENT

If the patient is collapsing and cannot be persuaded to stand, he must be lowered to the ground immediately.

The nurse executes the following moves. She:-

1. releases her hold of the patient

2. moves behind the patient (Fig. 20.9.)

3. opens her hands and takes one step back

4. allows the patient to slide to the floor (Fig. 20.10.)

5. lets the patient remain in a sitting position on the floor (Fig. 20.11.)

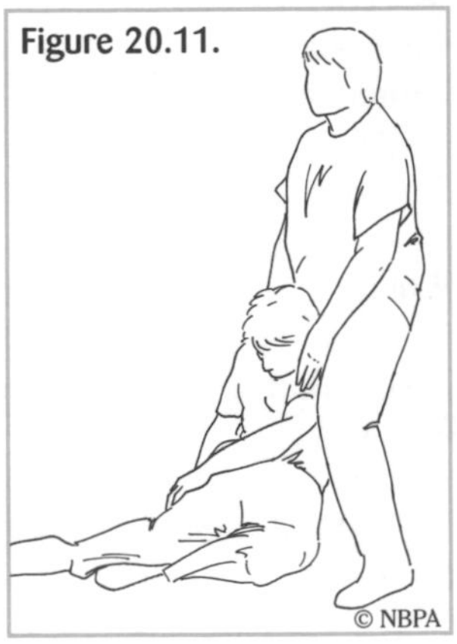

If the patient has fainted, then the nurse can kneel down and allow the patient to lie down. She then repositions herself to place the patient into a recovery position.

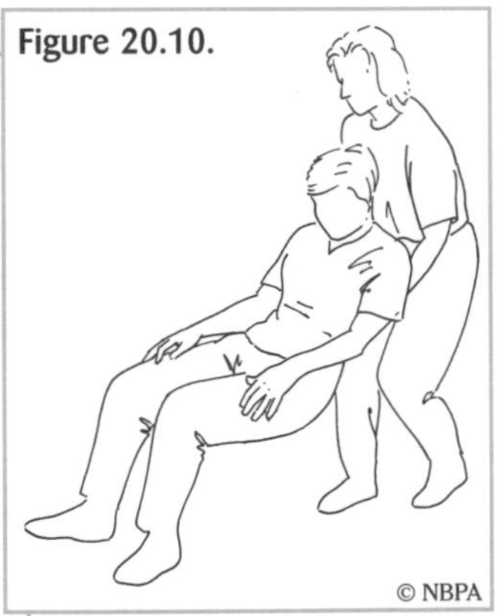

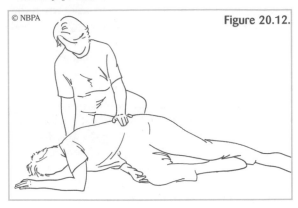

Figure 20.12.

N.B.

1. IT IS IMPORTANT TO PLAN FOR THE EVENTUALITY OF A COLLAPSE. THE PATIENT MUST NOT BE HELD OR SUPPORTED IN ANY WAY WHICH PREVENTS THE NURSE RELEASING HER GRIP.

2. THE NURSE MUST ALSO AVOID ANY METHOD OF SUPPORT THAT ALLOWS THE PATIENT TO GRAB HOLD OF HER

3. THE NURSE MUST NOT RUSH TO RESCUE A FALLING PATIENT. SHE WILL NOT BE CLOSE ENOUGH TO GET INTO POSITION IN TIME.

WARNING

The practice of the nurse pushing the patient's foot forward with her own foot or placing her foot under the patient's foot is dangerous. If the patient needs such assistance, he is not yet ready for walking practice.

Figure 20.9.

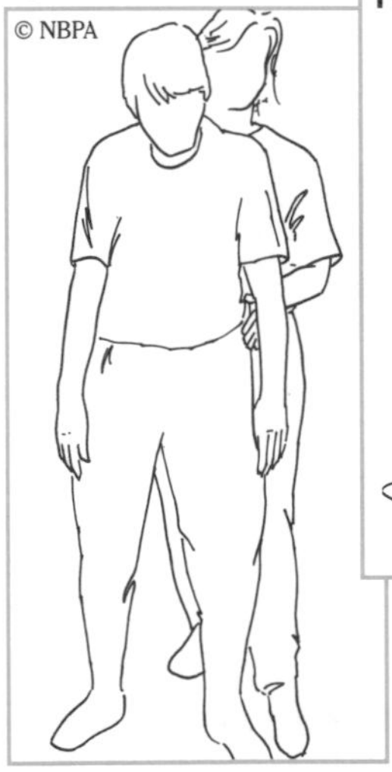

Figure 20.10.

Figure 20.11.

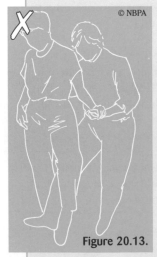

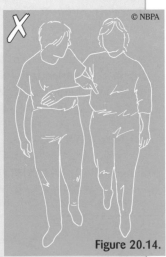

Figure 20.13.

Figure 20.14.

Walking arm in arm with the patient is dangerous. Because he is linked to the patient, the nurse is not in a position to let the patient slide to the floor.

THE FALLEN PATIENT

It is reasonable to expect that some patients in hospital, at home or in nursing or residential homes are likely to fall at some time. The nurse has to be aware of these possibilities and have planned solutions for moving a patient off the floor. The managers of all hospitals, nursing homes, residential homes and home care services must recognise that their staff will be faced with this situation. They must ensure that they have planned for dealing with fallen patients. They must have provided appropriate solutions.

Patients can and will collapse in all areas that they can gain access to. Plans must be made for dealing with them where they fall. Some of the more awkward aspects of this are discussed in the chapter on Emergencies.

When a patient is found collapsed on the floor, the first priority is to see if he has had a respiratory or cardiac arrest. If this is the case he must be resuscitated on the floor. ON NO ACCOUNT SHOULD THE PATIENT BE LIFTED UNTIL THE APPROPRIATE EQUIPMENT HAS BEEN OBTAINED. See the emergency chapter for a longer discussion on dealing with this situation.

Having established that the patient does not require resuscitation the nurse must establish that the patient is not injured in some way. If he is injured the nurse must decide if he can be treated where he is or if he can be moved before he is treated.

Having decided that the patient is ready to be moved off the floor, there are only THREE options that can be considered.

Lift using a hoist

Lift using an inflatable system

Guide the patient to get himself up.

Do not rush to get a patient off the floor. Calm him down and calm anyone who is agitating for him to be moved. Patients on the floor do make a place look untidy but, this is no excuse for injuring someone in rushing to get them up. The patient should be made comfortable. A pillow can be placed under his head and he can be covered with a blanket to keep him warm whilst the nurse prepares to get him up. If the patient can be sat up safely then he can lean against an upturned chair. Someone should be left to comfort him whilst the equipment is fetched. See Chapter 14 on techniques for sitting a patient up.

Getting a patient from the floor using a hoist

If the patient is in a confined area where the hoist cannot be operated the patient must first be moved out into the open. This can be achieved by rolling him onto a sliding sheet and sliding him out. This technique can be used even in confined areas such as between a toilet and the wall.

There are two different approaches to lifting a patient from the floor with a hoist. These are using a fabric sling or using a stretcher attachment. In general a fabric sling will be adequate. However, the patient may be injured in some way that excludes the use of a fabric sling. In this case a stretcher attachment must be used. (N.B. It is thought that a patient who has been resuscitated following a cardiac arrest must be lifted in a supine position. The use of an ordinary fabric sling will bend the patient. This creates increased abdominal pressure that may cause a further arrest.)

Lifting a patient from the floor using a hoist with a fabric sling

The sling can be inserted under the patient in two ways. The patient can be rolled onto the sling or he can be brought to a sitting position and supported by the back of a chair. In the latter situation the sling is slipped down behind the patient. These techniques have already been described in the section on handling the patient in bed (Chapter 14).

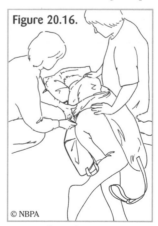

Figure 20.16.

Inserting hoist sling.

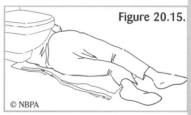

Figure 20.15.

Sling with long loops ready to be pulled.

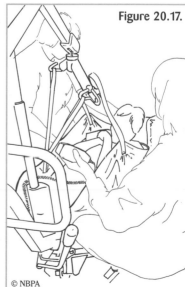

Figure 20.17.

Patient being raised by hoist

Lifting a patient from the floor using a hoist with a stretcher attachment

The use of this type of patient handling system has been described in detail in the section dealing with moving patients from bed. The problem is that most hoists are incapable of lifting the stretcher unless it is positioned across the legs of the hoist. It would be unsafe to manually lift the stretcher into this position.

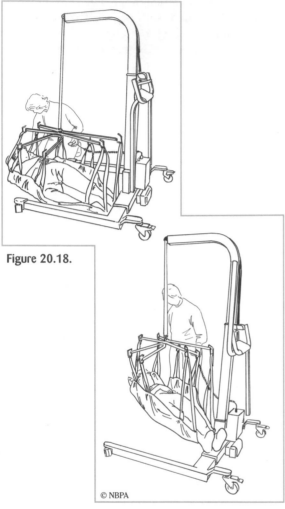

Figure 20.18.

© NBPA

Lifting using an inflatable system

There are a few inflatable systems that can be used to lift a patient from the floor. If the patient is reasonably aware and able to balance to some extent he may be able to use one of these to get to chair height. The patient is rolled to position the device under him. He is brought to a sitting position using the ELBOW TO ELBOW GRIP (see bed chapter). The device is then inflated and the patient is brought to approximately chair height. The patient can now be transferred to a chair or a wheelchair. If needed, a sliding system can be used for this final move.

Inflatable systems are particularly useful in situations where children or patients with learning difficulties are being cared for. It is possible to lift the client anywhere. These devices carry their own power so they can even be used in the middle of a field. They are relatively light so they can conveniently be taken about. For example, they can be taken on holiday with the client.

The current designs of inflatable systems are not suitable for patients who have no upper body control.

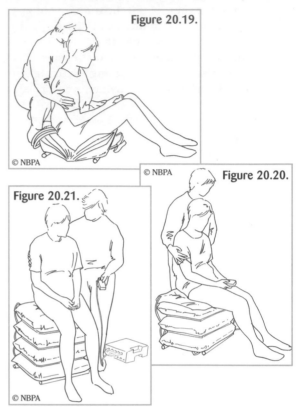

Figure 20.19.

© NBPA

Figure 20.21.

Figure 20.20.

© NBPA

© NBPA

Getting a patient to get himself up

Many patients who have fallen can be persuaded to get themselves up. This procedure must be carried out without the nurse or carer taking any of the patient's weight at any stage:-

1. Get the patient to half turn onto his side.

2. The patient then climbs up so that he gets his arms onto the seat of a chair or wheelchair.

3. He is then persuaded to go on climbing until he can turn into the seat.

4. In some cases the patient can make use of a foot stool as a first stage on the way to the seat of the chair.

5. Nurses should beware of the temptation to lift the patient into a final position once he is in the chair.

It is particularly valuable to teach this technique to people who are living on their own. It can greatly increase the confidence of a person with limited mobility to know that if he does fall, he can still get back up without having to wait for help to arrive.

CASE STUDY

The following case study illustrates the problems encountered caring for people with marginal mobility.

"Gone Off Her Legs"

At 4 p.m. one Friday, the G. P. visited Mrs X her home. She was increasingly difficult to manage as she had lost a lot of mobility. The patient was well known to the G.P. who had looked after her some fifteen years.

He wrote "Gone off her legs - please admit."

The patient was admitted to the ward later that evening. The records show that the lady was approximately 5 feet tall and weighed some 114kg (18 stones). She had difficulty in walking. She had her own wheelchair.

The nursing care plan stated that she was to be moved from bed to chair with the assistance of two nurses.

On the Saturday morning Mrs X legs nearly gave way and she almost fell. This was recorded in the nursing evaluation notes. However, the care plan remained unchanged.

On the Sunday night whilst the two nurses were assisting Mrs X into bed, her knees gave way and the two nurses let her slide to the floor. As she fell the patient suffered a compound fracture of her lower leg.

She sued the hospital for failing to take care of her.

Conclusions

Mrs X's fracture was caused by the fact that the nurses continued to expect her to stand even though they knew she could not do so with reliability. She had been admitted because she had "gone off her legs." Never-the-less the nursing staff continued to insist on attempting standing transfers. The patient collapsed on the Saturday morning. Again the nursing staff chose to ignore the problem and continued to stand the patient.

If this patient had been properly assessed it would have been realised that the patient was not in a condition to be stood or walked without external support. She was not in a good enough physical condition to be able to walk. She would not have passed the assessments described above. She was also far too heavy to

be supported by nurses. The only options were 1) to use sliding systems to enable the patient to slide herself across; 2) to use a hoist or 3) to use a walking support hoist. The care plan ought to have specified which of these options was to be used by the nurses. If this had been done the patient would not have been injured.

Because of this error, Mrs X apparently never recovered her mobility. If the nursing staff had used the correct techniques she would not have been injured and might have eventually regained some or all of her mobility.

FURTHER READING LIST

1. Chartered Society of Physiotherapists (1996)The Criteria for the Delegation of Tasks to Assistants C.S.P.

2. Chartered Society of Physiotherapists (1996) Guide lines for the management of physiotherapy helpers C.S.P.

3. Health Building Note 40 (1995) Common Activity Spaces Vol.4 Circulation Areas H.M.S.O.

4. Kendal H. O, Kendal F P, Wadsworth G. E (1971) Muscle Testing and Function Williams & Williams Baltimore London

5. Medical Research Council (1976) Aids to the examination of the Peripheral Nervous System H.M.S.O.

6. RCN (1996) Hazards of nursing Personal Injuries at Work RCN

EMERGENCY

By Danielle Holmes

SUMMARY

This chapter addresses the planning that is needed to stop emergencies being a cause for injuries amongst those who are trying to handle patients. Nearly all emergency situations are foreseeable, therefore, safe solutions can be put in place and further injuries to nurses and patients can be avoided.

INTRODUCTION

The following definition of 'Emergency' comes from Websters dictionary:

> **emer.gen.cy** \i-'mer-jen-sÎ\ n, pl -cies 1: an unforeseen combination of circumstances or the resulting state that calls for immediate action. 2: a pressing need

The emergency services take the view that operating without planning and training lead to errors and danger. It is for this reason that they have plans and exercises for major disasters. This chapter is based upon the view that most so called emergencies are foreseeable and can therefore be planned for.

FOUR REAL EMERGENCIES

There are four situations that can be described as emergencies. In these situations the victim must be moved to safety immediately and there is no time to get equipment or plan the move. Risks may have to be taken.

The situations are where a person is:-

in water in imminent danger of drowning

in an area that is actually on fire or filling with smoke

in danger from bomb or bullet

in danger from a collapsing building or other structure

These situations are extremely rare even for the emergency services.

In a situation where people are caring for others, emergency situations are foreseeable.

Patients will collapse in any part of the hospital or home that they are allowed into. They will also collapse in some of those places that they are not allowed into! Staff will also be subject to emergency collapses!

Fires and other events will force evacuation of buildings.

In the Accident and Emergency Department the treatment of badly injured and collapsed patients is the normal work.

The Ambulance Services have Paramedics who are equipped with a wide range of medical supplies to enable them to deal with a range of foreseeable situations where people are ill.

All of these situations are foreseeable. Therefore, the handling elements of these situations are also foreseeable. Plans can and must be made to supply safe ways of handling the patients without putting the nurses and carers at risk.

It is the manager's responsibility to ensure that all foreseeable eventualities have been planned for in advance.

Managers of nurses and carers must consider the working environment and identify possible emergency situations. They must create a plan for responding to each emergency. There should be plans for dealing with :-

Cardiac or respiratory Arrests

Collapsed patients and staff in a range of situations

Handling patients in the Accident and Emergency Area

Fire, bomb and Other evacuations.

Etc.

These situations should not come as a surprise. Each situation needs to be planned for so that the matter can be dealt with, without putting people at risk.

CARDIAC OR RESPIRATORY ARREST

Speed of response is essential when dealing with a cardiac or a respiratory arrest. Where a patient has an arrest in bed, the first response is straight forward. Treatment can be given immediately on the bed. However quite often the arrest occurs when the person is not conveniently on the bed. It is strange that some nurses will choose to spend the first half a minute trying to lift the person into a bed. Resuscitation should occur on a firm surface. There is no firmer surface than the floor!

Sometimes, the patient must be moved to provide enough space to attend to him but, there is no good reason for lifting a patient into bed before carrying out resuscitation.

If the person has the arrest and is on the floor in a confined place, the first problem will be to get enough space to provide resuscitation. Move furniture if possible. If the person is in a confined space such as a toilet the first action may be to pull him clear. If a sliding sheet is not available a stout rubbish bag is a good substitute. DO NOT TRY TO PULL A PERSON WITHOUT SOME SLIDING AID. See Chapter 20.

When the patient has been resuscitated the problem getting him off the floor must then be addressed.

Lifting the patient in a standard patient hoist sling can be a source of danger to the patient. The compression of the abdomen can bring on another arrest. Therefore, it is important to lift the patient without bending him. All stretchers are dangerous when lifting from the floor and are not therefore a safe option.

A ceiling hoist with appropriate attachments can be used to lift the patient providing that the rope or belt is long enough to reach to the floor. However, it will be rare that a patient conveniently collapses under a ceiling hoist. Sometimes such a hoist is available on a gantry supported by an A-frame. If such an arrangement is available it should be used. (In a large hospital this type of hoist is useful for other purposes and is therefore the ideal solution.)

Many makes of mobile hoists do not accept stretcher attachments. Even those that do have stretcher attachments are often not designed to lift a stretcher from the floor. In many cases the stretcher must first be lifted a few inches so that the legs of the hoist can be slipped under the stretcher. This would be an unsafe manual lift. One option that can be considered is to place the patient in a scoop stretcher and slide the patient and stretcher up a ramp of some convenient material.

At present, the Liko hoist is the only hoist that is capable of lifting a stretcher from the floor without any need to raise the stretcher. The patient is held in a fabric support under a full length frame. This will allow medium to short patients to be lifted from the floor.

COLLAPSED PATIENT, MEMBER OF STAFF OR VISITOR

People collapse for a variety of reasons other than Cardiac Arrest.

Before considering how the patient is to be moved, the first action is to find out what is wrong. The nurse must establish why the person fell to the ground in the first place. The nurse must also establish what damage was done by the fall.

CASE HISTORY.

A patient fell from his bed. Two nurses lifted him in a "top and tail" lift. The patient sagged in the middle and a taxi driver who had come to collect the patient had to come to the rescue and lifted the middle of the patient. One nurse suffered a permanent injury. If the nurses had properly checked the condition of the patient before they tried to lift him they would have found that he had a broken femur. The pain of being hauled up in the "top and tail" must have been excruciating for the patient.

The nurses made three errors:-

1 They failed to check the patient's condition before moving him.

2. They carried out a manual lift from the floor - All such manual lifts are unsafe.

3 They used an inappropriate lift. The patient was bound to sag in the middle.

The patient ought to have been lifted using a hoist with a fabric stretcher attached to a full length frame.

Methods of getting patients from the floor are discussed in the chapter on support in walking and the falling or fallen patient.

HANDLING PATIENTS IN THE ACCIDENT AND EMERGENCY AREA

It is foreseeable that an A&E unit will see people who are stretcher cases or who arrive in wheelchairs. This type of patient cannot be regarded as unusual. Therefore, the handling needs that they present cannot be regarded as an emergency which by definition is an event that does not occur every day.

The unit's risk assessment should identity a range of handling situations to be planned for. The risk assessment must identify the handling events that do or might occur. For each of these choose a safe solution. Everyone must be told about the solutions and must practice them to ensure that they are proficient.

Move from Ambulance Stretcher to A&E Couch or trolley	These moves must all be done by lateral transfers. See lateral transfers (Chapter 14) for details of options.
Move from A&E couch to trolley	These moves must all be done by lateral transfers. See lateral transfers (Chapter 14) for details of options.
Move from A&E couch to wheelchair	See moving from bed to chair (Chapter 14) for methods to be considered.
Move from car to wheelchair and vice versa	See Chapter 13 for methods of moving a patient from a car.
Move collapsed patient from floor	See Chapter 20.
Assisting patients to the toilet	See support in walking. As the mobility of the patient is not known with certainty, there is a high risk of unexpected collapse. If in doubt, use a wheelchair or a sani-chair. Go to a toilet with enough space for the wheelchair.
Get a patient from a helicopter	Consider how the stretcher is to be removed from the helicopter. Some helicopters are fitted with an angled load ramp that moves the stretcher out of the helicopter where it can then be transferred to a trolley. If the helicopter is going to land on grass, the hospital will need a trolley with big wheels that will go over this type of ground. This list is not comprehensive. Be alert for situations not described here. Managers must ensure that they have carried out their own generic risk assessment and made plans accordingly.

FIRE AND OTHER EVACUATION EMERGENCIES

All establishments must carry out fire evacuation drills. As these are drills, they cannot be emergencies. The need to carry out such drills allows the management to prepare a plan for evacuating the patient's and staff in an orderly manner.

The plan should show those situations that will be left to the emergency services and those that will be dealt with by the normal staff. Where staff are going to deal with a situation, they must be trained and equipped. The complete emergency plan must be published so that all staff are aware of how they will respond to an emergency. Exercises must be carried out to ensure that staff are familiar with the plan and to check that the plan works.

Evacuation of a Building

It is a requirement of the law that every building has adequate fire exits. When a building is being used to accommodate patients of any kind, consideration must be given to how they can be evacuated in an emergency.

There are three basic methods of emergency evacuation. These are, in order of priority:

Walking,

Wheeled transport

Sliding along the floor.

Walking

Where patients and residents are able to walk, they should be firmly told to walk to the assembly point. Some patients may have to be walked to the assembly point. See Chapter 20. This should then leave the staff to concentrate on those who cannot walk.

Wheeled Transport

Where a patient cannot walk, it is invariably safer and less physically exhausting to evacuate the patient on wheeled equipment. There are several items of equipment that should be considered.

Chairs

Chairs fitted with wheels make a good means of transport for many patients. Equipment such as wheelchairs, commodes on wheels, sani-chairs, and even easy chairs on castors can be pressed into service.

WARNING

Chairs with castors can only be used on hard floors without obstructions. On soft or uneven surfaces they will require too much effort to move and may even get stuck.

Beds

The bed, providing that it is on wheels, makes a useful means of transport to evacuate the patient out of the immediate area of risk. However, this method has its limitations. The bed can only travel over a relatively even floor. The bed or beds can create serious obstacles in corridors and at the top of stairs. Bed wheels need to be regularly maintained to ensure that they are free running. Nearly all hospital beds have three position brakes. The positions are Brake, free running and steer. In the steer position one pair of wheels are locked straight and the other pair will turn from side to side. This is the right position for pushing a bed along a corridor. Make sure that all staff know how to set the bed to this mode. A bed can be virtually uncontrollable in the free running position with all four wheels free to turn in any direction.

If the plan involves the use of something with wheels to evacuate patients, checks must be made to ensure that the wheels will go over the "ground". Try it out with a person in the chair or bed. Ensure that a nurse will be able to push or pull without exceeding the safe pushing and pulling loads (see appendix 1 Guidance on the Manual Operations Regulations [1992]). Check the whole journey. Will it :-

go across the carpet or other floor covering

cross sills to rooms

traverse the ground outside the building. (The patient will need to be taken to a safe distance away from the building.)

Make sure that castors or wheels do not fall off when the chair or bed is tilted.

Many wheels are not designed for this sort of journey. Do not rely on something that won't work when the real emergency happens.

THESE CHECKS SHOULD BE MADE BEFORE CARRYING OUT ANY TRAINING EXERCISES

Evacuation Equipment

There are some pieces of equipment that are specifically designed to assist in evacuation in an emergency.

Ski Sheets

This device is a sheet that is kept under the patient's mattress until there is an emergency. When evacuation is required straps are pulled out and pulled tight around the mattress with the patient on it. They are fastened together by a clunk click type of car seat belt across the patient's trunk and legs. The ski sheet itself provides a slippery surface underneath. The patient mattress and all are simply pulled off the bed onto the floor and out of the building. The mattress being included in the bundle provides padding so that the ski sheet can be pulled down stairs or over lips at doorways.

The bed should be put into its lowest position so that the mattress can then be eased off the bed onto the floor. The method of pulling a ski-sheet off a bed needs to be practiced. The pull needs to be diagonal. Take the feet off first and then pull the whole assemblage away from the bed so that it remains diagonal to the bed.

WARNING

Pulling sideways off the bed can turn the mattress and patient on edge. Pulling the feet straight away from the bed can result in the patient's head dropping suddenly off the bed.

The patient can then be pulled out of the area, along floors and even downstairs. The mattress provides some protection for the patient from bumps and knocks.

This method is physically very demanding. Two or more nurses should hold the handling straps at the foot and head.

WARNING

Do not **LIFT** a patient with a ski sheet. Not only is this a dangerous for nurses, it is also dangerous to the patient. The assembly is not rigid and can jackknife. At least one person had her back broken when she was picked up in a ski sheet.

The Ski Pad

The Ski Pad has been developed from the Ski Sheet. It is a ski sheet with extra padding. Therefore, the patient's own mattress is not used. The main advantage of the ski pad is that it can negotiate narrow stairways, sharp bends, and narrow, twisting corridors with greater ease than a conventional bed mattress in a Ski sheet.

The Ski Pad is usually wall mounted in a ward in its own bag. The Ski Pad is laid on the floor and unfolded alongside the patient's bed. The patient is then transferred from the bed onto the Ski Pad and wrapped in a blanket. The straps are fastened and the patient can then be pulled along the floor on its vinyl base. This pad will protect the patient from some knocks and bruises.

The problem with this device is that there seems to be no way of safely moving an immobile patient on to it. It may be useful for a limited number of patients who are unable to move any distance or have difficulty controlling their limbs. Such patients may be persuaded to lay themselves on the pad so that they can be evacuated.

The ski pad may be of limited use. It should only be purchased where the evaluation shows that it can be used safely.

Evac Chairs

This is a chair which can be used to push a seated person along on the flat and **down stairs** only. They have a special track mechanism that allows the chair to come down a flight of stairs in a controlled manner. Using the Evac, chair one person can safely steer a patient down a series of flights of stairs.

The Evac chair folds flat and can be stored against the wall in a convenient place

THE EVAC CHAIR MUST NOT BE CONFUSED WITH ORDINARY CARRY CHAIRS (SEE BELOW)

Dangerous Equipment

There is a wide range of equipment manufactured specifically for the emergency services. The design of the majority of this equipment leads to the lifter taking loads that exceed the levels recommended in the Manual Handling Regulations. This equipment is dangerous. It should not form part of any planning for foreseeable emergency situations.

Stretchers

Poles and canvas have been criticised for a number of years as being unsafe in bed to bed and bed to trolley transfers. Lifting a stretcher from the floor requires the lifters to adopt positions which are much less ergonomically and biomecanically favourable.

There are two stages to be considered in the use of stretchers.

Getting the patient onto the stretcher.

With some types of stretcher this can be achieved relatively easily. Scoop stretchers consist of two halves that can be used to slip under the patient from both sides and the clip together to form a rigid structure. There are also a range of stretchers that use a series of straps that can be slipped under the patient and then clip onto an outside frame.

Stretchers with wheels and those with padded surfaces are not so easy to use. The patient must be lifted bodily up by six to nine inches 15 to 25 cms to place him on the stretcher. This is an unsafe lift.

Getting the stretcher off the ground

The stretcher with the patient on it must be lifted up to about 24 inches or 60 cms to allow transfer into an ambulance or onto a bed. Some modern stretchers have gas struts or springs to assist in this lift. Unfortunately these tend to require quite a high lift to get the patient onto the stretcher in the first place. Most stretchers provide no means of lifting.

The load that can be lifted safely at floor level is shown in the Guidance to the Regulations to be between 5 and 10kg (11 to 22lbs) for a man and two thirds of this for a woman. This is trivial compared to the weight of a person on a stretcher.

Effectively, all stretcher designs currently marketed in the UK are unsafe in respect of the loads recommended in the Guidance to the Manual Handling Regulations. Unless the problems described here can be resolved the use of **any kind of stretcher should be excluded from emergency planning.** It is to be hoped that developments will be made that overcome these problems.

One way that has been suggested to solve this problem is to use two air bags slipped under each end of a scoop stretcher. The air bags are inflated to bring the stretcher up to a height where the patient can be safely transferred to a trolley using a lateral transfer system. The insertion of the air bags would have to be done carefully. An approach would be for two people to lift the end of the stretcher. They would have to do this using straps to enable them to lift in a standing position. When the stretcher had been raised an inch or so a third person would insert the air bag.

Carry Chairs

These must not be confused with Evac chairs. Carry Chairs are used by the emergency services and patient delivery services to carry patients up and down stairs. They are light metal folding chairs with a pair of wheels at the back.

Carry chairs are designed to be used to wheel a patient along on the flat and to carry patients up and down stairs. One person can push a patient along on the flat. Two people are needed on stairs.

The main problems with these devices arise when they are used to carry a patient up or down stairs. Carry chairs must not be used for the following reasons.

The handlers have to carry the whole weight of the patient. The weight of a patient will, in all but the rarest cases, exceed the loads in the Guidance on the Manual Operations Regulations (1992). This on it's own makes the carry chair unsafe.

The person holding the back of the chair is in stooped posture as he has to bend a long way forward to reach the handles. This will multiply the load that this person is carrying.

The person holding the foot end of the chair has to stoop to pick up and put down the load. Lifting a load in a stooped position is dangerous. Some lifters make the mistake of remaining in this stooped posture throughout the manoeuvre. This posture also has the effect of lowering the load and increasing the forward bend that the other lifter has to adopt to reach the top handles.

One of the lifters is required to move backwards. (This is usually the person at the foot end.) There is a danger that this person will trip, throwing both lifters and the patient down the stairs. At the very least, the lifters would be exposed to a jerking injury.

The Carry Chair is unstable and is designed to be tilted back when it is wheeled or carried. The patient feels as though they are being tipped out of the chair. The patient may react against this. Even though he is strapped in his movement could cause problems for the handlers.

This type of chair is dangerous and should only be used in one of the four real emergencies. Even then it should only be used if no alternative can be made available. See Evac chair as a safer alternative.

The Evacuation Sledge

These are rigid plastic stretchers shaped like a canoe. The sledge has six castors so that it can be pushed along the floor. The designers expect the sledge to be carried over rough ground or down stairs.

There does not seem to be any safe way of getting the patient off the bed into one of these devices. The carrying of the sledge with a patient in it in any circumstances would be unsafe.

Fire Escapes

Ordinary fire escapes are largely unusable for disabled and immobile people and can be very difficult for people owith restricted mobility.

Consider access to the fire escape and the exit at the end of the escape. The access must be on the level with no steps or sills to be negotiated. Some fire escapes are accessed through windows. Climbing up on to the window ledge to get through a window will exclude most patients. It will also exclude the use of the evacuation equipment identified above. Some fire escapes terminate in the American style drop down sections. These will again exclude most patients and most evacuation equipment. Ensure that there is level access across to a safe place from the bottom of the fire escape. Internal fire escapes often have some steps or a sill to be negotiated at the end.

The fire escape should be tested using a volunteer.

The exact fire regulations vary slightly from authority to authority. Some forces require nursing homes and hospitals to have a holding area on each floor where patients can be gathered in a fire proof area to await evacuation. This is a useful approach as it allows the nurses to help the patients out of the building one at a time with less panic. The escape plan must be discussed with the local fire officer. He will be able to help to assess the effectiveness of the plan. The fire officer will be able explain how much or how little time is available to put it into practice. He will be able to give the benefit of his expertise in many different areas. A safe plan will need to be drawn up with the fire officer.

When practicing fire evacuation a dummy should be used.

(In one exercise it was found that a six stone dummy was almost unmanageable. Make sure that the planned solution will work with the weights of patients that will have to be evacuated.)

Handling Principles

When speed is of the essence, the nurse is at greater risk of injury because there is no opportunity for recovery and the handling task cannot readily be pre-planned. This is the time when the normal principles of manual handling may be forgotten or disregarded because of imminent danger. For these reasons, employers must plan and then ensure that the plan is practiced. This ensures that should the situation arise, everyone is prepared.

For the purpose of the fire drill, all staff and particularly non-nursing staff should be given plenty of time to practice manual techniques under supervision before being required to use the techniques under pressure. The manager must ensure that drills are carried out completely, conscientiously and regularly.

"EMERGENCIES ARE EXCLUDED FROM THE MANUAL HANDLING OPERATIONS REGULATIONS"

It has been said that the Manual Handling Operations Regulation allows all rules and regulations to be ignored in an emergency.

The Guidance on the Regulations do allow the exclusion of emergency situations. However, this exclusion is not defined and has not been tested in the courts. It should be noted that this provision is not part of the Manual Handling Operations Regulation itself.

The situations described in this chapter are sufficiently foreseeable for plans to be made and for equipment to be purchased for the purpose. Therefore, it is hard to see that they are emergencies within the meaning of the Guidance.

If plans are being made for emergencies they must follow the principles of safe handling.

FURTHER READING

1. (1992) Manual Handling Operations Regulations, HMSO.

2. NHS Estates Health Building Note 40 (1995) Common Activity Spaces Vol.2 Treatment Areas, HMSO.

3. NHS Estates Health Building Note 40 (1995) Common Activity Spaces Vol.4 Circulation Areas, HMSO.

4. NHS Estates (1994) Firecode, Fire Safety in Health Care Premises, Health Technical Memorandum 83, HMSO.

DISABLED LIVING CENTRES IN THE UK

ABERDEEN
Hillylands Disabled Living Centre,
Croft Road,
Mastrick,
Aberdeen AB2 6RB.
Tel: 91225 68527
Fax: 01224 663144

AYLESBURY
Independent Living Exhibition,
Stoke Mandeville Hospital,
Mandeville Road,
Aylesbury,
Bucks. HP21 8AL,
Tel: 01296 315066

BECKENHAM
B.A.T.H.,
30 Beckenham Road,
Beckenham,
Kent BR3 4LS,
Tel: 0181 663 3345

BELFAST
The Disabled Living Centre,
Regional Disablement Services,
Musgrave Park Hospital,
Stockman's Lane,
Belfast BT9 7JB.
Tel: 01232 669501 Extn. 2708
Fax: 01232 683662

BIRMINGHAM
The Disabled Living Centre,
260 Broad Street,
Birmingham B1 2HF.
Tel: 0121 643 0980

BRISTOL
Disabled Living Centre (West of England),
The Vassall Centre,
Gill Avenue,
Fishponds,
Bristol BS16 2QQ.
Tel: 0117 965 3651
Fax: 0117 965 3652

CARDIFF
Disabled Living Centre,
Rookwood Hospital,
Fairwater Road,
Llandaff,
Cardiff,
South Glamorgan CH5 2YN.
Tel: 01222 566281 Ext. 3/51/3/87
Fax: 01222 578509

CARMARTHEN
Cwm Disability Centre for Independent Living,
Coomb Cheshire Home,
Llangynog,
Carmarthen,
Dyfed SA33 5HP.
Tel: 01267 241743
Fax: 01267 241874

COLCHESTER
Disabled Living Centre,
Occupational Therapy Department,
Colchester General Hospital,
Turner Road,
Colchester,
Essex. CO4 5JL.
Tel: 01206 832172 / 832173

DUNSTABLE
The Disability Resource Centre,
Poynters House,
Poynters Road,
Dunstable,
Bedfordshire LU5 7IP.
Tel: 01582 470900

EDINBURGH
Lothian Disabled Living Centre,
Astley Ainslie Hospital,
Grange Loan,
Edinburgh EH9 2HL.
Tel: 0131 537 9190

ELGIN
Moray Resource Centre,
Maisondieu Road,
Elgin,
Morayshire IV30 1RX.
Tel: 01343 551339
Fax: 01343 542014

EXETER
Independent Living Centre,
St. Loye's School of Occupational Therapy,
Millbrook House,
Millbrook Lane,
Topsham Road,
Exeter EX2 6ES.
Tel: 01392 59260

GRANGEMOUTH
Dundas Resource Centre,
Oxgang Road,
Grangemouth,
Central Region FK3 9EF.
Tel: 01324 6655546

HILLINGDON
Hillingdon Independent Living Centre,
Colham Road,
Uxbridge,
Middlesex UB8 3UR.

Tel: 01895 233691
Fax: 01895 813843

HUDDERSFIELD
Level Best,
Access Point,
Zetland Street,
Huddersfield,
West Yorkshire HD1 2RA.

Tel: 01484 223000
Fax: 01484 223049
Text: 01484 420926

HULL
National Demonstration Centre,
St. Hilda House,
Kingston General Hospital,
Beverley Road,
Hull HU3 1UR.

Tel: 01482 225034

INVERNESS
Disabled Living Centre,
Occupational Therapy Department,
Raigmore Hospital,
Old Perth Road,
Inverness, IV2 3UJ.

Tel: 01483 704000 Extn. 5477

LEEDS
The William Merritt Disabled Living Centre,
St. Mary's Hospital,
Greenhill Road,
Armley,
Leeds LS12 3QF.

Tel: 0113 279 3140
Fax: 0113 231 9291

LEICESTER
The Leicestershire Disabled Living Centre,
British Red Cross Medical Aid Department,
76 Clarendon Park Road,
Leicester LR2 3AD.

Tel: 0116 270 0515
Fax: 0116 244 8625

LEWES
East Sussex Disabled Living Centre,
47 Western Road,
Lewes,
East Sussex BN7 1RL

Tel: 01273 472860

LIVERPOOL
Liverpool Disabled Living Centre,
101-103 Kempston Street,
Liverpool L3 8HE.

Tel: 0151 298 2055
Fax: 0151 298 2962

LONDON
The Disabled Living Foundation,
Equipment Centre and Information Service,
380/384 Harrow Road,
London W9 2HU.

Tel: 0171 289 6111
Fax: 0171 266 2922

LOWESTOFT
Waveney Centre for Independent Living,
161 Rotterdam Road,
Lowestoft,
Suffolk NR32 2EZ.

Tel: 01502 538571 (Minicom)
Fax: 01502 538566

MACCLESFIELD
Disabled Living Centre,
West Park Branch,
Macclesfield District General Hospital,
Victoria Road,
Macclesfield,
Cheshire SK10 3BL.

Tel: 01625 661740

MANCHESTER
Regional Disabled Living Centre,
Disabled Living,
Redbank House,
4 St. Chad's Street,
Cheetham,
Manchester M8 8QA.

Tel: 0161 832 3678
Fax: 0161 8353591

MIDDLESBOROUGH
Independent Living Centre,
Occupational Therapy Department,
Middlesborough General Hospital,
Ayresome Green Lane,
Middlesborough,
Cleveland TS5 5AZ.

Tel: 01642 827471

NEWCASTLE UPON TYNE
Disability North,
The Dene Centre,
Castles Farm Road,
Newcastle Upon Tyne NE3 1PH.

Tel: 0191 284 0480
Fax: 0191 213 0910

NOTTINGHAM
Disabilities Living Centre (Nottinghamshire),
Lenton Business Centre,
Lenton Boulevard,
Nottingham NG7 2BY.

Tel: 0115 942 0391
Fax: 0115 942 0391

PAISLEY
Disability Centre for Independent Living,
Community Services Centre,
Queen Street,

Paisley,
Strathclyde PA1 2TU.

Tel: 0141 887 0597

PAPWORTH
Papworth Disability Resource Centre,
Ermine Street North,
Papworth Everard,
Cambridgeshire CB3 8RH.
Tel: 01480 830495

PORTSMOUTH
The Frank Sorrell Centre,
Prince Albert Road,
Eastney,
Portsmouth PO4 9HR.
Tel: 01705 737174
Fax: 01705 821770

ST. ANDREWS
St. David's Disabled Living Centre,
Albany Park,
St. Andrews,
Fife KY16 8BD.
Tel: 01334 412606

SHREWSBURY
Shropshire Disability Resource Centre,
Lancaster Road,
Harlescott,
Shrewsbury,
Shropshire SY1 3NJ.
Tel: 01743 444599
Fax: 01743 461349

SOUTHAMPTON
Southampton Aid and Equipment Centre,
Southampton General Hospital,
Tremona Road,
Southampton SO16 6YD.
Tel: 01703 796631
Fax: 01703 794756

STAMFORD
Disabled Living Centre (Lincolnshire),
33 Ryhall Road,
Stamford,
Lincolnshire PE9 1UF
Tel: 01780 480599
Fax: 01780 480603

STOCKPORT
Disabled Living Centre,
St. Thomas' Hospital,
Shawheath,
Stockport,
Cheshire SK3 8BL
Tel: 0161 419 4476

SWANSEA
Disabled Living Assessment Centre,
St. John's Road,
Manselton,
Swansea SA5 8PR.
Tel: 01792 580161
Fax: 01792 585682

SWINDON
Options Plus,
Marshgate,
Stratton Road,
Swindon,
Wiltshire SN1 2PN.
Tel: 01793 643966

WELWYN GARDEN CITY
Herts. Association for the Disabled,
The Woodside Centre,
The Commons,
Welwyn Garden City,
Hertfordshire AL7 4DD.
Tel: 01707 324581
Fax: 01707 371297

WEST WILTSHIRE AND BATH
Independent Living Centre,
St. George's,
Semington,
Wiltshire BA14 6JQ.
Tel: 01380 871007
Fax: 01380 87111

Comprehensive, unbiased and up to date product information can be obtained from the Disabled Living Foundation. Disabled Living Foundation Data-Off-Line and the DLF Hamilton Index contain full details of thousands of products used to move, handle and lift people. Handling people - Equipment, Advice and Information (1994), is a comprehensive resource that covers the legal perspective, ergonomics, different moving and handling environments, access, and transport, as well as product information and supply and provision criteria.

USEFUL ORGANISATIONS

Ergonomics Society,
Devonshire House, Devonshire Sq.,
Loughborough, Leicester LE1 3DW.

College of Occupational Therapists,
6-8 Marshalsea Rd., Southwick, London SE1 1HL.

Royal College of Nursing,
20 Cavendish Sq., London W1M 0AB.

Chartered Society of Physiotherapists
14 Bedford Row, London WC1R 4ED.

National Back Pain Association,
16 Elmtree Rd., Teddington, Middlesex TW11 8ST.

National Back Exchange
10 Cinderford Close, Boldon Colliery, Tyne and Wear NE35 9LB.

Centre for Accessible Environments,
Nutmeg House, 60 gainsford St., London SE1 2NY.

Accident Incident Centre,
Hannibal House, Elephant and Castle, London SE1 6TQ.

INDEX

Immoturn: 192.

Incubators: 199.

Individual care plans: 104.

Inflatable system: 214.

Injury:
    back: 10, 15, 16, 30 - 38, 41, 70, 74, 75, 84, 188, 198.
    benefits scheme: 11.
    cumulative strain: 9, 10.
    degenerative change: 10, 47.
    proof of: 9.

Intra abdominal pressure: 35.

ITU: 184.

Jacuzzi: 175.

Job design: 88.

Joints: 39 - 42.

Learning disabilities: 190.

Leverage: 49, 52.

Ligaments: 36, 39, 40 - 42, 44, 46, 47, 52, 53, 57.

Lighting: 18, 99

Log roll: 105, 140, 141, 147 - 150, 183, 184, 186, 192.

Lumbar spine: 40 - 46, 56, 57.

Maliciously aggressive patient: 191.

Manual lifting: 10, 23, 24, 35, 64, 184, 187.

Manual Handling Operations Regulations:
    3, 6, 7, 16, 23 - 26, 28, 60, 61, 64, 66, 67, 69, 75,
    85, 90, 95, 96, 112, 115, 130, 183, 221.
    Guidance to the: 96, 103, 183, 201, 220, 222.

Manual handling:
    assessment: 50, 55, 60, 65, 67, 69, 71, 90 - 92, 95,
            96, 103, 104.
    policy: 23, 68, 91.
    technique: 58, 59, 61, 68, 102.
    weight: 95.

Maternity: 186.

Mattresses: 132, 135, 136.
    inclinators: 134, 141.
    low loss air: 137, 152, 184.

net: 133.
    pressure relieving: 131, 136.
    servicing and maintenance: 136, 137.

Measuring performance: 69.

Mobiliser: 184, 185.

Monkey pole: 137, 149, 150.

Mortuary: 182.

Musculoskeletal disorders: 80.

Neonates: 199.

Nucleus pulposus: 40, 42 - 47.

Nursing on the floor: 186, 213.

Occupational health:.
    job and fitness criteria: 75.
    team: 77.

Operating theatre: 182 - 184.

Orthodox (cradle) lift: 9, 19, 35, 185.

Osteophytes: 40, 47.

Outer annulus: 42, 43, 45.

Pain-provocation: 39 - 41.

Hand blocks: 138, 145, 152.

Patient refusal: 24, 64, 109, 155, 190.

Patient records: 69.

Podiatrists: 187.

Poles and canvas transfer: 35.

Posture: 45, 46, 55 - 58, 68, 79, 80, 101, 103, 142,
    144, 147, 150, 172, 177, 184, 186, 188, 196,
    199, 211, 221.

Professional conduct: 14.

Questionnaire, occupational health: 74.

Reasonably practicable, (ALARP): 6, 7, 12, 13,
    15 - 19, 22 - 24, 26, 34, 35, 64, 70, 90.

Resuscitation: 23, 152, 184, 213, 217.

Rehabilitation: 12, 25, 26, 64, 66, 75, 76, 79, 81, 82, 118,
    125, 160, 173, 192, 193, 201, 208, 209.

A WORD ABOUT THE NBPA

The National Back Pain Association is a registered medical charity, founded in 1968. We:

- Operate a network of self-help branches countrywide, where people with chronic back problems can learn self care, and benefit from mutual support. Many branches arrange regular group hydrotherapy sessions.

- Run a Helpline supported by the Department of Health, where specialist nurses offer support and information to sufferers and their families.

- Produce self help literature for use by individuals and workforces in commercial, industrial and health settings.

- Publish a directory of our professional members – from both orthodox and complementary fields. All have a stated interest in treating back problems, and are listed by post code.

- Provide hospital trust and corporate membership schemes to support occupational health staff in reducing work related back pain.

- Offer membership for individuals, families and professionals. Members receive our quarterly magazine Talkback, with a supplement for professional members.

- Fund research into causes and treatments of back pain.

- Raise awareness: **National Back Pain Week** is our major annual campaign. Run in October each year, the week offers opportunities to provide the public with latest information and self help literature.

National Back Pain Week is also an opportunity to raise funds to support our charitable work. Hospitals can help us by holding raffles and other fund raising activities during the week.

In addition to the Guide to the Handling of Patients, we supply books, leaflets, posters, videos and teaching aids, specifically aimed at back care at work and in the community.

If you think we can help you or your patients, or you wish to take part in National Back Pain Week, please get in touch for more information:

National Back Pain Association,
16 Elmtree Rd., Teddington, Middlesex TW11 8ST.

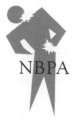